A Random Interruption

A Random

Interruption

Surviving Breast Cancer with Laughter, Vodka, Smoothies and an Attitude

Suzanne Zaccone

To order additional copies of this book, contact:
Xlibris Corporation
1-888-795-4274
www.Xlibris.com
Orders@Xlibris.com
58728

CONTENTS

"When we honestly ask which persons in our lives mean the most to us, we often find that it is those who, instead of giving much advice, solutions, or cures, have chosen rather to share our pain and touch our wounds with a gentle and tender hand. The friend who can be silent with us in a moment of despair or confusion, who can stay with us in an hour of grief and bereavement, who can tolerate not-knowing, not-curing, not-healing and face with us the reality of our powerlessness . . . makes it clear that whatever happens in the external world, being present to each other is what really matters."

~Henri J.M. Nouwen

"Without the strength to endure the crisis, one will not see the opportunity within. It is within the process of endurance that opportunity reveals itself."

~Chin-Ning Chu

"For last year's words belong to last year's language. And next year's words await another voice. And to make an ending is to make a beginning."

~T.S. Eliot

And I leave you with this: sometimes in the winds of change, we find our direction.

Dedications

Fear loses its power when it is shared and it almost leaves you completely when it is then understood. With that, I wish to extend my most heartfelt thanks in your willingness to join me on this journey. It would not have been as easy without you.

To all of those souls either experiencing cancer, or being a caregiver; this book is for you.

For Larry, the leading man not just in this book, but in my life. He has yet to read any of these chapters, as he feels that he lived the experience every day. As you read my words, you will come to know what a special man he is and how, without his presence and his love, I would have healed in all ways—but much more slowly and definitely without nearly as much laughter and love. I love you, Larry.

For Mom, Dad, Shere and Bob. You have always been a constant beacon of light, and a source of love and laughter in my life. The foundation of strength that you have provided has allowed me to happily persevere throughout life's inevitable struggles. Your care, concern and continuous positive energy have kept me from running off the road. I love you all.

For the Magnificent 7, all of whom are named below and introduced throughout this book. We made it, guys! We have two survivors in our group. Thank you for keeping me laughing, all the amazing dinners and your unfettered support. The first page of this book speaks the words that I feel in my heart when I think of you. It is a quote written by Henri J.M. Nouwen. Flip back and read it. I love you all, always and forever.

Acknowledgement to My Fabulous Friends

(Excerpts taken from emails written by Karl Zimmer)

Dearest Suzanne,

Of the many beautiful things you have manifested in your life, perhaps the most important are the people who have been such an integral and intimate part of this journey of yours.

Larry, Shere, Bob, your parents, and the other members of your family and closest friends; as well as the amazing team of doctors, nurses, and aids that have been there in so many loving and caring ways. They have been a stable and safe foundation for you. All the many others, though more physically distant, have also journeyed with you, supporting you and loving you in their own way. Each has provided prayers, loving blessings, affirmations and visualizations of perfect outcomes, positive energy, rays of loving light, requests for the presence of Angels at your side (the Angels have always been there with you, but additional requests can never hurt), kind words of support, and many other beautiful gestures.

At the risk of seeming a bit too flippant, I think the Mag 7 may have something about God wanting a few exciting chapters. Just think how boring the book would be if everything went smoothly; if there was no drama, if the entire experience was a cake walk, a piece of cake, and easy-peasy. No one would learn a damn thing and we'd all be wondering what the fuss was about.

But, NO! In typical Suzanne Zaccone fashion, all hell breaks loose, tears stream, hearts skip beats, and the world is treated to many more medical terms, valuable research and information, and eloquent descriptions of how an amazing, brave woman and the giants of support and love around her cope with and conquer this thing called cancer.

It is because of who you are that you have brought such wonderful and loving people into your world, and therefore into *our* world. For that and for so much more, thank you!

Brava, dear Suzanne, Brava!

I love you,
Karl Zimmer

(The following names are in the order that they appeared on the email list)

Mom—Loretta Zaccone; Dad—D.R. Zaccone; Dr. Shere Zaccone-Arnold, DVM; Bob Zaccone; Dr. Kurt Arnold, DVM; Lisa Zaccone; Jenny Bostick; Connie Insco (BFF); Christa Stankowiak; John Stankowiak; Donna Cannizzo (Mag 7); Debbie Donult (Mag 7); Carol Hendrich (Mag 7); Gina Woldman (Mag 7); Karen White (Mag 7); Marianne DePirro-Duitsman (Mag 7); Paul Myers; Yolanda Simonsis; Tommy and Marianne Matas; Kathy Welsch; Karin & Ferdinand Ruuesch; Kathy Pedroli; Donnell and Mike Buystedt; Linda and Steve Lee; Bill Podojil; Joe Schlesinger; Kathleen Scully; Jack Kenny; Ed Koznarek; Carol and Tony Lewandowski; Lori Levett; Pat and Marty

Marcuccilli; Michelangelo Capua; Yaakov Perry; Tomi Saas; Linda Failing; Jean Stanish; Hagai Ram; Jeanne Brommer; Katherine Stellatello; Judy Greiman; Sharon Rutt; Martha and Don Alexander; Cindy White; Mary and Peter Mulheran, Jeffrey Arippol; Debbie Forman, Julie and Frank Sablone; Terry Rowney; Michelle and John Hickey; Robert Biava; Eugene Matarese; Sophia Dilberakis; Ron and Katherine Harper; Dan Klobnak; Jennifer Dochstader; Mitch Karlin; Lesley and Brian Ludwick; Minna and Karl Zimmer; Mark and Cindy Wiercioch; Steve and Leslie Wiercioch; Bruce and Anne Wiercioch; Nancy Haller; Randy Thrall; Jeff Thrall; Jack Kraemer; John Kuhlman; Vince and Cynthia Di Trolio; Skip and Kathy Winnans; Richard Sinkuler; Ed Jospehson; Beth Lindahl, Kathy and Larry Tindell; Marta Cullen; Leslie Gurland; Lynn Syzmanski; Julie Chavez; Beverly Chavez, Barbara Otero; Gary Littlestar; Vince Allegra; Chris Pohlman; Ellen Rose; Jim and Claire English; Tony Scavo; Adam Laubach; Jeanette Hoag; Debbie and Jim Conrad; Corey Reardon; Hudson Young; Randy and Linda Buckley; Art Bowers; Cathy Parodi; Jorrie and Gary Gresko; Teresa Wouk; Karen DeRose; Adam Stock; Connie Zenawick; Tricia Laubach; Cindy Polster; Dean Littlestar; Robert and Angela Smithson; Brooke Thrall; Tom and Jonette Myers; Lisa Galyon; Karen Jackson; Toni and Walter Dow; Heloisa Jennings; Linda Tinman; Nadia Calfat; John & Beverly Mazour; Gerry and Teresa Gartner; Cleora Donaldson; Hao Nguyen; Renee Mazour, Elsie Menardy; Ken Solomon; Gerry Marting; Danielle Jerschefske; Karen Planz; Emily De Rotstein; Vicky Vasconcellos; Tammy Hemmingway (Trainer); Claudia and Glenn Cherney

Dr. Naheed Akhter, OB GYN

The Fruit Store; John Yurchak (my smoothie guru), Mick Yurchak and Jim Werderitch
Orren Pickell Builders; the entire team
Capri Restaurant; Phillip Ravito, owner; and Elton Kiaci, our favorite server
Moondance Diner; Theresa Manuele

The Chick Gang from Radiation
Rose Maza
Michelle Rosch
Jane Koulianos

Andrea Paula Borja; publishing consultant, editor, and an amazing writer herself. I first met Andrea in February of 2009. She quickly recognized the potential that this book had, to not only change but also improve lives. Her encouragement, suggestions, reminders of the rules of punctuation and positive energy propelled me to go on and helped to make this book possible.

This book was written in honor of my aunt, Joan Wiercioch; and my grandmother, Mitze Urban.

Introduction

BCD as Defined by Me:
Breast Cancer Drama

I used to find myself offering suggestions to God on what my life should look like. I am certain that God often laughed, and gave me precisely what I needed to experience. The universe has always been quite good at surprising me, and the end of 2007 and the beginning of 2008 came at me with a one-two punch.

This book started out as a series of emails that I sent to keep my family and friends up to date on what was happening with my destroyed lake house and with my breast cancer diagnosis. It was, in a sense, a coward's way out. It provided me with a vehicle in which to keep everyone informed, without having to answer the same questions over and over again. I had hoped that it would be a brief ramble, but it lasted just under two years and has turned into the book that you now have in your hands.

Throughout the process of writing, I was concerned that I would do meager justice to such a rich subject, and one that is different for each person experiencing it. The consolation was that while I tried to focus my thoughts to provide some value to someone else, it was also amazingly cathartic; it has been a great source of strength and laughter as I wrote what I felt, what I learned and what I experienced along the way.

I hope you find it helpful as well as hopeful.

Disclaimer

Please be cautious when reading the details I have described, as my cancer may be different from the one you are dealing with. I may have made an error in my literary translation, or technology may have changed.

I have learned a great deal during this two-year period. There are several types of breast cancer and they are all treated somewhat differently. There is also a very long list of physical and emotional side effects: nausea, hair loss, fatigue, diarrhea, constipation, mouth sores, a drippy nose, sexual dysfunction, dry eyes, depression and stress—to name a few. But it is important to keep in mind that medicine has come a long way. There are so many different types and degrees of surgery, chemotherapy and radiation therapy and they all produce different types and degrees of side effects. You may not get them all. Some are inevitable and many are temporary; the degree is based on each person. There are fabulous medications and techniques that are available for controlling side effects and the anxiety that the whole drama will undoubtedly produce. Use my experience as a guide but not as a suggestion that your diagnosis or treatment plan would or should be the same.

Each journey is unique; it's the experience that is shared.

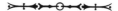

Dr. Song's Corner

While the word "cancer" does denote a certain set of universally shared and painful set of experiences, the types of cancer are not the same. In fact, cancer within the same organ sharing the same staging may not be the same experience for each patient. Conferring with your team of doctors will provide the best treatment plan for you and your family.

The Good, The Bad and The Ugly

The good

On Christmas Eve, we expected twenty-five people for dinner; twenty-nine showed up. It was fabulous: great food, plentiful spirits and it went on until midnight. Larry and I cleaned up a bit and then went to bed around 2:00 AM. We got up on Christmas Day, had a nice breakfast and then went to crash on the couch to settle into a good movie, with plans to clean up the rest of the place later, before going to Bob and Lisa's house for Christmas dinner.

Then the phone rang.

It was the alarm company and they were calling about the lake house. I had been getting calls the entire time I was in Florida the week before, visiting with Mom and Dad. The alarm company and I deduced that there must be a sensor that had been set way too sensitive, as the cops had gone around and looked in the windows and had seen nothing amiss. I'd just been there for an annual builder maintenance program before leaving town; everything had been working and in good operating condition at that time. I had the alarm company continually dropping off motion codes in some rooms during that week to stop the madness, and made an appointment with them to meet on the 27th of December, just after Christmas, to figure it all out.

On Christmas Day, the cop who had arrived after the alarm had gone off yet again, called immediately. The windows were all steamed up but he could see that the ceilings on both floors had fallen into the finished basement. It was eventually determined that the steam shower unit was at fault.

The ceiling in the living room and the ceiling in the basement were partially down, the master bedroom hall was wet, the office was trashed, the bar in the basement was trashed, and our beautiful kitchen and library cabinets were ruined. In effect, the following three weeks were spent moving out every fucking thing that was in there. The only unaffected rooms were the powder room, the blue bedroom, the bonus room, the purple bedroom, and the Jack-'n-Jill bathroom. Walls and insulation needed to be removed. Ceilings, floors, appliances, moldings, trim and cabinets needed to be reordered; and painting and beams must be replaced. A mold remediation crew would be called in to blast all spores away. It was a major mess and a loss of just over eighty-five percent.

No one was hurt and it's just material stuff. But I've gotta tell ya, I cried each night after the last person on the cleanup crew had left, as I viewed the scene in front of me. We had been acquiring special treasures on our travels over the last two years, and some of the items that were ruined were one-of-a-kind pieces that could never be replaced.

The ceilings displayed a pattern that was similar to a hardboiled eggshell after being cracked open. The wooden floor now resembled an accordion. All of our valuable and special pieces were eventually stuffed either in my car or at my parents' house next-door, taking over their bathroom because *their* furniture was stuffed in their bedroom, waiting for a refinishing of their floors. Things were at Bob's house, at our house in Hinsdale, at various cleaners or at the repair center or the storage center. It just went on and on. More things were packed in boxes in the garage for the movers to pick up later in the week.

The lake house was virtually destroyed. You won't believe the pictures. We hoped to be back in June.

The bad

Last Wednesday, January 8, 2008, I had my follow-up mammogram six months after my annual mammogram. They were watching calcifications. The calcifications had changed, but as the doctor said, that was now the least of my concerns. There was a mass in the twelve o'clock position in my right breast that had not been there six months ago. The doctor told me it was highly suggestive of a malignant cancer. There were irregular edges. I should speak to a surgeon. The next step after a biopsy would probably be a lumpectomy and then radiation.

I freaked out.

The doctor/radiologist had absolutely *no bedside manner*. He delivered the information as if he were dictating it to a secretary, to be transcribed into a document that would later be delivered by an actual human being. After Dr. Asshole blurted out the fact that I had cancer, I asked him if he was sure that they were my films. He must be asked this question a thousand times a day, as he quickly assured me that yes, he was sure that they were mine. He asked brusquely if I had any more questions. I said no, as I was too stunned to formulate a logical thought. I fled his office and the female breast cancer advocate followed me out, asking about when I wanted to schedule the biopsy. I said that I wanted to talk to Dr. Ahkter, my gynecologist, first. I got in the car, called Larry and went home hysterical.

Dr. Ahkter called the next day after she received the films and told me to get the biopsy scheduled *now* and to come in with Larry to see her that night. She said she had never experienced this particular radiologist use such definitive language on a report—and she sees many of his reports from other patients she works with. She was worried, and told me that I needed to act quickly. She assured me that we would take it one step at a time and we would look to a surgeon after the reports from the biopsy were in.

For the next four days, I never left the house except to go out for dinner on Saturday night. I had the biopsy on Monday. It was horrid, absolutely horrid. I stopped counting shots at seven and that little clicking sound of the biopsy instrument at eleven.

Hindsight is 20/20, as they say, but I am certain that I had an in-the-gut instinct that this mammogram would not go as all the others had before it. I remember doing every bit of laundry, paying bills in advance of due dates, sending off emails to the builder and the insurance carrier on the lake house flood, finalizing the inventory at the storage company and speaking to the myriad suppliers who were cleaning, destroying or fixing our things from the flood. I caught up on all the items on my to-do list around the house and at work. I was propelled forward at high speed, in a rush to get it all done. It was strange. As I look back at it now; the sense, the knowing that something wasn't right ahead of time was spooky.

I was compelled to voice this uneasy feeling to Larry in terrorizing detail, to explain why I was so scared. Being asked to come back in six months to check on something they were "tracking" or "watching" on your mammogram, is unnerving. Having those six months zip by as quickly as zipping closed a winter jacket forced me to face that another two seasons had quickly passed.

My godson, on leave from the Army, and I were to have lunch that day. I moved the time up an hour because I was too anxious and didn't want him to know my fears, as he was going off to risk his life the following day. He needed to concentrate on more important things, like staying alive himself. I was certain that once I'd had that mammogram, it would be a fast drive home. I desperately wanted to see my godson before he left. And I needed him to see me as the together, humorous, cool and collected Auntie Suze. So I did the Auntie Suze Fake Job and carried on with our plan.

The ugly

Waiting to hear what my heart was already telling me is true.

We got our answers later in the evening. We were just back from the doctor, and we had learned that I had an invasive

Ductal Carcinoma, Grade 3. The next few days would be spent scheduling appointments with surgeons and interviewing them. I wanted to make sure I found the best surgeon who could handle a patient like me. I needed to have a decision by Thursday and surgery within ten days.

I hoped I wouldn't embarrass myself too much throughout the journey and that I'd come through it with some modicum of grace.

Chapter 1

The Ultrasound-Guided Core Needle Biopsies

The night before the biopsy test was brutal. All kinds of terrifying thoughts emerged. Focus became different. In fact, there was no focus. Only a single-minded thought: *I have cancer.*

In my breast was a nasty glob of cells that were fighting silently within me, and yet I felt so good. My hair was strong and shiny and growing, and so were my nails. My skin was healthy, and up until recently I had been eating well and staying hydrated. OK, so I sucked at getting much physical exercise, but could I have been dealt these cards simply to teach me to get in the gym more than once every twenty years? Probably not.

I was constantly feeling my right breast; so often that it began to pulse. I was searching for those lumps. How had I missed them? Were they really that deeply set that I could not feel them myself? Had they moved to my lung? I took a sleeping pill and began writing. I knew that in forty-five minutes to an hour, the Ambien would finally kick in. I knew that as soon as I got up for something and began to walk into walls or cut a corner short, spinning myself around—only then would it be safe to go to bed and only then could I be certain that I could quiet my mind.

I woke up with my hand on my right breast. If last night could be described as brutal, then that morning could only be described as having heavy, abject fear. I got myself ready, popped a Xanax and put half of another in the pocket of my pants—all nicely wrapped in a Kleenex, which no doubt would also be used. I was told not to take any drugs to calm my nerves until after the consent forms and paperwork had been signed. No reason to change how I've always done things (which is *my way*), so I went ahead and pre-medicated. I have a high tolerance for drugs and I know that my body needs more time than most people for the drugs to take effect. I knew my body well enough to prepare myself way ahead of time. Because I wasn't going to be put out intravenously, and since I would be awake the entire time, I felt confident playing doctor.

Larry and I walked into the same place where I'd been given the diagnosis just a few days before. I'd been coming here for years to get mammograms but suddenly I couldn't remember the floor that the place was on and we needed to look at the directory. It wasn't the Xanax that had caused my memory to falter; it was the out-of-body feeling that I had. It was so textbook, so movie-like; like I wasn't really the one experiencing this whole event. I was floating above someone who looked like me and I was simply observing some medical program that I just happened to have a starring role in. Larry said that he wanted Brad Pitt to play him and Angelina Jolie to play me. But if we got Angelina, then he would be happy to play himself. You gotta love this man.

We arrived at the Breast Center. I was shaking like a leaf and Larry was pretty much leading—no, pulling—me through the door. We filled out masses of paperwork. I made adjustments and signed them and then the Patient Coordinator asked us to come into her office. She was the lady with me when the first doctor gave me his verdict. No, we had no questions at this point; I had been made fully aware of precisely what they would do to me here, today. She said this would be a good time to take the calming medication. I popped the pill I had placed earlier in my pants like a good, compliant patient. Then they took me away. Larry was not allowed to go further. He passed his strength on to me as we clung to each other in the hallway.

I was led into the changing room where I was given a locker and key for my things, and that ridiculous hospital gown that is open in front for easy access. I was crying like Niagara Falls. I asked if there might be a better place to have me wait so I wouldn't freak out the other women who may enter the room. It would not be fair to them to have to witness my emotional meltdown while they were dealing with their own demons at having to be there for probably just their yearly check-up. There was no crying room available, so I pulled myself together as best I could behind the curtain of the changing room. Afterward, I emerged somewhat calmer—or at least not as obviously freaked out, and I sat down in the room with the other women and waited.

My name was called and I followed the nurse into a part of the building that I'd never seen before. It was so far away from everything I was used to that I couldn't help but wonder if that was to put enough space between us to muffle the screams of those who must pass this far back. We walked into a room and the nurses explained once again what would happen today.

We started off with a digital diagnostic mammogram. A regular mammogram makes you as flat as a pancake; a digital mammogram presents more of a tortilla profile. OUCH! Then an ultrasound was taken and points that were important were digitally locked into, noted and marked on the screen image, frozen with a big red "X."

Fortunately, a different radiologist entered the room and placed his hand on mine. "I know you're scared, Suzanne," he said. "I'll do my best to make this as quick and as painless as I possibly can, but I need your help. We need to act as a team. Are you with me?"

I immediately liked him. I was relieved that he had approached me as a human; he had used my name, and he said he understood my fears. I felt better knowing that I was not just another right breast triple biopsy.

Next on the agenda were several breast numbing shots. Thankfully, a wall was on my left side. I'm still very flexible and my left leg was slowly inching up the wall as I braced for the pinch and then the sting. I attempted to remove from my mind the thought of getting needles stuck into my breast. They may be called breast *numbing* shots but that was certainly not how my body reacted to them. The radiologist made the first cut with the scalpel to gain access to the tumor for a core needle biopsy. I felt it and jumped a tad. I tried to stifle the sound of my pain by stuffing my fist into my mouth. He waited for the Lidocaine to do its job and then tried again. I still felt it. More shots were given. And then we just had to proceed.

I felt the needle enter me, along with a series of quick tugs. I heard a sick, disgusting *click, click, click* as they took out a piece of the tumor with the core needle. I was holding—literally squeezing—the shit out of the Patient Coordinator's hand who was there with me, trying to take my mind to other places.

Finally, we were through. The nurse had to keep a tight compression on the cuts for several minutes to eliminate the possibility of a clot that could eventually form into a hematoma, which is a collection of blood at the site of the biopsy. That's not all that comfortable either.

We walked into the next room, which was set up with all kinds of scary machines. One of them was the ultrasound unit that would find the tumor and offer the radiologist the best shot at getting to the heart of the matter as quickly and as accurately as possible. The ultrasound unit lay on a runner or rail system on the floor that provided the radiologist with the ability to move it to the precise spot where he needed it. It was placed under the table I would be on. The radiologist sat on a small moveable stool underneath me, doing his thing. This test was done while I was lying on my tummy on the strangest table that I had ever seen in a doctor's office—it had two holes in it; one for each boob. My right boob was hanging down through one of those holes.

The doctor told me that because my tumor was deep within the chest wall (that was why I couldn't feel it), they would have to work very close to my lung. I must not move, otherwise I risked injury to another organ. My natural reaction would be to bend my legs at the knees, in reflex to the pain and any needle sticks or knives that were slicing into my flesh. I asked if they could strap my legs down so that I wouldn't give in to that reflex. But there was nothing available to tie me down and they weren't willing to fashion something out of a hospital gown or several sheets. I must lie still and just deal with it.

The shots they had given me had finally reached their intended place in my body; suddenly, I felt no pain. I didn't feel the next two scalpel access cuts or the biopsy, although I could hear that nasty *click, click, click* sound—which was almost as bad.

It was over.

I hugged the doctor as he exited the room, rushing to get to the next patient.

I lifted myself off of the table and looked down stupidly. In the area where they had worked was a pile of bloody gauze, used instruments and small puddles of blood. The nurse quickly turned me away and began the compression on the cuts as we talked. I thanked her for taking such tender care with me and I gave her a hug. She was totally taken aback and I quickly apologized if I had invaded her space. She leaned over and hugged me back. No, I hadn't invaded her space but I had shocked her. She told me that there are three types of women who come in for these tests: those who are totally OK with the procedure and just sail through it; those who are terrified like me; those who are very mean; and sometimes it's a combination of the three. She told me that she had been kicked, bitten, sworn at, yelled at and hit by women who take their situation out on her, lashing out at her as if she were the cause of their suffering. I was amazed and appalled. But most of all, I was grateful that she came back every day.

I asked her how she does it. Surely, this job is more than difficult. It is life-saving, sad and emotional for all involved. She told me that she is committed to a cure and since that cure may not be found in her lifetime, she could at least be part of the prevention. I hugged her again and thanked her for continuing to be here for us each and every day. She was probably in her early thirties; a baby but a committed one.

In forty-eight hours, my life would change forever. But I did not know this yet.

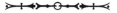

Dr. Song's Corner

Cancer is clearly a "me" experience and justifiably so, but there are others involved along the way who are there to help. It can be helpful to remember that the health care provider is also a fellow woman/man who may have gone through something similar. This is obviously more difficult when she/he has "no bedside manner." But nonetheless, their job is to facilitate your care.

Chapter 2

An Inconvenient Year: 1-20-08

I decided to call these updates the BCD: Breast Cancer Drama. In the world of scuba diving, a BCD is known as a Buoyancy Compensating Device. If you consider the metaphoric parallels, it rings comically true! *Breasts* and *buoyancy* . . .

I returned scores of e-mail to thank all of the people who had given me kind words of love and support. I cherish each and every one of them and I am keeping printed copies of every email, so I can read them during those dark moments in the day. That is a very strange place for me, but I never stay too long.

It is amazing how many people have told me that they too have had this disease touch their lives in some way. Many have suggested that an "email control center" is the most expeditious manner in which to keep everyone updated. I couldn't agree more. Being the medical midget that I am, I can promise that nothing too disturbingly graphic would be shared.

A diagnosis of breast cancer and the knowledge of all that is to come to get rid of it has become a shock to my mind and body. I am attempting to be very careful these days about paying attention to the words I use to describe the experience, as well as the body language I display in order to maintain a peaceful warrior attitude. Always having a "can do" positive outlook would now be put to the ultimate test.

I made a list of breast surgeons, radiologists, oncologists and plastic surgeons in the Chicago area. I added references that came to me that would help people in other parts of the USA, as well as a fairly comprehensive set of questions for each of these medical disciplines (the list of questions would be helpful to anyone in any city).

Then I considered journaling; writing it all down in a notebook. Not for me! My Type-A perfectionism would require too many notebooks, as there would be pages upon pages of ripped-out rewrites and edits. The computer was the only way for me, as I could edit and keep it all fresh and manageable. I decided to type the experiences that I encountered, in this format—and when written from a medical Chicken Little's point of view, it would hopefully be splattered with humor. I want these words to help someone else get a faster start on their journey. If you learn of a lady or a man in need, as always, send them my way.

This week, I had an appointment with a breast surgeon every day except Thursday. One more appointment may be made next week if we were lucky enough to get on their schedule. Surgery would follow quickly after that.

In Chicago, it was cold and snowing. I checked the weather station and Australia and Brazil were warm and sunny. It was rainy in Rome, London and Switzerland; overcast in Amsterdam; and snowing in Germany. Everything was normal. But it wasn't—I have cancer, and yet the world continues to spin.

Chapter 3

First Opinion

I was melting into small puddles. Once in a while, I found myself in a dark and dreary place; one that I'd never visited before. A place where there were no faces I recognized. I always knew that everything happens for a reason, and very often that reason would not be divulged or discovered until you were at the other end. God generally placed people or events in my life for me to teach something or to learn something; occasionally, I got both. I couldn't help but think that I was to learn something REALLY BIG on this journey and teach something REALLY CRITICAL to someone else. Why else would this be happening? A singular awareness seemed selfish and such a waste. I hoped it would come as a fast lesson this time.

I was literally fucking scared to death. Not the crying, *boo-hoo-hoo*, snotty, messy, snorting kind of crying—but more like Niagara Falls; constant.

The entire drama, so far, had been hard on Larry. He had taken control of the situation, as he clearly knew that I was just not capable at that time to do much but sit like a vegetable, either completely empty or embroiled in turmoil. He was keeping me strong, focused, laughing, and feeling loved and still desired. He was heading up the team, running for films and prescriptions, talking to doctors, coordinating with Bob and Shere, keeping the whole family up to date, making sure I ate something, making the best Grey Goose Cosmopolitans in Chicago—which have been renamed "Larmos"—and pretty much leaving his business behind, and not at the best time either. It was such an odd place for me to be: submissive in a way, completely willing to give up full control. I absolutely could not have done it without him.

We had—*I* had, really—been going through the "losing the boob" thing, too. Larry is an ass man but that does little to enhance my sexual self-image. Just last Tuesday, I completed walking this trip through hell with a friend of mine from high school. There are seven of us that still get together every month and go on a yearly vacation. Carol Hendrich had been diagnosed with breast cancer and had decided on a double mastectomy. She'd been visiting hell since last April. Could I avoid that drama?

Larry, Bob and his wife Lisa, and I were all going to these appointments, so we had many ears closely listening. Here is my take on the next steps, which for me and a lot of other women seem brutal and completely unnecessary. And please don't bother with the expected platitudes like "You have to do it." I completely understand that. But there is also a compromise that should and can be made. Somewhere, somehow, with someone, I will find it if it is out there. And if it isn't out there then I guess I'll head up the charge to change it.

I needed to get two tests before I could be properly assessed. But at this point, the first doctor's opinion was that a lumpectomy and then radiation with possible chemo were in order. It all depended on my MRI results (a needle would be plunged into my vein, shooting radiated glowy crap into me so that they could see if there was cancer any place else, and if it was spreading). I could find a way to get through that one. But the worst test I'd ever heard about was the sentinel node test: a series of four needles would be stuck into my nipple to push radioactive fluid that would advise the doctors which of the nodes was probably cancerous and therefore, which needed to be removed. The sentinel node technique was introduced in the early 1990's and was now the standard of care for staging and treating patients with localized cancers who were at significant risk of having a metastasis to their lymph nodes. The theory was that cancer typically would spread through the lymphatic system by first moving through one or two sentinel nodes. These are the nodes that the tumor drains into, so they are the first place wherein cancer cells would appear in the lymphatic system. This test provides the surgeon with enough knowledge to remove *just* those nodes during a future surgery and not the whole lot, in order to determine if cancer had spread.

For the sentinel node test, I must be awake. I told the first doctor we met, Dr. E—who was about six months pregnant—that I would absolutely *not* do those procedures awake. If necessary and if they would not accommodate me, I would pre-medicate myself. I was willing to accept only solutions to taking care of this requirement in a more humane way. End of story.

I wasn't moving.

She wasn't moving, either.

I needed to find an MRI gal/guy who would knock me out (twilight sleep; not a full intubation with an anesthesiologist) or I might end up knocking him/her out. It would be a reactive impulse.

"OK, here's the first shot in your nipple and just three more to go."

NOT A CHANCE.

If they can put someone in twilight sleep to stick a camera up their butt for a colonoscopy, why the heck can't they do the same for a part of a woman's body that is pretty darn sensitive and isn't meant to be poked like a pin cushion?

This is not acupuncture!

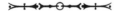

Dr. Song's Corner

The patient will first go to the Nuclear Medicine Department to have a radioactive dye injected into the skin. An X-ray image will also be taken. This image helps us to visualize roughly where the sentinel node is and how many there are.

During surgery, the doctor will inject the tissue around the nipple and areola with a blue dye. This substance travels directly to the sentinel node. Through a small incision made in the axilla, the surgeon can pick out the node (sometimes there are two or three) that turns blue from the dye and/or emits a radioactive particle, which is then detected with a probe like a Geiger counter. The blue dye and the radioactive tracer are used because the "sentinel node" is not always easy to find.

The pathologist then very carefully and meticulously examines all the cells in that sentinel node under a microscope. The sentinel node procedure, therefore, has the added advantage of being accurate and the oncologist will have a clearer understanding of the status of your lymph nodes. If the sentinel node is "negative" for cancer cells, we will know that it accurately predicts that the rest of the nodes are negative.

The theory that is now well-accepted is that breast cancer cells travel along the lymphatics if and when they metastasize. Instead of biopsying the entire axilla to find out if breast cancer has metastasized to the area, the thought is that biopsying the sentinel node or the first node will give us an accurate picture of whether the tumor cells have invaded other nodes, thus precluding the need for a full axillary node sampling, as has been previously done. Cancer would have to go through this sentinel node first. Several landmark studies have shown this to be true.

Chapter 4

Second Opinion

I was really mad about the nipple test. It provided me with renewed energy and something important to fight for. Along with the pink boxing gloves that my cousin Bruce and his wife Anne had brought over last night, I was ready for battle. Once I made a decision on a doctor, those gloves would travel with me everywhere. There had to be a better way to take care of this sentinel node test. If it was out there, I would find it.

I spent the morning talking with many of my friends. Those talks have been so helpful. I also talked to way too many "ologists" to count, insurance people, nurses, scheduling staff; and I'd just completed filling out the third medical history form of the week. I'd come to cringe at the word "ectomy" anything.

By the third form, I was going wacky. To me, so many of the questions appeared either obvious or totally ridiculous, especially in this context. A few examples—

> Q: Describe your symptoms.
> A: Abject fear
> Q: What would make this problem/condition better?
> A: Waking up in six months after it's all over
> Q: What would make this problem/condition worse?

A: Being awake for the next six months while it is all happening

Q: Change in sleeping habit or appetite?

A: Come *on*. Are you serious?

The second doctor we met was Dr. D (Carol's doctor). He recognized me but I had to remind him how we had first met. I really liked this guy but he is a general surgeon and not a breast specialist. His opinion was pretty much the same as Dr. E's; only, Dr. D tended to think that a mastectomy was a better choice, as the size of the mass to be removed would be a minimum of 2.5 inches plus whatever they needed to take in addition to that, to get to clear margins (there are two trouble spots that are close but not connected). This was the same thing that my sister (Dr. Zaccone) and her husband (Dr. Arnold) had been preparing me for since last week.

I asked Dr. D what he would recommend to his wife and his answer was delivered without hesitation: a mastectomy. Because of the two spots that spanned a large area; one being cancerous and appearing to be a very hot spot that was quickly growing and was invasive and the other, an insitu tumor—localized but colonizing that could quickly turn into cancer.

The question now became—

Do I have a lumpectomy then radiation and deal with a potentially large depression in my breast, with a chance of additional breast reduction caused by radiation, and fret over a potential recurrence? Or do I get it all over with and have a mastectomy, maybe chemo if it was found that I had lymph node involvement, and probably radiation later?

Those were very, very difficult questions. But there were three more opinions to come. A little over the top with five opinions, but I wanted to hit the big three hospitals, all having breast cancer centers and specialists in their midst, as well as two local doctors who had been referred.

The encouraging issue for today was that I think I got through to Dr. D. He had *never* been asked to alter the nipple test for the sentinel node before meeting me, go figure, but he was willing to look into it. Here is what was really driving me to make a big stink out of this: the reason why I must be awake is that the radiation department of the hospital is over here, and they are not set up with anesthesiologists or even twilight sleep options that are really quite simple (think dentist's office). The staff that handles anesthesiology is over there, at the other end of the hospital. It is simply too inconvenient for them.

I am now the self-appointed High Priestess of Breast Cancer Ease and I am strongly considering setting up the FBPA (Federal Breast Protection Agency). I will find a way to make this test less barbaric and find a hospital, a doctor and an anesthesiologist—whatever and whoever is needed—who can do the procedure in such a way that the patient's terror, pain and anxiety are reduced. I was fighting for me, for my goddaughter, my nieces and for you who are reading this and may experience breast cancer in the future. We must find a better way.

The best thing that happened today was that when we all came home from this doctor's visit, my sister Shere was at the house waiting for me, fresh from New Jersey. She had left her practice and her family to visit her older, wimpy sister. It was a fabulous surprise for me. I hated the thought that she had to leave them but I loved her for just showing up. We are very close, and she would be a rock for Larry and me, especially since Bob would be out of town for the next two meetings. Bob had been taking notes so Larry and I could focus and listen and ask our questions. Mom and Dad wanted to come home, but we convinced them that there was really nothing much to do until surgery and then—*wail*—I WANT MY MOMMY AND DADDY!

I had an appointment for a Breast MRI with contrast (needle), an abdominal MRI with contrast (needle), a chest X-ray and a bone density test on Friday. Bob made all the appointments earlier in the week as I sat by the computer logging them in like a robot. Shere made the appointments for me for this last series of tests. She even gave them the myriad medical details and regular patient details that they ask you before you get that appointment. I was amazed at how much she knew about me, medically speaking.

What a change from the Suzanne of just a month ago.

Tomorrow, we would add Lisa to the caravan. I was feeling guilty about putting my family through this. But without them, I am afraid I would still be staring at the doorknob in my office at home, alternating between empty and terrifying thoughts.

Chapter 5

Third Opinion

We met with the Breast Cancer team at Rush Hospital: Dr. A, Dr. B, Dr. C and Dr. D—a surgeon, a breast oncologist, a radiologist-oncologist and a . . . a . . . crap, I can't remember the last "ologist," but it would make the final list.

Picture this: Larry, Lisa, Shere and I were all cramped in an examining room with all types of creepy-looking machines. I was checking out the labels, nameplates and panels through a silent veil of tears, looking for names and addresses for our sales team, when the first person dressed as a doctor walked in.

She introduced herself as a psychiatrist.

OK.

This was just too much, and I laughed so hard I almost choked. I looked at everyone through my laughter and tears and asked which one of them had asked for this. They all assured me that it hadn't been any of them who had asked for the psychiatrist to be there. Maybe it was because I had been crying through the blood pressure cuff test and height and weight measurements that they figured I was more of a nut case than I really, truly am. Evidently and thankfully, this was their protocol with cancer patients. And I suppose I looked as though I was suicidal.

She was a very nice lady and she quickly understood that I was as solid as they came except for the medical stuff, that I had the most support any human being could ever hope for in my friends and family, and that I had nothing but high hopes for the future. I told her that I simply wasn't crazy about seeing a stethoscope within five feet of me. We had some laughs. She left.

In walked three more doctors. They asked me to tell my story and what I knew. Then we had to do three (flipping *three!*) breast exams. They each wanted their own shot at copping a feel. I hated this. Just where was I supposed to keep my eyes at that point? More talking ensued. They left. We waited again, this time for the surgeon to make his entrance. He was a likeable man and appeared to be compassionate. I immediately trusted him and felt that I could work with him. He quickly understood and accepted my fears and was willing to play along with my sense of humor, so we too had some laughs. His suggestion was that I could go either way but that due to the size of the tumor and the fact that there were two rather large spots, a lumpectomy would probably leave a rather large "site." I took that as: not the "sight" you want to be looking at every day.

I noticed a few meek smiles when I went through my thoughts about the nipple biopsy for the sentinel node. They know this has to be a hard one for most women. But the surgeon was having none of it. It was clear to me that we were not going to have a balanced discussion about this issue.

We talked about a mastectomy which, in the long run, he felt would be my best option. This method would eliminate the need to have the sentinel node test. What a relief; but where does that leave those who don't meet this particular team? I asked him about lymphedema; a surgical complication that is caused by removing too many lymph nodes, causing your entire hand and arm to swell and pulse. It required a surgical type of undergarment be worn to keep things tight, and you would need to do certain exercises for the rest of your life in order to obtain relief. Lovely! I loved his answer though: "You have a slender body frame and that is generally a plus factor for not getting this disease." Good to know that while I was taking care of one disease, I was not walking into another. The "slender body frame" comment earned him extra points, as well.

I ranked these doctors as the best (so far) because they are experienced breast specialists. They work as a team, therefore eliminating my need to find the next doctor in the drama, interview them, coordinate appointments and medical records, receive referrals, and keep everyone up to date. The entire process of sending things back and forth between different groups of doctors would be eliminated with a team approach. They were very compassionate and loving and they all had a personality. I could easily work with this team.

We talked about the other tests I was scheduled for on Friday in the suburbs. He cautioned me that the tests I would be getting at the group I was scheduled for would only be accepted by the doctors' group who had originally ordered the test. Therefore, should I decide to go to another doctor, they'd need to do it all over again, as they would not take responsibility for treating a patient that they had not done the complete work-up on. That made perfect sense to me. I canceled those tests and appointments without batting an eyelash.

My fear was doing a lumpectomy now and worrying every day when and if cancer would come back. A ticking time bomb was not something I would like to wake up to each day. I already had calcifications that they could further study, but they would always be a risk factor for me. If cancer returned, a mastectomy would be my only option. The "girls" were still fairly perky, so I didn't want a brand new perky boob next to one that was a much older cousin. And I didn't want to have one pointing west while the other was pointing to the heavens when I was lying down. What a look!

So, a mastectomy with plastic surgery immediately to follow removal may be the way to go. To me, it sounded like a gross process.

The hard part in selecting this hospital would be my memories of being here many years ago. It was where I remember going as a little girl. Mom would pack the three of us kids in the car, pick up Grandpa and drive him to Rush Hospital to get his radiation treatments for lung cancer. I hated going there because I was terrified of the place. He always felt awful when his treatments were finished for the day and it continued for many hours and many days after we returned home. Even before this issue had come up for me, simply driving through the highway and nearing the hospital—my first instinct was to quickly look away. Things have changed and improved in forty years but memory and association are strong forces.

Chapter 6

Free Day!

It's a free day; no medical stuff!

At 8:00 AM, hand-carrying the pathology slides, Larry met Romella Lee, Operations Manager for breast cancer, who coordinates appointments downtown at the University of Chicago. Larry somehow talked her into rushing things through. We had an appointment for next Wednesday with Dr. Connolly.

A long-time friend (kiss to John Kuhlman) who is prominently involved as one of the Board of Trustees, was using his pull to make that happen even sooner. It had been confirmed by this hospital that any tests that would be needed must be given by the hospital that would ultimately do the final work.

Important side note: Larry gave this hospital's cafeteria a high rating.

Chapter 7

Fourth Opinion

We met Dr. B at the Lynn Sage Breast Cancer Center at Northwestern Hospital. He had been highly recommended by several people, including Marianne's friend, Yolanda Simonsis, Mayor Daley's wife Maggie and several others. Dr. B is a very compassionate, gentle man who was willing to share his knowledge in a very clear-cut and organized manner. My options remained the same but I would be under twilight sleep while this doctor did the sentinel node test. He was waiting for the radiologist's report and the estrogen progesterone tests but I doubted that this would change his opinion strongly, one way or the other. I liked his style, his demeanor and his office.

This doctor also works with a team, and they have all of the required facilities at this location, although radiation could be done closer to home. Dr. B told us that he would be able to manipulate the breast tissue surrounding the lumpectomy site; therefore, reducing the size of the indentation, deformity, hole, disfigurement—take your pick.

It had been a month since Christmas Day when we learned of the flood, and seventeen days since my diagnosis. The Christmas tree was still up, although we had stopped turning on the lights. It was too embarrassing to announce to the neighbors that we still hadn't been able to organize ourselves enough to take it down; they weren't aware of what was happening.

Lisa decided to remove all of the ornaments and placed them carefully in the boxes for safe-keeping until next year. If she hadn't taken care of this, I fear that the tree would have been up until next Christmas.

The last appointment would be next Wednesday at the University of Chicago Hospital.

Chapter 8

Estrogen-Progesterone Test

I tested positive for the estrogen and progesterone test, and the tumor was well differentiated. This was a good thing; I should respond well to drugs after surgery. Shere explains this much better than I ever could, especially in person, but here is a recap of her explanation—

A positive result on these tests means that the tumor has receptors on the surface that interfaces with estrogen. Think of the "lock and key" theory. Estrogen helps the tumor grow. Since we don't want that, we put the patient on an estrogen receptor *blocker* like Tamoxifin or Arimidex. These drugs sit on the receptor site so that the estrogen cannot. This doesn't really have a whole lot to do with prognosis; it simply aids the doctors in evaluating what drugs your tumor responds to. Also, "differentiation" refers to what your tumor looks like under the microscope. A well-differentiated mass has breast cells that look mostly like breast cells. A poorly differentiated mass has mostly cells that do not resemble normal breast cells.

This leads to more questions for the surgeon and his team as to the risks of taking bioidentical progesterone to help keep things in balance.

Chapter 9

Fifth Opinion

The entourage met with Dr. Mark Connolly at the University of Chicago, which is another very highly rated hospital.

He, too, was charming, professional, knowledgeable, and compassionate. He had a great personality, which further compounded my decision in our search for "The Exalted One." I would be placed in la-la land when all of the scary, brutal tests would be done. *Whew!* He felt that I could go either way but that I was a good candidate for a lumpectomy.

Dr. Connolly used a team approach to treatment. Every Thursday, there is a Breast Cancer Conference, where new and current cases are discussed with three to four cancer surgeons, radiologists, pathologists, oncologists, and plastic surgeons—all of them breast cancer specialists. Once they are selected by the patient, these folks review the entire case, and they decide as a group on the options available and the treatment plan. If there is more than one option, then the patient decides. Pre- and post-surgical decisions are reviewed as a team throughout the process.

Dr. Connolly would become my breast cancer doctor for life; every three months for a year, then six months for a year and then once a year thereafter for the rest of my life.

If I had a lumpectomy, there is a procedure that I couldn't be sedated for, which completely freaks me out. It involves the insertion of two very thin copper wires that the doctor uses to isolate the cancerous tissue. Once inside the breast, all tissue looks the same, and only through this radiological test would the bad cells be seen. The radiologist would take a scan, and insert the wires on both sides of the tumor so that the surgeon would know precisely where and what to remove and how far to go, to hopefully get to clean margins.

The wires are supposedly small; less than a needle used for a blood sample. I *clearly* remember the radiologist telling me the same damn thing when getting the shots for breast numbing when I'd had the biopsies over a week ago. Those "miracle drugs" had taken forty-five minutes to work—along with my self-prescribed dose of 1.25 mg of Xanax that I had taken an hour before arriving for the test, to "calm my anxiety." I finally "didn't feel a thing" after forty-five minutes and several more breast numbing shots before the second set of biopsy tests. So forgive me if "a very thin needle," as described by anyone in medicine, is just a tad hard for me to believe. Especially coming from a doctor who sees and uses needles on other people all the time and is trying to ease my fear.

Dr. Connolly said *he* never had one of these tests but that "it shouldn't hurt." I wanted to whack him. I suggested that we do the tests together, side-by-side so he could experience it all firsthand and be able to tell his patients *exactly* what it was like. He smiled a little and then quickly changed the subject.

Towards the end of our meeting and after having answered all of my questions, Dr. Connolly said, "Look Suzanne, you will no doubt receive excellent care no matter where you decide to have your surgery. What I can tell you is that I do breast surgeries every day and I am a very, very good surgeon. I will take excellent care of you."

I loved that answer.

He didn't rip up the competition, yet he had confidently stated how he viewed his skill set and its results. And he had looked at me squarely in the eye.

We now had several different opinions from all of the doctors we had met, as far as testing and treatment were concerned. Tomorrow would be spent in research mode and I would compile a list of questions for each of the top two contenders and then await their responses.

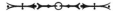

Dr. Song's Corner

Each individual will react differently to sedative medications and anesthesia. Particularly those who have had previous experience, have consumed alcohol on a regular basis or are genetically pre-conditioned. The same dosage of sedatives for the same height/weight individual may be received and may act quite differently. Discuss your lifestyle openly with your doctor, as this will help her/him to modulate the dosage more clearly for you.

Chapter 10

The Facts I Am Considering as Key after All Five Opinions

The rate of life expectancy is the same with a lumpectomy, as it is with a mastectomy in my case. They would be closely monitoring the lumpectomy breast and would be able to catch a change early. If a change would be detected, tested and found to be cancer, then I'd be left with the option of a mastectomy or a further disfiguring lumpectomy. Taking a little at a time until it's just best to take it all.

It came down to what my personal risk tolerance is (high), what my odds might be within the current percentage numbers (or my luck factor, I suppose, as you won't know until a few days after surgery if they need to go back into surgery to get to clear margins) and what my tolerance for multiple surgeries is, if it were to come back (low). How the sentinel node test was accomplished is also of great importance, as are the overall esthetic results.

As far as after-care is concerned, I've learned that there is a method of radiation wherein a balloon is left in the breast right at the "site," which is attached to a tube that lies outside of the breast. Twice a day for five days, your tube is hooked up to a machine where a seed is blown into the balloon and the tissue closest to where the tumor was, is radiated. This method, more focused, saves radiating healthy tissue.

The option that is most used is to radiate the entire breast every day for six or seven weeks. I wasn't sure that I wanted my healthy tissue radiated; unless, of course, that was my only choice. One doctor said that I was a candidate and another said that I was not. One doctor said that he could manipulate breast tissue to fill the cavity on a lumpectomy and another said that it wasn't a good idea. What a set of choices—dealing with not just the tumor but also with a part of me that is erotically mapped and esthetically marked, as all external organs are.

It was going to be a thought-provoking weekend.

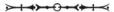

Dr. Song's Corner

There are very few absolutes in medicine. Place ten expert physicians in one room and give them the same clinical problem, and multiple different and correct answers may be rendered. Medicine is not like other scientific disciplines such as mathematics, in which there is often a universally correct formula or theorem; there are many variables and even more unknowns in medicine. To get the best outcome for you as an individual, find a set of doctors that you trust—and then trust them.

Chapter 11

The Decision

The doctor we had selected was Dr. Mark Connolly at the University of Chicago.

It was a very close and difficult decision and it had all come down to the fact that I felt a stronger connection to him than the second runner-up at Northwestern. I suppose *location* had absolutely nothing to do with this one. I would have preferred the hospital at Northwestern because if I were to get the right room, on a high enough floor, I could see Escada and Chanel from my window and I would be two blocks from fine dining. What a source of inspiration that would have been to break out of the hospital! Shopping for me, and eating for Larry. Like I would really need a reason to break out of a hospital. Or like Larry would ever have a problem feeding his always-hungry tummy!

University of Chicago, on the other hand, is near Cottage Grove at the edge of a questionable neighborhood. I went with my instincts, which have always served me well, and my heart, and I left my wallet at home for a future shopping trip. The University of Chicago has been named one of the top leading hospitals in cancer treatment and research in the world and it is the only one in Illinois to have ever made the list.

The next steps would be—

On Monday, I would have a series of MRI's, ultrasounds and needle sticks. A few days after that, they would know if the cancer had spread to other areas of my body. At that time, a date for surgery would be given.

I found a handy little flashlight to get me out of those dark places. It's called an operating plan. Only it was quite a different type of "operating plan" from those I am used to working on. As I'm certain you can imagine, the meetings these past weeks had been unbelievably hectic and emotionally demanding, but also informative and occasionally reassuring. It looked as though some of the experts I'd seen were not just doctors but also, at least potentially, caregivers and maybe even healers. I was playing the odds, baby—once again rolling those dice. We were going to take it one step at a time with a lumpectomy and we would fight this random interruption with everything we've got. Only this time, the outcome would be out of my control. Another new one for me!

Channeling Frank Sinatra and "Doing It My Way."

Chapter 12

"Prenderla Giorno per Giorno"
(Taking It One Day at a Time)
MRI's and the Ultrasound Tests

Monday, February 4th

We arrived on time at 9:00 AM. Why couldn't we have been delayed by the usual traffic jam or a surprise Chicago snowstorm this morning instead of the night before? Four inches of snow had fallen last night. More was expected tonight. Today was just cold. But I know better than to delay the inevitable, so I took a 1mg dose of Xanax before leaving the house this morning. This provided some assurance that I could at least walk in the hospital door without being dragged. It is probably more dignified to be drugged than dragged.

I had a magazine, my glasses, my iPod, driver's license and medical card. All metals and jewelry were left at home and I was in sweatpants so that I could more easily persuade them that there was no "metal anything" in them, on them or around them.

We are here for breast tests and nothing else, thank you very much.

Do you think they will let me keep my pants on?

I signed more forms than a customer would sign to get into our manufacturing plant for a tour. Surprising myself, I thought of Ed Josephson, who has been the family lawyer for a very long time and was my first professional crush when I was around ten years old. He was a young guy then who had a corner office and whose name was on the letterhead and the door; he was part of the corporate name and identity. When you spoke to him at his desk, the view out of the floor-to-ceiling windows was the skyline of Chicago. How could you not be impressed? I was. Through the years, he had become someone I've come to call a friend, as well.

I drive the man absolutely nuts. I read every bloody word of any contract or document that he sends me. I correct spelling and punctuation errors, question legal terms, change things a lot, and pose challenges to him that he tells me he's never been asked to do before. Together, we've come up with some very creative and downright fun things regarding my will. I wish I could be alive to witness it all because it would be so much fun to be involved. In short, everything I have ever signed has been thoroughly reviewed, understood and adjusted if necessary before my signature hit the bottom line.

Sit down for this one, Ed.

I skimmed it all, every last hospital form I was asked to sign. My skimming is like most normal people's reading but it still felt odd not to take the usual time in reading each and every word.

Jeanette or Paula, please give him some water and an aspirin.

The staff at the hospital was absolutely amazing. I am in awe of the things they do every day, dealing with all of the varied emotions that each patient brings along with them. And still, they carry on, smiling. They didn't make me feel bad about being the human version of Niagara Falls. They were gentle and caring but alas, I still hate stethoscopes. Don't get me started on needles and machines.

I shall spare you the details of the process. It wasn't pleasant for me in any way but now it's over and it's simply another speed bump that I've traversed—landing squarely on my feet and running down the halls afterwards, as fast as my body would move to get the hell out of the place.

My friend Gene Matarese recently told me, "You decide what you want to make of this experience. It can be woeful or it can be transcendental. It has a beginning, middle and end. If it doesn't, then you are in the morgue! The world will go on as if it doesn't miss you."

I continue to do my best to "Live out the String," as singer and songwriter Marc Cohn says—live out the string!

Note: regarding who won the battle of the sweatpants being left on—I did. I'd sensed that there would soon be *something* that I would need to adjust for. I'm sure that occasionally, even Sinatra had had to understand and accept a compromise. And because I prefer to place a positive spin on things, I'd rather lose a battle or two in order to win the war. This time, my pants had stayed on—but then there had been that pink thong with the tiny blue bow at the top in the back that wasn't coming off, even if the pants had had to. That would have marked our first compromise.

Chapter 13

Notes of Clarification

Note of Clarification #1

Since my diagnosis, I have only just begun taking Ambien for sleep and Xanax for anxiety. I'd never needed either one before that. It was suggested to me by Carol Hendrich, my friend since I was thirteen, who is almost done with her breast cancer drama. I'm glad I listened to her. In fact, as soon as she learned of my diagnosis, she had come over with Marianne DePirro-Duitsman and handed me a few pills in little plastic bottles. The doctor was not surprised at all by my request for my own prescription. I am far from an expert on these drugs, so be sure to discuss the pros and cons with your doctor. Now as for "Larmos" (Cosmos), I know *everything*. (I am being very cautious when taking drugs and drinking a cocktail but even the doctors say a few won't hurt me.)

Note of Clarification #2

I appreciate all of the emails mentioning how "brave" I've been. In truth, that isn't accurate at all. I continue to have a difficult time the night before anything medical, the morning of and occasionally during the "free days." I sink into this place that finds me very complacent and just kind of going along. Well, going along most of the time, at least.

It is easy to be glib when writing. My intent for these chapters is to update, educate and humor you. That's about it. I am not taking it lightly inside, as it might at times sound or look like, but I am trying to react to it lightly on the outside. You'll have to watch the news for what some fireman, policeman or EMT team did—to look for true and honest bravery.

Note of Clarification #3

No, I did not do it alone. Larry, Bob and Mom were there the entire time. Five hours of their day. Two hours total traveling time and three hours sitting around a hospital waiting room, in the Oncology Department no less, amongst people with portable IV's and oxygen tanks; some sitting up on their own while others were slumped in their wheelchairs or beds. A few people were bald, some were balding, and several displayed thinning veils of hair. All of them ensconced in their own horror as they waited for their name to be called.

I have an amazing family.

Chapter 14

MRI & Ultrasound Test Results, Second Round BCD Results

Monday

During the ultrasound test, the radiologist kept digging around one specific area in the pit of my arm, closest to the breast side; and it was becoming hugely uncomfortable. I asked him why he concentrated so deeply on that spot.

"You have enlarged lymph nodes," he said.

I asked him what that meant.

"Not a good sign," he replied.

A professional would not say this without knowing precisely what he was saying, and the effect it would have before a confirming test was made. But he was being honest with me, and that was one of the deals we had made early on.

The MRI wasn't bad at all—*after* they had done the needle, injection and radioactive dye thing. The sounds were unbelievably loud but that was easy to get past, as they had provided ear plugs.

My mind was telling me to prepare for that first compromise, which I sensed I shall need to surrender to very, very soon.

Tuesday

The doctor's nurse sent an email stating that I needed further biopsies of the lymph nodes under my arm. The doctor would call me after 2:00 PM on Wednesday. That was a day before they convened for the weekly Thursday patient review. I was supposed to hear from him before that meeting.

I was literally scared out of my mind.

Wednesday

Dr. Connolly's nurse Donna Christian called. Dr. Connolly would be calling me tomorrow after the council had met to review my case. At that time, I would have more details. But at this point, she was able to tell me the following—

I had two choices to make. Get a core biopsy of the axillary lymph node under my arm, where they would remove tissue samples from the enlarged lymph node; this would determine if the cancer had spread. This must be done *awake* and even Donna would say that it was not a pleasant test to have, based on where this node is located.

Or, I could wait until the night before surgery when I would receive an injection of a radioactive isotope, which is placed around the nipple in four places. This is not the sentinel node test but yet another barbaric medical test. It would slowly filter radioactive dye into my lymph nodes. It is done in nuclear medicine. I must be awake.

The following morning, I would return to nuclear medicine. They would place wires through some camera-guided gizmo that positions one wire at the top of the mass and one at the bottom. This would guide the surgeon to the precise location. And I must be awake.

From there, I suppose Dr. Connolly would guess how much margin to take out once he got in there during surgery. I would *finally* be put to sleep for surgery after this procedure.

Option No. 2 was a great deal more accurate, and it would ensure that the right nodes would be taken. I was praying that

Nurse Donna's last positive thoughts would come into play for me. These enlarged lymph nodes may simply be white blood cells reacting or congesting at the trauma sites of the earlier biopsy episodes.

I was having a very hard time with these two choices and wishing I could simply hibernate this winter and wake up healthy again in the spring, just like a bear.

Thursday

After a day of *real* business meetings, a few doctor's appointments and basic running around—there was still no call from Dr. Connolly. It was 6:00 PM and we had decided to leave a message for the nurse, telling her how to reach us. For a change, Larry and I were hungry at the same time. At home after dinner, we noticed the message light on the recorder. We wouldn't be hearing from the doctor until tomorrow.

I was practicing my skills in the art of negotiation.

Friday

For the past seven years, we've gone on an annual vacation with a group of Larry's business friends. We both look forward to this trip, not only because of the locations we go to but because of the people who attend. They are hard-working, entrepreneurial, positive, happy and fun people to be around. Not a bad one in the bunch.

For weeks, I had tried to persuade Larry to go without me so he could have some fun. It would be silly to be on vacation and deal with the very real possibility of my spontaneously starting to cry, bumming everyone else out. He needed this break more than I have ever needed one, even now. Other than my drama, his assistant is battling leukemia and her attendance at work is spotty; his dad had had a heart attack two weeks ago and we'd just learned that his mom had been diagnosed with emphysema. He was carrying around quite a load every day but he was handling it with amazing ease and grace.

It was almost unbearable for me to say no to this leisure trip.

Giving up the opportunity to earn frequent flyer miles pissed me off. It was bizarre to hear my own words: I was "afraid to be out in the sun." Afraid to be out in the sun because of an upcoming surgery—for cancer. Wait a minute, surgery like this had never before been mentioned in the same sentence with my name! Missing out on potential scuba diving was really making me sad. Thinking about having time alone with Larry and away from all the usual noise of our lives, was so tempting. Hell, I really must be sick!

Well, as cavalier as this may sound, and as out of sync with the gravity that this random interruption in our lives had become, we had decided to "Live out the String." We were going. End of the story—at least for now.

All of the above was written late last night after having a long heart-to-heart talk with Larry. Today, the doctor called and reality changed things a bit.

The MRI confirmed that I had an invasive cancerous tumor, and it further enhanced other things going on in there. They had found that the insitu mass had grown very large. It was now at five to six centimeters. Both tumors had to be removed. The end result was a chunk the size of a baseball—the doctor's analogy, not ours. I must have the core needle biopsy test under my arm to further determine if it had spread to the lymph nodes. Based on how those results would come in, I would then have the lumpectomy-versus-mastectomy decision to make—or they could tell me that I didn't have a choice.

To further complicate things, they may not be able to do reconstructive surgery immediately after the first surgery, like others I've known have been able to do. If radiation would be required, it could harden the implant and cause further issues down the road.

Barbaric Test No. 3 would be next Thursday. Depending on the results, surgery would be on February 20th.

I never packed for the trip. I think that deep down I had known that Hawaii was out for me. I was still hoping to get Larry packed and out of here for tomorrow morning's flight. He fought me big time, but I think I was slowly denting his armor of resistance.

Chapter 15

It's the "Me" in Medical that's the Problem

I recommend a good scream now and then. I just go into a room and *scream*. I sometimes worry that I will never stop and that I will be forever rolling on the floor like one of the supposed witches of Salem. Never happens. I scream and then I go into the bathroom to brush my teeth. I just need to let it out. Maybe I release endorphins in the process.

I think the real challenge about this ordeal is that in the end, I'm left with me. My body. My decision. My fight. The *me* I never knew or wanted to know. The *me* that I had forgotten about or had pushed aside when I was so busy distracting myself with life, with others. The *me* I've come to like and dislike for all of my self-judgments about what is good and what is bad about me. Simply reckoning with the fact of being me, and accepting whatever that feels like in that moment. No first impression management or pretense. I'm *me*.

Finding those moments that separate me from others, also make me realize what I share with the human race.

Some say they find God. In my experience, that has been true but I've also found a higher sense of myself. Frankly, it isn't all bad and a lot is quite good. I am learning to forgive myself when I think about mistakes that I felt I've made. Now I realize that based on the information that I had at hand, I would probably have done the same thing again.

I grapple with what you grapple with: *Who am I?* What am I becoming because of this experience? Will I allow myself to explore and experience all of the parts of me, physically and emotionally and without apologies? Will I like the new me? What was, or will be, the true purpose for my being here on this earth?

The most difficult issue that I confront a great deal is: do I love me enough to forgive or at least be compassionate with myself?

If ever there had been a moment when I needed to be fully aware, it was now.

I am trying hard to live in the moment. Straining to listen for that higher-pitched sound; attempting to recognize a soft flutter of air passing by, or to see the flash of light that often precedes enlightenment. I am trying hard to stop speeding through life at two hundred miles an hour on the hood of a car's bumper. The speed of my life as it was has ended and thus the process starts all over again until I figure out just what it was that I was put on this earth to accomplish.

No future to plan for beyond the next "medical thing," a fabulous past to reflect upon but an excruciating present that I cannot avoid. I'm at a fork in the road without a map and no gas station is in sight. But the engine keeps on purring.

Chapter 16

Something Else We Need to Change:
How They Track Research

While at Northwestern University Hospital during my opinion gathering stage, I was given a thick document to read at my leisure. It explained the research program they have, using tissue samples collected from patients who agree to become involved. Loving any kind of research, and fully recognizing the importance of this type of research, I eagerly read on.

I reviewed the documents at home. I discovered that they would not remove any more tissue than what was needed to remove the person's cancer; but if there was any tissue left over after the required testing, they would use those samples and place the slides in a database. So far, I was good with that.

This database would be connected by a code number. That code number would be connected to my name, address, birth date, phone number, medical history (past, present and future) and Social Security Number.

I fully understand the need for most of these statistics; but in this age of fraud, giving out a Social Security Number is darn risky. I am certain that all of us have heard of hospitals, universities, insurance companies and corporations where someone had breached their "secure" database. And what a perfect database to breach: a list full of cancer patients who may or may not be in remission and may or may not have the time or the energy to fully recognize early on that their credit is now SHIT.

Fast forward to the University of Chicago, where I had elected to have my surgery and treatments. Just before having the MRI and ultrasound tests last week, a young researcher had come over to me and explained the purpose of their similar document. I asked about the need to relate it back to a Social Security Number; she had no answer that satisfied my concern, so the document was not signed. Her disappointment was so obvious that my heart simply ached. I explained how much I appreciated and fully believed that what she was doing was crucial. I told her that I knew her projects were important to so many people, and that if they could rewrite the contract, I would sign it in a minute. She understood and did not pressure me. But I could tell that this was not the first time she had been turned down, and probably for the same reason.

This is total crap! If the goal is to track the mutations, cellular baselines, statistics, demographics, eating habits, ages, medical results (past, present or future) and medical history for this much-needed research to help eradicate this awful disease—*why* in God's name is my Social Security Number of any relevance?

My list of things to work on changing that are related to this disease seems to grow each week. Am I missing something? Being too protective? Rhetorical questions here, folks—because frankly, I don't see myself changing my mind on this one. Personally, I feel that the requirement has absolutely zero merit. The research that these teams are doing require tissue and medical-based patient details. They could give a crap if they have a Social Security Number or many of the items noted above.

This makes me very sad and very mad. With my personality, one does not cancel out the other; they simply fuel the fire.

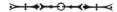

Dr. Song's Corner

Clinical trials and studies that patients will be asked to participate in are extremely valuable as a means to gather prospective data on the efficacy of treatment plans, drugs and other therapeutic or diagnostic modalities. But it should not come at the compromise of an individual's set of circumstances. Ask the questions, seek the reasons behind each and every trial, and ultimately trust your instincts.

Chapter 17

Test No. 3:
Core Needle Biopsy of
Axillary Lymph Nodes

Thursday; February 14, 2008

Happy Valentine's Day!

Dad, my very first Valentine arrived home last night. Now both parental units could fret over me and while doing that, and doing it very well, hold each other up like they always do.

Once the core needle biopsy of my axillary lymph nodes was over, it was hard to keep my right arm close to my body with all of the bandages. Sleeping on or near that area was very uncomfortable. The bandages couldn't be removed for forty-eight hours.

When a nurse tells you that a test won't be pleasant, multiply "not pleasant" by ten and you are closer to the truth. When I arrived, I learned that the nurse and radiologist for today would be the same ones from last week. I was so happy about that.

When Diane Pruitt, Registered Nurse walked into the room, I was visibly relieved. She recognized that relief. I said that she was probably disappointed about having to go through this again with Chicken Little. Instead she said, "Come on, we'll get through this one together, just like the last time."

She held my hand throughout the entire process and talked to me about everything. I remember answering her in short, precise sentences, desperately trying to keep myself alert to what was happening around me. When it was necessary, she would explain the next step in the procedure.

As soon as I was on the table, I was asked to lie on my left side and place my right arm up and over my head. My first reaction was to move into the fetal position. It just felt right.

"Girl, you are scared," Diane commented. "Moving into the fetal position—my, my, my. Give me your hand."

I was holding her hand so tightly that I needed to ask if I was hurting her. She told me to squeeze as hard as I needed to. They remembered my drug tolerance being high and waited a little longer than the last time to let the shots take their proper place in my body.

Then the radiologist began his work. I heard the most aggravating sound of paper being crumpled and gradually realized that I was creating the noise. My shoes were digging into the paper over the table I was lying on, making shreds of it and creating quite a mess.

When the radiologist was done, I gave him a hug. He wasn't ready for this at all. He stood as stiff as a board but gave in to it in the end. Then I noticed that I had left a large spot of blood on his white coat. We shared a brief laugh as I implored him to change his coat before he went to his next patient. I would have flipped out if he had walked into my procedure all bloody from the last one.

Diane and I had a nice chat as she cleaned me up. Then I got dressed. This time, she gave me a hug before I could give her one. I loved that!

You've all heard of people who lose a limb and sometimes feel as if that limb were still there. It's called *phantom limbs*, *phantom feelings* or *phantom* something or other. I had a different twist to that one. I had this odd sense that now, while still whole, it was already gone. It was creepy, terrifying and very sad.

This disease is something that I can fight but not control—not yet, at least. So I attempt to move on, separating myself from

74

the control part and suiting up for the fight. Doing my best to take the moment for whatever that moment is, and seizing it. That is not quite the right phrase for me these days: "seizing it." But, oh well—you know what I am getting at. We all know that there won't be another moment like the one that just flew past. Frequently, I find myself relieved to know that many of those moments will never be the same, as these past weeks had been filled with some pretty frightening and painful stuff.

However fragile or strong we think we are, we learn to bend or to gain a stronger backbone; to let go of whatever it was that we felt so concerned about. At least, that is what I keep telling myself.

I remember all that I am grateful and happy for because I know that the future can change in an instant. *Whoosh!* In an instant.

Time to try and sleep . . .

Chapter 18

Hear Me as a Woman and Not as a Cancer Patient

It is my breast.

Yes, my breast!

Something you might have taken notice of at one time or another; maybe not. A part of me and one that I've lived with and have become quite attached to over these last fifty years would soon be gone.

I see them each day, wash them, and smile at their still-perky attention; thanking God for fabulous genes. Sometimes, I attempt to hide their emotions, which are not always reflective of "the moment" or are—at best—poorly timed. Whether your boobs are perky, droopy, engorged or deflated; breasts have a way of attracting attention, getting in the way, providing pleasure and nourishment and for generations, have caused quite a stir.

This is a hard one to explain, and therefore understandably difficult to truly digest for anyone who is not a woman or who in some way, however large or small, can't identify with the fear of losing one or both breasts. The issue for me is altering my sexual image—"my" being the operative word.

I am certain that many people, even in my incredibly close family and among my treasured friends, simply don't understand the big deal. I get that, when I consider it from their perspective.

But consider it from mine.

My situation does not end with the fact that I have an invasive cancer. That is where it begins. I will not insult you by suggesting that I might enlighten you with profound thoughts culled from the depths of despair. I simply ask that you look at things from the viewpoint of where it is all happening: in my head, on my body and with my boob.

I've traveled the globe. Attended fabulous events, given speeches in three languages (all professionally translated), attended all kinds of parties, and taken part in many traditions that were outside of my own. I've dined at the finest as well as the worst of restaurants and stayed at some of the biggest dives as well as the best hotels in the world. I've seen sights and experienced things that will be forever etched in my memory. Some of those experiences have become the stories of my life. And I have met and loved so many people who cannot possibly be fully described in the time that any of us have on this earth.

I am not concerned about how you will see me. That will be something you will need to work out for yourself.

My fear is how I will see *me*.

How I will accept me.

Now, for the first time, I wonder how my body will appear in those glorious gowns, those classically tailored business suits. Will a strategically draped scarf help shield things? Or maybe a modified neckline will hide the varying levels of my chest wall? That's an easy one to figure out. So, let's go a bit deeper. What about the man I have undressed in front of for twenty-four years with blissful freedom and ease? In the fat times and in the thinner times, when I was bloated and when all was as flat as a pancake. Soon I shall be a different topography; one that is unfamiliar, not just to him but unfamiliar to me.

Stop. Think. Feel it with me. Now we are in bed, and while he may be seeing *me*, I am thinking about the *new me*. The mind and body connection had carried me through to this point. It had helped me to overcome such trembling fear. How could I deny its power now?

Chapter 19

Results of Test No. 3:
Core Needle Biopsy of
Axillary Lymph Node

Test results

The overachiever in me had struck yet again.

Cancer had progressed and had spread to my lymph node system. This means that a right breast mastectomy and removal of lymph nodes (Level 1 and Level 2 with a maximum of three levels) was now the order for Wednesday. All intramammory lymph nodes that the doctor could scoop out would be removed in that area. Approximately one week after the nodes have been removed, I would learn if it had spread or metastasized to other parts of my body, and I would then be precisely staged for cancer treatment follow-ups.

I would go home with a drain, which would hang outside the surgical site that would drain all of the unnecessary fluids from my body. Dr. Shere Zaccone would be coming in tomorrow so she would handle all of that medical stuff, as I was certain to pass out if left to my own devices.

I canceled the two trips that had been planned for March. This would be the first time in my history that I would miss a TLMI Association meeting—damn, I could have set a record. The most important trip I would miss was Kurt's fiftieth birthday party. Kurt is Shere's husband and my brother-in-law. That one really hurt to miss.

The surgery would be two to two and a half hours in length. I was scheduled to arrive at 8:00 AM and surgery was scheduled to begin at 9:30-9:45 AM.

It was really happening, wasn't it?

Next steps: This was the Go Forward Plan

Tuesday would be spent getting mentally prepared and packing for the hospital (but being the Type-A person that I am, I was already packed). I was required to take some pre-operative measurements prescribed by the nurse to render my body germ-free. They would do the same germ removal thing all over again, once I arrived the next day for surgery.

I planned to finish the laundry and pay bills in advance of next month.

Our bedroom had already been set up with what I thought I might need, so it was close at hand. I didn't know for certain how long they would keep me in the hospital. It was supposed to be only overnight. I was persuaded to leave the computer and PDA at home, so I wasn't sure when I would write again but it wouldn't be long after I was allowed access to a computer. I had practiced a little; typing one-handed, as my right "wing" would be rendered useless for a while. Thank God for spell-check. Having Larry's talent at being ambidextrous would be quite helpful now. Oh, the many talents of my Larry.

Marianne DePirro-Duitsman (one of the Mag 7) came over that night to bless me with holy water before surgery. I pulled open my shirt and she proceeded to bless lefty. I didn't have the heart to tell her that it was righty that needed the blessing—until I stopped laughing. She started again. Marianne would continue to do this throughout my drama. I had been given two bottles of holy water from Lourdes in France. One was from Mike Fox, a business associate and one from my parents' dear friend, Heloisa Jennings. I was using both bottles liberally.

Everything was now ready.

I was told on the instruction sheet to "get a good night's rest." I wanted to slap fucking silly the person who had came up with that helpful little hint.

Imagining how Wednesday morning might play out

I imagined that I was all rested now. Right, just like the pamphlet suggested. I arrived bright and cheerful (uh-huh) and ready to get my boob lobbed off (nope, I was still not quite ready for that).

I wasn't able to eat or drink anything since midnight the previous night. No problem; late night eating is Larry's challenge, not mine. I was not allowed to take anything to calm my nerves on the morning of surgery, and it was too frightening to pre-medicate myself, like I've done before—as the anesthesia that I hoped they would give me would be strong. I did not want to have a bad reaction, and I did not want to mess up any plans for a full load of anesthesia.

I'd learned that the two really nasty tests where you need to be awake wouldn't be necessary for me, as I would be having a mastectomy and total removal of axillary lymph nodes. A little of that silver lining was trying hard to break through. I made the best attempt at savoring the moment. It's ironic, though, how suddenly those dreaded tests didn't seem so bad; considering that the need for them would have meant a better prognosis.

Everything must go, but Dr. Connolly would "attempt to save some skin" to assist in the reconstruction that wouldn't happen for at least another year at best.

Larry would be allowed to be with me up to the point where they take me into the operating room. That was a comforting thought for so many, many reasons but especially because he is so much stronger than me and would not allow me to flee the premises.

I would be placed under general anesthesia, and then . . . off it would come. I agonized, mourned, cried, pinched myself and realized that yes, I was really awake and this was my reality. Never before had I had such a struggle in facing my reality. I stand in awe of those who have walked this road before me, those souls who have been able to handle this without crying every day for six weeks and who have faced the world with such ease, such strength and such grace.

I pretty much stayed close to home, writing volumes of literary brain diarrhea. I did a great deal of research and then wrote some more. But I am satisfied that at least I continued to be true to myself. I did the research, chose the best solution for my disease with the knowledge that had been learned and that I could understand. I had selected what I hoped to be the finest hospital, nurses, anesthesiologists and doctors that I could find. I'd surrounded myself with a top-notch team; and now together, we simply needed to execute the plan.

That is very important to me: remaining true to myself in all ways, under all circumstances. Although I wondered how simple it would really be to execute this plan.

Chapter 20

The Night before the Next Two Days

My thoughts before drifting into sleep

As of tonight, I had begun to crawl off of the car's hood and bumper. The usual two hundred miles per hour journeys had slowed a bit in recent days. I was finding it easier to feel comfortable enough to hang out for a while. Throw my head back. Spread my arms wide, close my eyes and feel the moon and the stars warm my face and light my journey.

I let the breeze travel wildly through my hair and didn't care if it whipped around and stung my eyes because soon, it wouldn't be there to brush or comb or sting. And the sting in my eyes would be replaced by something else.

So I took a breath and I savored the moment.

I was nearing the driver's seat as I moved off the hood and strained to reach towards the open window and slide my body in. I've always preferred to look at life through the windshield, and I am working hard trying not to look in the rearview mirror too often. My friend Yolanda Simonsis reminded me of something I'd once said to her in an interview a few years ago: "I don't look backwards because we aren't going that way."

I am signing off for now and looking forward. But first, I must sleep.

Chapter 21

And Then There Was One, Which Is Truly the Loneliest Number That Can Ever Be

Wednesday; February 20th, 8:00 AM

I filled out more paperwork, signed several consent forms and as usual, I made adjustments as to what I would and would not allow. (i.e., *yes* to students being present but *no* to them doing the operation and *no* to pictures. If it wasn't going to be Playboy, it wasn't going to be a medical journal or a slide in a college lecture, either). I answered the same questions over and over again for nurses, doctors, anesthesiologists and sundry others who approached us in either a blue or white coat.

I changed into the hospital gown they had provided me and put on the slippers and socks. But I didn't put on the stupid little hair net. At least I could look decent until they took me into the operating room. Who would want to sit here looking completely like patient material at this point, I wondered.

As I slipped into the gown, I looked in the mirror at the "girls," together for the last time. A huge lump settled in my throat. I glanced over to where Larry was sitting. He looked so worried, so scared that it broke my heart. He was with me the entire time up until surgery. In fact, he would continue to go as far as they would allow him to go.

He made it to the operating room doors.

The surgical team was a wonderful collection of people: the anesthesiologist from Israel, the second doctor in command who hailed from Australia, and Dr. Connolly. I know he is Irish Catholic but I think he was born here in the United States. Larry and I had had a chance to talk to them all before surgery but we were not able to meet the other nurses, doctors and anesthesiologists who would be in attendance.

They told me that I did well in surgery.

As expected, the doctor came out to the family when it was all over and told Larry that they had had to " . . . really snow her under before we could start." Why do doctors doubt me when I tell them I have a high tolerance for drugs?

I had nothing on but one of my favorite thongs, of course, and those ridiculous hospital gowns. Before surgery, Larry and I had joked about whether the thong would still be there when he saw me next. It was!

Dr. Connolly came to see me in the recovery room. I remember Larry being there, too. The doctor was dressed in a suit and on his way out of the hospital to give a speech. He asked me if I could feel *this*—and he pinched my arm, hard. I said yes and shot him an aggravated smirk. Next he asked me to shake his hand, which I did. And then I remembered. Just before surgery, when Larry and I had been waiting for me to be called in, the doctor had stopped by to see us and I'd asked if he could please be very careful and try not to nick my muscle so that I would still have feeling in my arm in the future. I was concerned, as well, about something called a "winged scapula," with which the shoulder blade would stick out instead of remaining flat when you extend your arm, causing your head to tilt like a marionette doll, bobbing off to one side. Dr. Connolly wanted to show me before he left the hospital that he had done his job well. At least I was not going to experience those problems.

Then off he flew.

Like Superman.

Able to whack off cancerous boobies in a single bound!

After surgery, I remember seeing Larry, Mom and Dad, Shere, Bob, Lisa, Karen White and Donna Cannizzo and then *poof!*—it was nighttime before I knew it. It was too late to order dinner.

Order dinner?

Just where the hell did I think I was? At the Plaza Athénée, the Ritz in Paris or the Marriott Marquis on Broadway in New York? Shere somehow persuaded the nurses to find something for me to eat; I couldn't have cared less, but she was vigilant in her efforts to look after me in every way. At around midnight, I was finally given a sandwich that some amazing nurse had found after she had gotten the rest of her charges settled.

I couldn't sleep a wink, and not for lack of trying. The room was incredibly hot and my roommate and I were perspiring as if we'd just run a marathon. As soon as we realized that no, they were *not* hot flashes—we got the room temperature adjusted.

I wasn't in an "Oh my God, I am going to beat my head against the wall" kind of pain. It was more of an occasional stabbing and constant throbbing when the drugs started to wane in my system. The best description would be *hugely uncomfortable*. It felt like the pain ran a circuit along the area that was traumatized. Around and around the circuit it went, and it fired off quite a nasty sting.

A drainage system had been placed in the wound to collect blood and other liquids. The part that was inside of me was attached to a long tube that was attached to a pressurized bulb where all liquids were collected and later measured and discarded. Most of the system hung outside of my body, so it needed to be pinned to my clothes. A wrong movement caused a tug against the stitches that anchored it to my skin, and gave me a great shock of searing pain.

They wrapped up my right side very tightly and were diligent about keeping me comfortable.

There were a few surprises during the night. I thought my roommate was playing solitaire and that she liked to shuffle the cards a lot, as there was this incredibly loud sound coming from her side of the room. The drape was closed between our beds and I was hooked up to all sorts of stuff, so at first I just dealt with it. We were sharing a room and she had rights, too. After two and a half hours, I was not only getting a tad aggravated but I was curious as to what was going on over there. I unplugged my IV system from the wall, took off both pressure cuff boots that were wrapped around each leg and made my way out the door, dragging the entire IV stand along with me.

She wasn't playing cards or snoring; she was grinding her teeth! Her *false* teeth. And they were moving in and out of her mouth with each breath.

I walked through the halls for a while, found a chair, hooked myself up to an electrical outlet so that the IV would remain effective, and sat. The nurses accommodated my new sleeping arrangement because they had heard this loud and unique sound themselves from the previous three nights. There were no other rooms available, so I had to tough it out. Soon enough, the discomfort that I experienced from the sitting position far outweighed the noises, so I went back to my room. My iPod was acting up but the noise-cancelling headphones were a big help.

Nurses took vital signs throughout the night. My drainage bag needed to be emptied, and of course the meds had to be dispensed. Sleeping in a hospital is an event you grab when you can. Hating hospitals as I do would have made sleeping a big surprise, anyway. I wasn't expecting to give blood twice but I did. It became more than I could handle when the nurse came by in the morning with a long-ass needle that was to go into my arm and not through the IV, as everything else had up to that point except for the blood tests.

I respectfully declined.

The drug was Heparin, and the doctor had ordered it to thin my blood. It is given to patients who have undergone surgery and are unable to move around freely afterwards. It helped to ensure that there were no blood clots forming. The nurse accepted the fact that there would be no further discussion about this. She admitted that she had heard from the nurses on the last shift that I had been walking around most of the night. We agreed that I was probably clot-free.

Thursday, 11:00 AM

Dr. Connolly was in surgery the next morning, so a colleague removed my dressings. It was uncomfortable, as the tape had stuck hard to my skin and the dressings had become a security blanket. They kept everything tight and safe and in place.

I surprised myself yet again. I was certain I wouldn't have the strength to look—but once the bandages were off, I had to. It was a quick drive-by look but I saw enough. I melted, and off went Niagara Falls.

I cried like a baby.

It was hard to look at. Parts were sunken in, other parts protruded. The edges of the wound were particularly sensitive. Soft and tender in some places yet hard and tender in others. Once Shere arrived and was able to inspect things more closely, she said the doctor had probably used a cauterizing knife, and for lack of a better term, had "seared" the tissue and blood vessels as he went along. The drain tubing was clearly visible, all coiled up inside of me. I cried and cried and cried.

There were to be no more hospital IV-administered drugs. I had passed all of the discharge tests. Once the doctor had left the room, I began to dress for the trip home. I was so ready to end my twenty-three-hour drive-by mastectomy.

Shere and Larry arrived just after the dressings had been changed. Shere later told me that as soon as she saw my face, she knew something weird had happened. The nurse was still in the room when they arrived and I told her that I felt like I needed more support than these new bandages were providing me. I was absolutely serious and only later, when I reflected back on the day, did I understand why she had looked at me a little oddly. Support? What exactly was I hoping to support? Yet she went and found larger silk bandages and gently placed one on top of the other, carefully taping them all in place. It really moves me as I look back at how sensitive, how human, how utterly kind she had been in that simple action. And she had never said a word to make me feel bad; she had just smiled and gone about her work.

It must have been those *phantom* feelings that I was experiencing once again.

During that second unveiling at the hospital, Shere and Larry were there and were able to see the surgical site. My sister is a doctor; she performs surgeries every week on all kinds of animals, and she has seen more blood and guts and gory things than I will ever see in my lifetime (thank God!), but this was her *sister*. It was different for her. Larry and I watched her turn gray, and Larry noticed that she had suddenly broken out into a sweat. He began fanning her. He grabbed her around the waist when he realized that she was going down. She realized it, too and she simply pushed me aside on the bed and crawled in with me. There we were, the two of us in bed, feeling sick and dizzy, leaving Larry to wonder what he was supposed to do next.

We received directions from the nurse and doctor for post-op care at home.

Once at home, I slept the better part of the afternoon while Larry, Shere and Bob kept an eye on the drainage bag and kept track of and dispensed all of the drugs. Shere would remove and re-dress the bandages in two days, and then I would see Dr. Connolly late next week. This was when I hoped that the drain would be removed and when I would learn if the cancer had spread and what my next course of treatment involved.

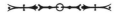

Dr. Song's Corner

Drains are a necessary evil. After surgery, the damaged blood vessels and lymphatic vessel that need time to heal will leak fluid into the surgical site. If a drain is not used to evacuate this accumulating fluid, the fluid can build—and at the very least, be uncomfortable; at the very worst, can become infected, which may lead to further surgery. We all hate drains, but they are employed judiciously and when necessary. Unfortunately, after a mastectomy, they are almost always necessary.

Chapter 22

It All Comes at Me at Once

The first four days after surgery were an incredible personal discovery of the body's ability to deal with healing and trauma. It had been a rough couple of days and for me they all blended together as one very, very long day.

I know how a junkie feels. I found myself all too frequently asking Shere and Larry, "How long until the next pain pill?" I couldn't believe how slowly time seemed to move. The doctors had prescribed some very potent stuff; Oxyconton and Oxycodone being two of the drugs. I was told to strictly adhere to the pain relief time plan so as to stay on top of the pain. This type of pain would be much harder to catch up with than to stay on top of.

While Shere and Larry are completely aware of my high drug tolerance, we all talked about it and agreed that these were not drugs to fool around with. In other words, the bottles were left in *their* control and not mine. I was totally OK with that.

Those first four days were filled with pain or what I *perceived* to be pain, and the pills only provided relief for three to four hours. I was searching for a totally pain-free, blissful experience and the morphine drip was unavailable. This time I was uncharacteristically afraid not to take the pain pills. I wanted to be sure to stay ahead of the potential for more pain and I knew that only through these drugs would I find relief. Things were so out of whack for me that left to my own devices, I might easily have popped just one or two more pills before the prescribed time and it would probably have been way too soon or in some deadly combination that I was not aware of. Trusting Larry and Shere as I do made it easy to give up this control. They had it all written down in a notebook: drainage output, date and time noted, drug given, date and time noted, and all the side effects that I'd experienced. Shere had also made a key at the bottom of the page of their log book to show which drugs could not be mixed together. I now had my very own personalized PDR (Physician's Drug Reference).

They were in a much better place to handle this than I was.

Larry, Shere and Bob changed my pajamas, the bedding, and the zillions of pillow cases on the pillows used to prop me up in different positions, at least half a dozen times today. I couldn't seem to regulate my body temperature. I got extremely cold and shivered uncontrollably, turning an odd color gray; and then it all shifted and I quickly developed sweats and heat flushes of which I'd never experienced before. My pajamas and sheets were literally soaking wet every few hours. By this time tomorrow, I was certain that I would be no more than a puddle.

The thought of eating turned my stomach in knots.

We named my new accessory "Dickie the Drain." Getting up and moving in any way increased the volume of liquids that flooded into the drain. We proved it. On two occasions, I thought it was OK to be downstairs with the family as Mom was making dinner. Perched high on a bar stool at the island in our kitchen proved to be a dizzying experience, so I sat most of the time in a chair at the table, comfortably positioned a tad lower to the floor, firmly anchored by my feet. The problem was that it was hard for me to be sitting down while everyone else was moving about keeping busy. I continued to get up to do something or move something or just *move*. After being yelled at continually, I would remember and quietly sit down.

The drain filled up during those active times much faster than when I was at rest. Since the doctor wouldn't remove Dickie until there was less than 30 cc of liquid measured over two consecutive days, I tried to keep my activity down to a minimum. Taking the drain out any sooner risked that fluid would continue to collect at the surgical site and then it would need to be drained in a most uncomfortable way: by a series of needle aspirations.

I was becoming used to Dickie. Not particularly attached to him, but used to the damn thing, so another few days would be worth the wait in order to avoid another medical anything. I started out at 165 cc output on the first day after going home and I still had a long way to go. Therefore, I needed to learn to be at peace in a new way. I needed to add a speed or two to the gear shift, as the days of running with two speeds, two hundred miles per hour or parked—had ended for me, at least for the time being. Coasting is not in my DNA. This would be a challenge.

Saturday was the hardest day so far, after surgery.

I was delirious. I had not slept or eaten much in at least four days. I would get some rest here and there and then my body and mind would push back towards the surface like a swimmer coming up for air, and the drama would begin all over again.

My body clock was messed up. The temperature changes as noted above were in full swing, and I ached all over. I had been in bed for so long that it actually hurt my left lung when I lay down. There was no way to sleep on my right side or on my chest, so my left side and my back had to be used exclusively. My lung would get so heavy and full inside of me. I could literally feel it just lying half-inflated on the floor of my rib cage. This was a completely new kind of pain and one that I'd never experienced before. It was a dull, slow, and pulsing ache that pierced through with each and every breath.

Shere changed the dressings that day. I cry even now while reliving those moments as I write this chapter. Two sisters, who are very close to each other, sitting in one of their bedrooms, removing surgical dressings after one of them has had a mastectomy. Trying to be gentle, trying to be brave, all kinds of thoughts whirling through each of their heads. The dressings were off. I was at home with my sister. It felt safe to do more than just a drive-by look. So I looked. I *really* looked, and I liquefied a little more. Niagara Falls started up again. Shere said she wanted to see things from my perspective. From behind me, she placed her head on my shoulder. She saw what I saw. She told me that I was beautiful and that the doctor had done a fabulous job and had left me with a lot of my own skin for reconstruction. She was rocking me in her arms and kissing me on my back and neck. I didn't even feel like it was me. How could it possibly be me? But it was. I started to shiver. I was going to be sick. Thankfully, a garbage can was nearby.

She cleaned me up and settled me back into bed. We talked for a long time. I was so very tired. I had rings under my eyes and my facial muscles were unable to muster any expression at all. Blank. We agreed to skip the pain pill so that I could take a sleeping pill, as they cannot be taken together. I prayed for sleep to come. It finally arrived. I savored the moment and allowed the drifting numbness to possess me entirely.

Finally, there was no more terror and no more pain as the night swallowed my exhausted body; my last memory before drifting off to sleep having been conjured in hell.

Larry and I became very dependent on Shere. Mostly *I* had, as she had covered so many bases. I was blessed with a live-in doctor, who not only looked after me but also helped us navigate the medical details. She was my sister, my friend, my confidant and someone with whom I could be true and honest. I held nothing back from her.

She never stopped moving once she had arrived at the house from New Jersey. Today was her husband Kurt's fiftieth birthday—and she was here. That's so wrong. I didn't want her to go next week, although I knew that she must. Her sacrifice, her family's sacrifice and her practice's sacrifice had been huge. It was time.

This has been very hard on my family. I constantly wondered if I was being a baby. Have others responded similarly, physically? It is hard to compare emotional responses, but aren't physiological responses supposed to be more closely aligned? I agonized over my responses. I agonized at being the cause of my family's pain.

Chapter 23

Short Takes

Sunday, four days post-surgery

When Larry had done the house rehab a few years back, he had designed our incredible bedroom suite. It includes an enormous bathroom, two closed closets and a huge walk-in closet with an island of drawers in the center. It is a suite that takes up most of the third floor and is all by itself.

It is my dream room.

Larry had put in a huge steam shower—I counted the days until I could use it again—and the biggest and deepest Jacuzzi bathtub we could find that is surrounded by a marble landing. That landing was really helpful, as I could sit on it and more easily enter the water. Being a shower girl, I had finally come to appreciate the luxuries of a bath. It was my second bath since being home but this one I could linger in and enjoy for a little bit. The drugs from the hospital and the drugs from home were finally leaving my body.

I needed to be careful, as the bandages couldn't get wet, which made a shower an impossibility. After the bath, Shere gave me a luxurious shampoo in that deep, warm tub—which is equipped with a removable spray handle (*ahhhh!*). She changed the dressings, and finally . . .

Sleep.

I felt like a quarter million bucks!

Monday, five days post-surgery

The nurse called to check in on me. I was reminded that Dickie the Drain must be at 30 cc for two consecutive days before I could kiss him good-bye. I had a fairly good sense that this constantly changing accessory that was adding to my daily ensemble would probably be around for a little longer than I had hoped. I've already mentioned what happens if we rush things, and there is still fluid present around the surgical site. *Yuck.*

I've always been a girl to accessorize, so I would adapt well.

It was a rough morning today, emotionally. I slept all afternoon. But overall, I had a wonderful day. There was less than 70 cc in the drain and by 11:30 PM, I felt like a half million bucks.

Tuesday, six days post-surgery

Before Shere left for home, I had another bath, shampoo and bandage change. Mom was there so she could see the way things were. It was important for me and for Mom to have her involved in this new kind of unveiling. It wasn't easy for her. The pain in her eyes kept the tears in mine at bay. It was very difficult for me to see my mom in any kind of pain. I know that she feels the same way.

I'd decided to write the book that several of my friends had suggested. Now that this was the plan, I'd begun adding to the chapters. Things that you wouldn't necessarily want to know about, but someone you know or may meet will—well, *might*—want to know about. Those additions were added as thoughts came to me; but they were available, even in their current rough format, for anyone who might have needed them, whenever they might have needed them.

I am not vain enough to consider ever getting published by a well-known publishing house, but I am also one who believes strongly in dreams. I have been dreaming with my eyes wide open since I was a kid; some call it "visualization."

I read constantly and am forever amazed at the current level of talent that I come across. I am also quite certain that the numbers they speak of in publishing are true. Less than twenty percent of submissions are even read. This means that you, my friends and family and those we meet along the way who might be helped by this story, are the publishers (under my name, of course. Come on. I haven't had a pain pill in twenty-four hours. I'm coming back).

Tomorrow would be a big day, as we would be seeing Dr. Connolly. It would be precisely seven days after surgery. I was up all day and had even accomplished something of value for the office.

I felt like three quarters of a million bucks!

Chapter 24

My Body Sends Me Two Important Signs,
Two Days after Surgery

Flashback to the Friday after surgery: a familiar flush of heat and heaviness came to me in regular rounds throughout my lower abdomen.

It was my period. Two days early.

I was elated. Elation is not something that generally occurs when my period comes. My body, while still a bit messed up from surgery, was showing me that it continued to operate. As anyone at fifty can attest, having a period two days early or two days late is nothing out of the ordinary. Many women were in full-swing menopause by now but I was still getting regular monthly periods. I welcomed and I savored all of the crap associated with a period and celebrated in silence (until now) that I was still working.

Then the best surprise of all arrived on Saturday morning. Those flutters of soft and gentle wings that slowly build, and the flush of heat that rises and ebbs like ocean waves and when all combined, signal quite clearly that you are horny.

Oh, my God.

Dad, maybe you should turn the page. Mom, you'd better read this first and approve it for daddy consumption.

I was amazed. I felt like shit physically—again, I was certain from the way too powerful drugs—but I was *horny*. I'd just had a boob cut off! How could this be?

Calm down, I told myself. It must have been an excellent dream.

I took some deep, lung-filling breaths, savoring the moment that never seemed to end. It would be hours later, and every once in a while that little wink would come back. I was quite pleased with the whole experience. It was a constant craving with no relief in sight, or energy if it were, but I was thoroughly enjoying every damn minute of the tease.

I told Larry, Bob, and Shere. It was pretty obvious that they thought I had completely lost my mind. They smiled and looked at each other, nodded their heads and one of them said, " . . . uh-huh, get some rest, Suzanne." I am certain that each one of them was silently betting on who would be the first to crack up laughing once they had left the room. But I was dead serious. My body had shown me twice within twenty-four hours that it was fighting back!

If things truly come in threes, hell, I almost couldn't wait to see what was coming next. And no, I was not hoping for a bowel movement. I'd already climbed that mountain successfully on two consecutive days. (Cue the Rocky song!)

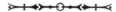

Dr. Song's Corner

Oftentimes, the stress of surgery will initiate menses early. Don't be alarmed; it can be seen as your body "working," as Suzanne writes. But if the flow is heavy (heavier than normal), it should be something that you share with your doctor. Remember that surgery involves blood loss and of course, so does menstruation. Too much blood loss can cause dizziness, headaches, a fast heart rate, palpitations and in its extreme can be life threatening. Ask your doctor about iron replacement and notify your team about long or heavy menstruation.

Chapter 25

A New Twist to Living out the String

Once Dr. Shere had left for home, Larry the Warden elevated the status of the remaining staff and re-established responsibilities and watch times. I imagined the keys to the cell had been relocated and the secret password had been changed. This was really quite beautiful to watch, but confusing to the sole inmate who had felt perfectly fine since about 8:00 PM Monday night.

Here we were on Wednesday. I was planning my breakout very carefully because these guys were slick. One left, and *poof*—another quickly appeared.

I'd stopped taking the pain meds on Sunday and had felt progressively better with each passing minute. I highly caution anyone taking these two drugs to consider a gentler alternative. I am convinced that they were partly to blame for the temperature changes and overall disgusting feeling that I had had after surgery. And, not knowing just what to eat when I had taken them was definitely part of the cause of those physical reactions during earlier days.

The Warden left the house at around 5:00 AM after checking on me, filling up my water pitcher and visiting with me about his day. I would be free until 9:00 AM when Officer Bob would arrive. The parental units were scheduled to arrive at 11:00 AM and then we would all reconvene at the house and leave for the doctor's appointment. Dr. Connolly would either love the audience or simply attempt to give me the general once-over. It's going to be so much fun to see this one play out. They *never* get away with a general once-over with a Zaccone.

Today, I was accompanied by Larry, Mom, Dad and Bob. My name was called and five people got up and followed Nurse Reanetta Reed. She seemed to love the company, so it started out really well. I was no longer crying through the weight, height, and blood pressure tests and we were able to share a few laughs. I reminded my family that for the rest of my life, my right arm cannot be used for a blood pressure test, a blood test, IV or even a finger prick—as lymphedema and infections are now a huge problem for me on that side.

We were passed on to Donna Christian, Dr. Connolly's head surgical nurse. She told us that there was good news today and proceeded to take off the bandages and check everything out. Dr. Shere had done a marvelous job in keeping the wound and drain site totally clean, clear and free of all contaminants. Donna reminded me to carry my bag, briefcase, luggage, groceries and anything else heavier than a gallon of milk on my left arm, in order to maintain proper blood flow and not restrict lymph fluid.

My mom had already experienced this visual, so she knew what to expect. Yesterday, I had asked my dad how he felt, just before he had fallen asleep next to me, and I knew he was curious as well. Larry had seen a quick drive-by at the hospital that first day but had wanted to wait for the final unveiling until he felt I was feeling better about it. I would have showed him immediately but I am sure he was respecting my anguish, recognizing his own fear, or possibly both. In any case, this is not something to push on anyone. I tried to convince Bob that I would be all covered up and that he would not be seeing his sister in any way that anyone would or should consider odd. It's not like I was naked. I was uncovered on top but only on my right side; a surgical site. He was uncomfortable, though, and stayed behind the curtain, which provided me with the perfect response every time he spoke: "Do not pay attention to that man behind the curtain."

The exalted Dr. Connolly entered the room and we learned the following things: out of twenty-eight intramamory axillary lymph nodes that had been removed, only one was cancerous. If there was any cancer remaining in my body, it should be taken care of by the chemo treatments that I would undergo. The Doc was able to get a clean margin, which simply means that all the cancer in what used to be my breast is history and nothing had been left behind.

I could drive again, immediately. I couldn't lift anything or overexert my right arm for a few more weeks and I needed to be very careful until the drain was removed. The physiological reactions I had experienced were definitely due to those very strong drugs. I could have a martini or two as long as I was not taking any pain meds.

"Are there any restrictions with sex?" I asked Dr. Connolly. "Is there anything to be careful of? Anything we should expect or avoid?"

If he had a shocking moment that day, that would have to be it. He looked around the room and said, "Suzanne, your father is sitting right here!"

To which my father answered, on perfect cue: "And sex is what brought us all together today. Go ahead, answer her question."

Larry immediately spoke up. "Look, Doc," he said. "I had no idea about any of these questions and particularly not *this* one. I swear I had nothing to do with this."

Of course, I had carefully printed out everything in a document and was prepared and looking forward to some kind of reaction. "Larry," I said simply, "if you had known the questions in advance, you might have silently wondered why sex was the seventh question asked and not the first. Doc, you can talk about this stuff in front of my family if I ask the question in front of them—and besides, Larry is an Irish Catholic. I believe I can assume that you are, as well. Need I say more?"

Dr. Connolly smiled and said, "No restrictions," although he felt we should wait for the drain to be removed and suggested that we refrain from bouncing off the walls for a while.

No problem.

I mentioned that the landscape of my arm, underarm, upper chest area and back had been altered. He said they would go back to normal in a few months. As would some but not all of the entire area which was totally dead or numb and did not feel part of me until I moved the drain wrong, and then *yow* . . . it hurt. He seemed quite pleased at the mobility I demonstrated in my arm, but asked that I refrain from exercise until the drain was removed. The drain output had really gone down. Yesterday, it had topped off at 60 cc and today it had ended up at 41 cc. I estimated that by Saturday, I could say farewell to Dickie the Drain.

Due to the size of my tumors, their Grade 3 status, rapid growth rate and the fact that I had a cancerous intramamory axillary lymph node that they were aware of before surgery; I walked into surgery with cancer at Stage 2. I prepared myself to hear today that I was at Stage 3. I ended up at stage 2-B.

The doctor told me that they were going to hit me hard and fast with a full court press for several months of chemo. I would lose my hair. I would be very, very sick. But I would survive. Then another set of less caustic rounds would be administered, but that would bring forward other side effects such as bone and muscle pain, to name a few. Radiation was an unknown at this time.

I felt that with this terrific news and the two fabulous surprises I had noted in Chapter 24, we had experienced the best ending—or a beginning—that was possible.

Lymph nodes are aligned in a string and now I can truly "Live out the String." (Kiss to Sophia Dilberakis, Marc Cohn and Shane Fontayne)

Due to good behavior, I was hoping for an early release from the Warden and his ever-efficient and well-loved staff.

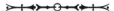

Dr. Song's Corner

After a mastectomy, patients most likely will have temporary numbness of the remaining skin, chest and even of the arm. This is because as the breast is removed, so too are the nerves that innervate the breast and the skin of the breast. There is also a nerve called the intercostal brachial nerve that supplies sensation to the underarm and inner/upper arm, which can be bruised during surgery. Sensation typically starts to return within several weeks and can be painful at first, like tiny electrical shocks. This is a sign that the nerves are growing back into the skin. If sensation doesn't start returning in several weeks, don't be alarmed, as everyone is different—but clearly discuss this with your doctor.

Chapter 26

The Disengagement of Dickie the Drain But First, My Tribute to D2 (D-Squared)

Before we get to the disengagement of Dickie the Drain, I failed to mention in the last chapter that I told Dr. Connolly that I was writing a book. I would either use his name or would change it in some way so as not to identify him directly if that were to be his wish. He replied that using his name would be perfectly fine with him. Bingo!

Now, the hard part faced me. I needed to get inside this team of doctors and nurses heads; really understand it from their perspective. I mentioned to Dr. Connolly that I would like to interview him, get the real deal from his perspective. What wasn't working? What was needed? How could things be made better? How are insurance rules and regulations affecting his team's real work? How can we make the barbaric tests more comfortable for the patient? I told him that at this point in my life, I finally had some time, that I was blessed with a vast worldwide network of caring and influential people and a burning desire to change things up a bit for the good of all. And so I suggested lunch one day, since we'd be seeing so much of each other over the next thirty years. He said he'd do it, and I had witnesses!

I gave him a big hug.

My tribute to D2 or D-squared; some would know him as Darrell Dochstaeder. I've cast the line out as far as I could reach. The snap of my wrist was tight and strong and I listened carefully to the sound as it sliced through the mist and then plunged into the waters below. I knew it would travel far; the whip of the line against the breeze had assured me of that.

Plunk.

The line landed clean and deep in the marsh and the bait was quickly taken.

We've only just begun D2. The doctor is on board.

Friday, February 29th

It's Leap Year!

The amount of measurable liquid in Dickie the Drain went down to 20 cc this morning. I called Nurse Donna to schedule the disengagement party. Monday at noon, Dickie would be history.

Note: the Warden, Officer Bob and the Parental Units had determined to release me early due to good behavior. This afternoon, my girlfriend Donna Cannizzo stopped by for lunch and Carol arrived at around 2:30 PM. Other than that, I had the whole day to spend as I saw fit. There was so much to catch up on: paperwork, paying bills, insurance for the lake house flood, insurance for the boob, organizing my office and clearing up the clutter.

I loved it; the busy craziness of my days. Life was coming back to what I was calling "the new normal" once again.

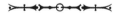

Dr. Song's Corner

Healthcare delivery in our country today (August 31, 2009) is one of the main—if not *the* main—issue that is being discussed by the leaders of our government. Access to healthcare, proper delivery, trimming waste and increasing efficiency should be concerns for all of us. It is my belief that everyone should have access to proper healthcare and in particular, timely screening for breast cancer. This includes, first and foremost, a breast exam by a

105

healthcare provider, timely mammograms and regular follow-up exams. Insurance companies need to realize that preventative care in the long run decreases costs, and thus can increase net profits. The gauntlet of paperwork, phone calls and appeals for approval needs to be streamlined—as this process and the human resources it takes to implement this process necessitates a huge cost structure. Without getting too political, universal healthcare administered by the government, in my opinion, is not the answer. Government-run programs, in general, have not worked as well as free market industries. Furthermore, defensive medicine needs to be curtailed. Currently, many physicians order more tests than are always necessary as a means to protect themselves from malpractice lawsuits. It is a daily occurrence that physicians will order tests not because they crucially need that information to make a decision, but to protect them from being sued if a result is contrary to what was surmised. There must be a better method of protecting patients from bad doctors (yes, there are bad doctors) without having the entire country of doctors ordering unnecessary tests to prevent frivolous lawsuits.

Despite the media coverage of what is broken in our system, we should take a critical look at what is working. We still have the best doctors and the greatest innovative research and development machine in the world. More attention needs to be paid to how we can make our system better. This means streamlining, providing efficiencies, allowing doctors to be doctors and restoring trust. Patient advocates and navigators should be better equipped and empowered to centralize care information, prevent redundancies and extraneous actions. Finally, patients need to take their health into their own hands. Prevention of obesity by proper diet and exercise would be the single greatest budget improvement for not just our healthcare but for our entire economy. If everyone walked more, ate less and exercised and became more accountable for their own health, we might not be in this position now.

Chapter 27

Pictures: Ladies, These are for You

Right after my diagnosis, Larry and I were sitting at the island in our kitchen, talking about—what else?—my boob. It was what consumed our lives for those six weeks before surgery. It was all that I was interested in. He would take me out and plan a romantic dinner and I would play along and joyfully enter the topic of the moment and somehow find a way to spin it back to my boob. How pathetic is that? How self-centered and mean? Before me was a man I had known since I was thirteen years old—and I was adding to his agony. I wasn't being very fair.

I was attracted to him from afar in high school. He was the hot, cool, bad boy; very popular, athletic, so good-looking and one of the three biggest catches in the class for the entire four years. I had never even considered him as a possibility. I was popular amongst my own group (we were a class of just over one thousand kids; still a leading record today), I was on the Pom-Pom squad and Drill team and helped put together the yearbook. I was as far west of "Good Girl" as he was east of "Bad Boy."

We both had many different groups of friends from all of the cliques in our class of one thousand; and because of that, we would frequently meet up at parties before and after graduation. Larry was sensitive to the feelings of others even then, as I have always been; looking to protect the underdog. I love that about him to this day.

After high school, we grew up quickly without seeing much of each other. Then the ten-year reunion arrived and we met up again. He'd calmed down a bit and I had opened up a bit . . . but I digress. Long story short, I pursued him and it became a fabulous explosion that has lasted for twenty-four years. We've tumbled forward through so much good and through so much pain and we thought we had experienced it all. Good times and bad times and those heavenly in-between times. Times we had to be apart due to my traveling or his. We never imagined that this, *cancer*, was to be the big test.

He had never let me down once throughout this drama. He never said the wrong thing. It seemed that he always knew what I needed, either before I knew it or at the same instant. It was mesmerizing to see this synchronization for the first time from such a selfish and self-absorbed place: my newest perspective; floating above the living of life and observing more clearly than ever before all the nuances from a safe distance. This synchronization has always been there and I've always known it. In the process of writing everything down, I was reminded of it in so many little ways. I simply needed to stop a bit to think about it, really think about it. The phone calls when I would know it was him from the extra beat of my heart when I heard the phone ring. The laughs we shared each and every single day we've been together. Much like living with Shere and Bob when we were kids; a nonstop fabulous ride filled with laughter and fun. I was totally satisfied with the things we are so much alike with and OK with the things we are on opposite poles of the world on; in the end, we agreed to disagree. I'm very lucky. Twenty-four years. My godchildren, nieces and nephews have known us as a couple all their lives. We are a matched pair. Could this shitty disease mess up that synchronicity?

Getting back to the island in our kitchen right after my diagnosis, I wanted to mark with pictures the upcoming changes in my body. Thank God for the digital times we live in! We could view pictures without the photo guy or some teenager that the girls know at high school, also possibly seeing them while working at the local photo-mart. I wished to chronicle "the girls," not just now but throughout the entire process.

I anticipated that Larry would be pulling out the equipment faster than I could complete the thought, but he seemed to look at this idea as something other than I had expected. I mean, really, it was totally something other than I had expected his reaction would be. Believe it or not, it never happened. For him, it wasn't for the right reason. I could not enlist him in taking pictures for the reason I wanted to have those particular pictures taken. I never did take that last picture of "the girls" . . . together.

Sunday, March 2, 2008

Dickie the Drain would become history tomorrow. Call me a sicko—I don't care, because at this point I could handle having that moniker added to my bio. I wanted to remember what it looked like to have a drain coiled inside my breast, around the skin left from the skin-sparing mastectomy, causing me to look like the beginning drawings of Barbarella or Madonna on her big musical tour. I didn't want to forget the drain tube spewing out of my side, attached to the drain hose that is attached to the drain bulb that was forever getting caught on something, catching any and all residual blood and ooze and unknown liquids spinning around the trauma site.

Off I went. Larry was cleaning up his office and I was moving between reading a magazine, pacing, writing this book—and then the thought came to me. I had little time left to mark this last step conquered. I went to the bedroom with the camera.

Self portraits are difficult to do well; and after many attempts, I finally captured the best images that I could, considering the angle, and got several shots that I was satisfied with. Artistic masochism, for posterity's sake! They looked like mug shots, only with a boob and a boobette as the main feature instead of a face. One perfect and one—let's say, under construction. A little bit of neck, some strands of hair and no torso. Tomorrow, or one day soon after, I would mark the same change with another photograph or two. These would be of me without Dickie the Drain.

Why do this? Why chronicle such a painful experience?

I want women to feel comfortable with what has happened to me. I want them to be comfortable with what is *still* happening to me. It could only help me to become more comfortable with what has already happened and is still about to happen to me. I want to have proof and to be able to show them upfront, up close and personal, not to be scared like I was, to forget about what a mastectomy used to mean. A short decade ago, the surgery would have left you disfigured. It's different now.

Ask me to show you.

Chapter 28

Dickie the Drain is History

I have another clarification to make regarding the meeting we'd had with Dr. Connolly on the Wednesday after surgery. He had ordered Vicadin for my pain relief at home but upon my release from the hospital, I'd looked at the script and freaked, knowing that this stuff didn't really do much for me. Since I was unable to take the morphine drip home, I wanted to be sure to have something really strong available. I had tried Vicadin after dental surgery and all it did was make me constipated. The doctor, covering rounds for the floor at the time of my release, looked at my chart. No doubt he noticed my high drug tolerance and the amount of drugs needed to put me out for surgery. He prescribed Oxyconton and Oxycodone. I was elated, knowing that this was strong stuff. I quickly bolted for the doors before he could change his mind. I was now feeling much better about separating from my friend the morphine IV drip.

It was a very bad choice, as I had not yet learned the correct combination of food required to be in your system before taking these drugs. I learned very quickly. I strongly suggest that you consider taking it slow until you learn the balance of what types of food products need to be in your system for each drug prescribed, or you could get mighty sick as I did. These three drugs are also highly addictive.

I suggested that Dr. Connolly add "artist" to his bio, as he had really done an amazing job. He then told me that he *is* an artist, and that selling his art had helped to finance medical school. He said he would show me some of his artwork at one of our future meetings. If I didn't know better, were a little younger and did not have my right top side exposed to him after he had just hacked off my boob tissue—I'd think he had just delivered a pick-up line. But I know better, and we are very close in age. Enough said!

Friday, February 29, 2008

Dr. Connolly called me on Friday afternoon to check in, make sure I didn't have questions, and to go over what had been discussed at the team meeting yesterday. He felt that the chemo oncologists were right-on with their plan but that the radiation oncologists were being far too aggressive with the radiation program they had planned for me. He strongly suggested that I get a second opinion on the pros and cons of that treatment.

"Suzanne," he said, "I really don't think that radiation is necessary for you. But listen to what they have to say, do your usual exhaustive research and get that second opinion."

He made this an issue twice in the conversation. I wanted to explore this topic with him in greater depth and in person. But the signal was loud and clear: I needed to question the prudence of radiating healthy tissue since he felt quite strongly that the cancer had been all but removed through surgery, and any residual cancer cells lurking about my body should definitely be killed off during chemo.

I love the relationship I have with this doctor; yet I still sweat the details.

Monday, March 3, 2008

I'd taken care of Dickie the Drain for the past week since Shere had left. Bob and Larry had helped on occasion but for the most part, it was Dickie and me. Lots of things were becoming less gross to me; yet, I still have an unquenchable dislike of all things medical. Stethoscopes, needles and stainless steel paired with porcelain continued to be an issue but I could finally walk into the hospital without being dragged or drugged.

Progress for me has always been a swift forward movement. This medical stuff continued to slowly inch forward but was getting much better.

Dr. Shere called it accurately once again: the alcohol wipe that was used to clean the drain site area on my side, stung. The *clip, clip, clip* of the stitches holding the drain stable against and inside my body felt odd but did not hurt. When I was asked to take a deep breath and slowly let it out, I felt a *whoosh* as the tube slid smoothly out of my body. It was very weird, not painful at all, but oh-so-liberating. As each inch left my body, I could feel a huge release of pressure and immediately found air space. Larry said it was amazing to see it slither out, nice and clean and easy. I was shocked at how much had been coiled inside of me. No showers until Wednesday, but I was getting used to baths.

Chapter 29

A Boutique Like Most
Have Never Seen Before

Yesterday, after Nurse Donna had removed Dickie the Drain, I asked her to ask Dr. Connolly to call me at his convenience sometime this week. I stressed to her that I was not in any pain, was having no problems whatsoever, I had no complaints and there was absolutely no rush. I just had a few questions. The most important question being: "Where do I go for a second opinion with a radiation oncologist when I've been to the top five hospitals in the area just to find you and your team? I'm a marked boob! They'll know me as soon I pass through the door!"

Dr. Connolly called this afternoon and asked me where I lived. He suggested that I set up an appointment at Loyola University. Of course, the next question I had was if he might recommend a specific doctor at Loyola. He couldn't. He also works out of St Joseph's Hospital in Lincoln Park but he thought that would be too far for me to travel.

Was he kidding? Lincoln Park—shopping—people-watching—fabulous dining—near the Magnificent Mile with *more* shopping! These words were a favorite melody in my ears. But I said coolly, "Lincoln Park would be no problem for me at all."

So Dr. Connolly gave me the name of a colleague at St. Joseph's Hospital.

I asked him how we would get the required films, reports and documents over to this guy without pissing off the radiation oncologists at the University of Chicago. He said he would take care of that once I had set up the appointment; and he would make sure they all got back in my file, safe and sound.

Hmmm . . .

Maybe a chapter on the dueling radiation oncologists would add some spice?

Tuesday, March 4, 2008

After Dickie and I parted yesterday, I was brought into a "boutique" of sorts that was located right in the hospital at the Breast Center. They were set up with everything like bras with hidden trap doors—kind of like a secret compartment all ready to slide a prosthetic boob in. This is the kind of bra that is worn while a woman waits for reconstructive surgery, or used if she has decided to leave things as they are but desires a more balanced look when dressed.

It was a cornucopia of boobie accessories. And these ladies know their stuff! Tsiona Bittin, the owner of the boutique, was in that day and I was fortunate enough to work with the breast priestess of prosthetics. She took one look at me naked, made a quick measurement, turned on her heels and waved me on. And with one breast leading the way, I followed her.

She immediately locked on to a beautiful black bra. She whipped out a drawer filled with all sizes of prosthetics, selected one and deftly placed it into the hidden compartment in the bra. I tried it on. It was a perfect fit. First shot out of the proverbial box.

I needed more than one, though (bra, not prosthetic). I mean, come on; Victoria's Secret has a small outlet in my dresser drawer at home. I needed a white and nude color, at least.

The amazing part was that I was out of there inside of fifteen minutes. And best of all, you would never know the difference if you looked at me or hugged me. I'm a hugger. I tested it out several times today, and it passed my test. The prosthetic that you slip into this compartment in the bra is so strategically placed and so very well designed and manufactured that it is truly foolproof and even *feel*-proof. It is made of a very soft, life-like and malleable plastic, and moves around like a firm bowl of Jell-O. It also resembles a skinless, boneless, uncooked chicken breast—but with a better shape. It's a strange analogy but actually quite accurate.

Chapter 30

Taking Control of How I Lose the Rest of Me
But First, How I Met the Auditor

Over the last eight weeks, I'd only been at the office four or five times; partly because I am now semi-retired and I work just two days a week. Those days, I worked at home, mostly because of the BCD (Breast Cancer Drama). Every time I am at the office, either for a meeting or to stop in to pick up mail and drop off other documents that I've worked on, I feel so much positive energy and have so many laughs that I wonder if I should apply for a full-time position. Being in that environment is definitely good for my health.

Today, several of the girls at the office were interested in seeing the "real deal." As I've mentioned in a previous chapter, I would be willing to do an unveiling. So off to the ladies' bathroom we went.

I've grown up with many of these women. Kathy Welsch started the company with Bob and me twenty-four years ago and she and I had worked together for at least four years before that. These ladies are extensions of my core family.

Unable to cram ourselves in a bathroom stall, we just kind of hung out in front of a large bank of sinks. Being that we were in the ladies' bathroom, we were confident that we would not be interrupted by any of the guys. Knowing that, I was pretty open about the whole thing. I was in the throes of my newfound medical knowledge, explaining and showing all that

I'd learned—when in walked a new face. I assumed she was a new employee, and I apologized for having to meet her in this rather awkward way. She told me that she isn't an employee but an auditor.

Shit.

An auditor!

I turned green and wondered which of our customers I had just shown my breasts to. She quickly explained that no, she's not a customer; she was there along with our regular ISO Quality Auditor and was assisting him with training a group of our staff to become internal quality auditors.

Now that I understood that she was helping us train our staff (read between the lines: we are paying them) and that she was not a customer, supplier or tax auditor, I decided to have a little fun and mentioned that we are very strict and totally compliant with our quality system and that she could now say that she had witnessed our quality standards herself, from top to bottom. Quality control all the way.

I'll bet this customer visit will be in her trivia box of not-to-be-believed ISO audit classes for the year 2008.

I found hair everywhere. On my dark blue winter coat, my sweater, on the bathroom floor, the kitchen floor, the couch, the carpet. Larry even complained that it seemed to appear frequently in his car and on his clothes. My hair is very fine, but there is *a lot* of it. Long, light-colored hair all over the place. This *shedding* was quite normal for me, and I hadn't even started chemo. I shuddered to think of what it would be like when it really started to fall out.

I have a habit where I constantly play with my hair. I twirl it around my fingers and run my hands through it a zillion times a day. I have pins, clips, scrunchies, headbands, barrettes, decorations and all kinds of brushes, combs and electrical gizmos. I use them all. A good hair day makes anything seem possible first thing in the morning.

To add to my dilemma, my hair is a very odd color. It's an unusual color match of varying shades of browns, blondes, silvers and platinums. I've no idea where it came from but I rather like it. I only hope that this is the color that returns after chemo. I've been told that right around the second chemo treatment, your hair starts to fall out. It falls off very quickly and dramatically. Not the little strands that end up in your brush or on the floor of the bathroom after blow-drying; but clumps, gobs, more than what is normal.

It would be hard to lose my hair.

I'd been told, and I had seen for myself that there are ways to take control of this inevitable occurrence. An opportunity to turn the tables after all these months, and a chance to decide under whose terms it would fall out: mine or cancer's. So, off I'd go to find a wig that was as close to my color as possible. And then I would shave my head—on the day I chose, in the method that I chose to lose it.

I hoped for a normal-shaped head.

Stay tuned!

Chapter 31

Shaving My Hair Off

Many women would agree with me on this: finding a talented and likeable hairstylist is like finding a talented and likeable gynecologist. It is absolutely, positively priceless.

I've been blessed with one of the best in the city. Tony Scavo works downtown at the Marianne Strokirk Salon. It is one of the well-known, hip and chic salons that cater to our local TV news anchors; Hillary Clinton and Maria Shriver among others, when they are in town. I just love Tony. Plus, she is Italian and we share common family ideals, celebrations, traditions, morals and ways of looking at life. I asked her if she would come out to my house for a styling/shaving party, and without hesitation she said that she would.

A group of us had done this with Carol several months ago when she had decided to shave her head and take control of losing her hair as well. We had made a party of it then, and we would make a party of it now. Carol's was done at a salon, after hours, very private with just us girls. We imbibed on fabulous food and several bottles of wine that night.

I planned on changing it up a bit in a few ways. I would do it at home, and anyone who wanted to be there would be welcome. It should prove to be an evening worthy of many good, hearty laughs. Everyone would be able to eat and drink to their heart's content, and we have plenty of room for overnight guests. Bob and Lisa have an alcohol breathalyzer, and all the teenagers who go over to their house are made aware of this fact. We would borrow it that night, and keys would be confiscated from those who would be unable to drive.

The plan would be to cut my hair a little at a time, all in the same evening. For weeks, I gathered pictures of different, shorter hairstyles from magazines. We planned on starting with the longest cut and would keep going until I looked more and more like a boy. We hoped to do some funky cuts if there would be enough hair left to do that. This would provide me with an opportunity to see what styles might work when my hair grew back. I would soon be able to present a photograph of me, Dad and Bob: the bald Zaccone trio.

I suppose I would look like a boy named Sue for a while, although I prefer a boy named Suzanne. The big date for the unveiling of the true shape of my head would be decided once I had spoken to the oncologist on March 10th and learned the schedule for chemo, what Tony's availability for the party was, and when the wig would be available for her to style beforehand.

Chapter 32

A Family Connection: Through All the Clutter and Noise, I Hear Her

March 6, 2008

I've had a huge fear throughout this drama. It's a fear, as well as a continually nagging thought that constantly knocked at my head and would not be quieted. That's generally a sign for me to pay attention. What was happening to me appeared to be a repeat performance with a strong family connection.

My Aunt Joan died of breast cancer at age seventy; but she was a mighty young and vibrant seventy. Ask anyone who had known her. She was diagnosed with the exact same breast cancer as I was, in the exact same breast.

In the beginning, there were three things that separated us, as far as statistics go. She was diagnosed in January of 2001 at the age of sixty-five; I was diagnosed in January of 2008 at the age of fifty. She had had a small tumor, Grade 1; I had one tumor that was two centimeters and one that was five to six centimeters, Grade 3. Two tumors and a Grade 3—which was a faster growing, flaming cancer—and I am fifteen years younger.

I'm scared.

I asked my cousins to find all of her pathology reports, history of treatments and prognosis, any documents they could find. They even found slides of Aunt Joan's tissue for me to review (like I would really know what I was looking at). For a while, I actually had pieces of her with me that were smashed solidly between two pathology slides. It was sad and oh-so-bittersweet for Shere, Bob and I to be looking at a slide that had once been a part of her. She had been one amazing babe.

One night, Shere, Bob and I were poring over her documents after I had pulled together what I believed to be the pertinent information from a banker's box that was filled to the brim with documents. We wanted to compare Aunt Joan's stats to mine. Shere was able to explain all of the confusing medical mumbo jumbo. There are many unanswered questions, and depending on whom you ask in the family, you will come up with several theories on what had taken Aunt Joan away from us.

She had died five years after being diagnosed with breast cancer, which means that her cancer responded precisely the way the statistics show. If you live for five years after cancer treatment, you should be home free; it's that time in between that is so dangerous for a potential recurrence. The cancer had spread or metastasized to her bones, liver, lung and brain. My prognosis was worse: I was fifteen years younger, I had two tumors with a higher grade and a faster growing cancer. Would I be dead in five years? At fifty-five years old?

My God, help me.

Was it because she had chosen to have a lumpectomy and not a mastectomy, and a nasty little cancer cell had snuck out and hadn't been killed off by her chemo treatments? Was the chemo cocktail not strong enough or taken for long enough? Did she continue as required with her recommended chemotherapy? What about her radiation therapy? Did she fail to take proper follow-up care?

I know my cousins had done everything humanly possible to save her life. They had done everything from hiring a cook to provide a macrobiotic diet to seeing every doctor who was out there. Who fucked this up and why did she die?

It's so easy to become confused with all the medical mumbo jumbo. I'd read through so much stuff that I actually started to believe that I really understood it all. I called Dr. Shere today to catch up, and to get her take on my pathology report as compared to Aunt Joan's.

I was far from understanding what I thought I understood.

Reading very quickly through the buzz of unpronounceable medical terms, I read that I had a typical cell in my breast tissue that surrounded the cancerous tumors. Cool, it's simply a typical cell. That was what you wanted in a case like this, right? Something that was typical? No, that's not the exact medical fact at all. The report noted that there were "A-Typical" cells—*not* normal cells—which meant that even after the tumors were removed, there were still bad cells in the surrounding breast tissue. A lumpectomy for me would have been a Band-Aid temporarily covering a future problem, and they probably would never have gotten to a clear margin.

Should Aunt Joan have had a mastectomy? Her pathology report, post-lumpectomy, shows that they got clear margins and that she didn't have these nasty cells in her other tissue like I did. She had gone through some chemo and radiation. I am not sure she completed the recommended cycle; that is an open question for now. But why did she die? And how can I prevent that from happening to me?

I made a list of all of her stats on the left side of the paper, and mine on the right. I attached the documents that supported my comparison. These would be brought to the oncologist appointment. Maybe *she* could find some clue to the mystery.

So, there you have it. My fear started with learning that I had CANCER, moved to losing my breast and all the associated mental anguish and physical changes associated with it, to now tracking down why Aunt Joan was not here on earth with us today. It's a cycle that needed to be broken, or at least understood.

Then I had an "Oh My God!" moment. I had been thinking about my aunt all day but had not made an immediate connection with the date. I talked to Shere about our pathology reports and wrote this chapter. I wanted to confirm if Aunt Joan had died at age seventy or seventy-two, so I sent an email to dad—her best friend and her brother. Dad responded that she had died today, two years ago, on March 6, 2006 at the age of seventy.

That day two short years ago, Larry, Bob, Lisa and I had been at a TLMI Association meeting. We had packed up and left for home the next morning. Bob was at this year's TLMI meeting as I wrote this chapter. I began to see many similar family connections running throughout this drama; important medical connections, as well as little insignificant connections like an association meeting. But when they were all strung together, they became a tad freaky.

Aunt Joan was talking to me today, through whatever method was available to her because she couldn't be here in front of me now. She broke through all the noise and clutter and reached out to me.

I have questions. Maybe she does, too. We will get our answers. I get so angry that she is gone, but then something like this happens and I remember that she is still here and always will be, as long as she is remembered. She will *always* be remembered.

My cousin's wife Leslie's response:

> Suz,
>
> I'm sitting here reading your last chapter, with Joan's records (the ones you gave to me) right next to me. The fact that you are thinking about all of this and are seeing these similarities around the time of her death is very much something that would have intrigued her. She would have called it fate. All these little "co-inky dinks" (her term again) that all of us encounter she would say were some type of intervention. She felt and saw many signs of Frank after he passed away. I actually saw a vision of him sitting in my car one day. Maybe Joan is trying to reach out to you; maybe you just have her tucked away in the depths of your brain. Either way, you should take away the strength that she is passing on to you.

However, please don't make yourself crazy with comparisons. Nobody fucked anything up. The course of Joan's life followed the path she chose, as did the course of her death. The difference between you two is that she quietly accepted it as inevitable (fate), while you are fighting with both pink boxing gloves on.

Joan was a very private person and did not let us into her fight the first time she was diagnosed. Even then, it was quietly done and the choices she made for her treatment were hers alone. Whether or not she finished all recommended chemo and radiation, I don't know. Maybe there should have been different or better follow-up care. Again, these were her choices and she accepted what was told to her. You are questioning everything and everyone around you and then going back for more. She knew something was not quite right, long before she was diagnosed the second time. We could not convince her to check it out. She kept saying that it would just go away, or it's just aches and pains. By the time she was diagnosed, she already knew in her heart that death was her fate. I remember riding in the car with her and Danny after one of her many scans and asking her if I could read the reports from previous ones. She said, "Yes, why not." When I finished reading, all I could say was "wow" softly because I could see what a battle this would be. Her answer was: "There you have it." She knew before any doctor told her that she only had a few months and she made up her mind not to do any treatment. Yes, we investigated alternative things (Bruce worked day and night at it) and she was okay with trying a few of them. Ultimately, though, she did these things because it gave her kids the feeling that they were doing something. She told me that she didn't want to die but that when it's your time, it's your time (fate again). She also told us that she never expected her husband to go first. So she went along with some of the things that Bruce found and saw many doctors and looked at many treatment options, but always on her own terms. She made all the choices. In fact, the only thing she got mad at was anyone telling her she had to do something. She brought us into her journey of death and showed us how to go peacefully and with dignity. She wanted her children to know that it wasn't hard to do. She was a great mother until the end.

So, that is why she isn't here with us. She didn't make the choice to question and talk and question some more. She did not choose to investigate those aches and pains. She did not ask whether or not her follow-up X-rays were enough. If she is trying to reach out to you, she might be telling you that she was willing to accept her fate but that it's not time for you to go yet, so you should not follow the same path she did. That is why you are fighting and questioning and researching and writing. That is why you will be here a long time.

Love,
Leslie

Leslie, my cousin Steve's wife, is a nurse and was intimately involved with Aunt Joan's care. I know these things are true; about the whole event having been Aunt Joan's decision. I know she was a private person. I, on the other hand, am out there screaming to the world, researching, questioning, and fighting like mad to live. She'd had so much life to live yet. I can't believe she really wanted to leave.

I believe in fate, too. But I also believe that you can adjust it, and sometimes even mold it, into something fair and not just manageable.

I know she was reaching out to me today. I kept thinking the chapter was done but I was continually urged back to the computer to write more, read more, question more. I was sitting there weeping, knowing how hard she had worked to break through. But she had done it "her way" and had found a path that is now open for us to connect through again.

Then my cousin Bruce chimed in:

Hi Suz,

I need to stick my two cents in here and clarify a few things.

First, yes there are parallels between Aunt Joan's cancer and yours. Same type of cancer, same breast but that's where it ends.

You mention a cycle that needs to be broken or at least understood. Well, you my dear cousin are on the verge of doing both! The reason why you ARE, HAVE and WILL overcome this is because of your willingness to share your experience with the rest of us! Just look at the extensive list above of all these wonderful people who all have expressed their love and encouragement throughout this journey.

My mom took a different approach and tried to deal with her affliction from within because she felt it would save the rest of us anguish. Was it right? She thought so. And that's what mattered most.

You, on the other hand, have graciously invited us all on this journey. And what a journey it's been. Let's be honest, we have seen the lowest of lows and the highest of highs through these last several months. The pendulum will continue to swing for just awhile longer and it's refreshing to know that EACH and every one of these people above are sending positive energy to YOU, SUZ (one very special person indeed)!

Here is the most important parallel between you and Aunt Joan: you both have taught us something along your journeys. My mom left us with a powerful message when she was dying and this was just a day before she passed on. I quote, as her eyes were closed and she pulled us all close to her, she said in a serene and peaceful voice, "If this is dying, you have nothing to fear." As my cousins and brothers already know, she taught us many things about life and now she was teaching us about death. That was powerful and will stick with me forever.

You, on the other hand, are teaching us about life through your emails and the responses that are generated from this list. We all take away something positive. Granted we all get something different out of each chapter and each response! But rest assured it's all good.

I think I can speak for everyone here when I say thank you for inviting us along on your journey. Because of your willingness to share (*everyone's* willingness to share), we have learned many things about life and the people who touch our lives, and we are all better people for it.

Couple all this positive energy with your persistence to understand, learn and question everything, we are in store for one happy ending.

So, Suz, you keep writing. People, you keep responding and we all KEEP learning!

Love to all,
Bruce Wiercioch

Chapter 33

Kind of/ Sort of Meeting the Chemo Oncologist

March 10, 2008, 8:00 AM

We met first with a nurse who took the obligatory vitals, height and weight measurements. I had prepared a list of thirty-five questions for Dr. Rita Nanda, my chemo oncologist. I was certain that many of these questions would be answered when she went through her treatment plan, but I had them ready just in case one was missed. I didn't want to have to call back later, as one question and its answer can so easily lead to another.

We met next with Dr. Lucy Chen, a fellow in hematology/ oncology; two very scary words that had never previously held much meaning for me. Dr. Chen and Dr. Nanda worked together. While Dr. Nanda was otherwise busy, we started with Dr. Chen.

We began with the usual surgical and drain site exam. She felt the lymph nodes in my entire upper body, as well as my other breast. She said I was healing well, things looked good and my range of motion was more advanced than they expected after just two and a half weeks post-surgery. She told me that even though I was getting regular periods, the type of chemo that they planned to give me would certainly throw me into early menopause. They called it "chemically induced menopause" and there was absolutely no way around it. Because I was getting regular periods, I was still ovulating and estrogen was the king of the castle. Now estrogen was my enemy. Because I was pre-menopausal, I would need to take a drug called Tamoxofin for at least a year after chemotherapy while they continually monitored my hormonal responses. They would eventually switch me to the drug Arimidex or Aromasin or whatever the next new "hope in a pill" would be at that time.

My concerns with Tamoxofin were: developing uterine cancer, bothersome hot flashes, and new calcifications developing in the other breast, not to mention lung clots. Arimidex and Aromasin are somewhat milder and do not carry these risk factors. They are mostly used by post-menopausal woman. Evidently, the positive reasons for me to take Tamoxofin far outweighed the risk factors involved. I will have more information in a future chapter after I research those drugs.

The chemo cocktail would travel everywhere that my blood does. It would hopefully kill all the microscopic cancer cells that may have escaped surgery or may be lurking around somewhere in other parts of my body and were, as yet, undetectable under current technology. The chemo treatment they had planned is the latest drug cocktail available. Evidently, it packs quite a punch. The facts all pointed to hitting this one hard and fast and strong; due to my young age, the size of both tumors, lymph node involvement (even though it was only one lymph node), the fact that they suspected that there were microscopic cells that had entered my blood, and the fact that the largest tumor at five to six centimeters was closer to the margins than they would have liked.

All of the above considered, the breast cancer counsel recommended a more aggressive chemo and then radiation therapy be employed. A virtual "Full Court Press." I still wanted to seek a second opinion on radiation, based on Dr. Connolly's concerns with the University of Chicago's treatment plan being more aggressive than he felt was warranted for me.

They expected my side effects to be intense, due to the mixture they planned to employ and the frequency of treatments (every two weeks instead of three). They expected nausea to affect me, so they would probably provide a set of variable steroids to fight it, in addition to the anti-nausea medicine given with each chemo treatment. I should expect to get very, very sick. And I would definitely lose my hair.

This specific cocktail is particularly hard on your heart, so they would be giving me a "Mugascan," which is a scan (with needles, of course) that looks at the muscles in the heart, as well as its ability to pump regularly. This would be the baseline test before chemo started and I may need to have one of these tests every few weeks during chemo to keep an eye on things if trouble began. The baseline test was scheduled for next Wednesday.

Additionally, they would need to monitor bone marrow effects due to the potential of low white blood cells, red blood cells and platelets—which are side effects seen quite often during chemo. I would receive GCSF or a growth-stimulating shot to help regenerate and grow bone marrow. They are called cyto protective drugs, which help to protect normal cells. I could take these shots in the arm, leg, thigh, the tummy or the butt. In the butt they shall go, where they would be farthest from my mind and eyes.

The doctors are always concerned during treatment about their patients getting an infection, as most of the normal and healthy cells would be greatly compromised and many would be killed off during the treatments. If I developed a fever of 101.5 or higher, was sick for more than two days, had any change in bowel habits or had diarrhea more than twice in four hours, developed sweats or shakes, bone aches, back aches, recurring headaches, mouth sores or thrush in my mouth—they needed to be called immediately.

I also needed to be watchful while out in the sun. Most chemotherapy treatments will make you a great deal more sensitive to the sun's harmful rays. They suggested that I avoid sun exposure and wear a broad-spectrum sunscreen and a hat when I needed to be out in the sun.

Until I knew just when my body would start to react after a chemo treatment, they preferred that I did not drive for the first several treatments. If after a treatment or two, I found that I got sick hours or days later, I could drive myself on future visits. I had no restrictions with driving, working, exercise or sex but I needed to be very, very careful about being around anyone who was sick or was starting to feel that way, as I would be particularly prone to infections. My immune system would get weaker with each chemo treatment that passed. If I were to be exposed to a virus or infection, it could delay the chemo treatments or land me in the hospital.

It was noted during a May 2007 scan that there was a nodule detected on the intra mammary lymph node (located between my breasts). But from May 2007 to date, this node had remained stable. It would be closely monitored and chemo and radiation therapy should deal with any potential future problems. Currently, no additional biopsy was recommended.

I would need to wear a compression sleeve to fly. This is very important, particularly during long flights when blood clots may occur all over my body, but especially in my right arm. Therefore, while up in the air, I am supposed to walk around frequently and make stretching movements while seated.

The compression sleeve would also be a requirement when scuba diving, and there was a possibility that a sleeve would be needed when I worked out, but only time would tell for that potential. I was told that this would become a part of my ensemble for the rest of my life when I am flying and or diving. I was also warned that I would need to be particularly diligent about wearing this sleeve to ward off lymphedema.

The bad news was that there could be weight gain in this chemo set.

The good news was that I could have a few Cosmos on Friday and Saturday nights!

If this chemo cocktail didn't work, there were alternatives, but Dr. Chen was confident that the treatment selected would do the job very well. She suggested that once a day, I take a multiple vitamin, calcium with magnesium, zinc and Vitamin D. I was assured that getting the non-smoking pill Chantix would not be a contraindication to these vitamins or the chemo cocktail.

I would meet with a Genetic Counselor at the halfway point to learn about the tests that I would like to get; tests that would tell me if I carried a cancer gene that my nieces and sister needed to know about. They were called the BRAC1 and BRAC2 tests. My HER2 and NU test markers were negative, which was good; otherwise, additional treatment would have been required.

The names of the chemo cocktail were Adrimycin, Cyclophosphamide and Taxol. The first two drugs would be given together for the first four treatments and would pack the strongest punch. The last drug would operate by itself for the last four treatments. It would be a tad less caustic.

I would begin chemo on Monday, March 24th. The last four chemo treatments involving the drug Taxol would continue to provide me with a steady and familiar bout of all the above side effects, but could possibly include numbness and/or tingling in my fingers and toes. If the tingling were to be present during the next treatment, I would need to advise the doctors so that they could dial back the dose. This drug could damage nerves in the fingers and toes for the long term. That symptom is called neuropathy.

I would need to allow for a half day (five to six hours) to get all the blood tests, shots and a full dose of poison inside of me. I could read, listen to an iPod or work on my computer or phone, as they are set up with a wireless connection. A blood test would be given prior to each session to confirm that my blood counts and blood sugar were acceptable. I should be done by June 30th if I'm able to keep to the bi-monthly schedule, and as long as none of these issues arise: blood counts that won't be strong enough to get a chemo treatment per the schedule, any potential associated heart issues, getting sicker than my body can handle, or being hospitalized.

My latest goal was to execute the plan precisely as described. We had scheduled a major family vacation for everyone on July 23rd, Mom's birthday. I was *not* going to miss that trip.

This afternoon, I had canceled the trip to Paris for the FINAT Association meeting in June. I had now missed *five* trips that were planned for this year—and it was only March 10th!

I asked if there were other drugs or treatment plans (other than chemo) that had been known to respond well to my type of cancer. Dr. Chen replied that chemo should definitely be considered. Without any further treatment, statistically forty-nine percent of women are fine after ten years; add chemo and the numbers go up to eighty-one percent.

Breast cancer has a bi-modal distribution; this means that there is a clear statistical recurrence recognizable on two humps on a graph over time. One hump deviates around the five-year mark and another hump deviates around the ten-year mark. If you make it to five years, you are responding terrifically. If you hit the ten-year mark, you are probably as safe as anyone else—if not better—for having undergone chemo treatment.

Our appointment with Dr. Rita Nanda was for 8:00 AM. We were, as always, on time. We had seen the nurse and the doctor's medical fellow, Dr. Lucy Chen. It was now 11:00 AM and we were done with all of our questions.

Where was the doctor?

Dr. Chen had left the room several times to find Dr. Nanda. I was beginning to get peeved. I had been told to allow an hour for this meeting; I had allowed an hour and a half to accommodate my list of questions. Because of their delays, I had already missed two appointments in the breast center downstairs and now I was getting dangerously close to being late for a meeting back at the office. It was clear to me that Dr. Chen was covering for Dr. Nanda's tardiness. To make matters worse, no one apologized for the time we had waited for the doctor who would be in charge of my care. In the same circumstances, you may ask yourself: "Now what do I do?" I did.

My questions, as well as Larry's and Bob's, were answered. Before we left the hospital, I was prepared to set up with the scheduling group the dates for the required heart tests and then chemo. I refused to have Larry's, Bob's and my time further disrespected and abused without so much as an honest explanation. I got dressed and we walked out of the examination room.

We ran into both Dr. Chen and Dr. Nanda in the hall.

Dr. Nanda asked if we might return to the examination room along with Dr. Chen and Nurse Gehring. Dr. Nanda apologized and asked if she could please examine me. Of course, I said yes. She asked and answered a few questions. I had a sense that she wouldn't be late again. She was apologetic but made a very lame excuse that she knew Dr. Chen was with us and that I would have a lot of questions. I could see that she knew I was not buying into that one.

I said simply, "We had an 8:00 AM appointment with you, Dr. Nanda. While meeting with you, Dr. Chen and Nurse Gehring would have been wonderful, as it would be important for your entire team to hear and answer my questions, I do not have time to go over this again. I've already missed two appointments at the breast center and I am in danger of being late for a business meeting for a company that I have an ownership position in. You are the doctor that we had an appointment with three hours ago, and my questions should have been addressed by you."

The meeting ended well, as we are all professionals. But now everyone seemed to understand more clearly the boundaries that shouldn't be crossed without an explanation, and certainly with an explanation given much sooner than three hours after a scheduled appointment.

On the other hand, I understood their constraints. These poor doctors were constantly running from one patient to another. They needed to be chameleons, changing their presence and their delivery to match the individual. An hour allotted for a visit could easily be extended to two hours because of issues that neither the patient nor the doctor had anticipated. How do they do it? It would drive me mad.

I mentioned the book. I couldn't resist. I wanted to measure their ability to bounce back, and I was curious to gauge their true commitment, their professionalism and their feelings towards me; in that specific order. I told them that the books I had read on breast cancer were either a personal story without many details or suggestions, or a medical book. My plan was to combine all of it in a book that looked at breast cancer from both perspectives throughout the entire journey. Tying it all together and hopefully helping the newly diagnosed patient gain a more complete understanding of what things looked like from both the medical and the individual point of view.

They all seemed to appreciate the need for this book, as they did not hesitate in agreeing to assist me with their medical perspective or to have their real names used.

I now had a script for a cranial prosthesis (wig), a script for a heart monitoring test with needles, and a script for the first three chemo treatments. They didn't want to schedule too far in advance, in case there would be developments with low blood counts, my getting sick or changes with this heart issue that they would be monitoring.

I left Dr. Nanda with Aunt Joan's stats and the comparison model I had made, as well as my recent blood test results and a full body CAT scan test result—all of which had been taken within the past six months.

I had a week and a half to get a mountain of things taken care of at work, at home and at the lake house; and there were two more doctors' appointments this week. Wednesday, I had that icky heart test, and another five days after that to prepare for chemo.

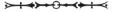

Dr. Song's Corner

There are now several models and online tools that help us to calculate risk. Input of age, stage of tumor, nodal involvement and the other details of one's cancer are placed into a model formula that then helps guide the doctors in prescribing the right treatment. Oncotyping further adds to this. One should also be armed with knowledge of these models (e.g., Gayle model). Ask your doctors.

Chapter 34

The Second Opinion from a Radiation Oncologist & My Get Out Of Jail Free Card

Wednesday, March 12th, 11:30 AM

On Monday, at the University of Chicago, we met the chemo oncology team. We had yet to speak with their radiation oncology team, although we knew their position.

Dr. Connolly made it a point to advise me that a second opinion was warranted in my case, as it related to radiation treatment. He also made sure that Dr. Timothy Hollister, his suggested radiation oncologist, had all documents, films and pathology reports necessary to provide an informed opinion in advance of our appointment.

Evidently, after a mastectomy that presented my statistics there were equally compelling reasons to have radiation therapy versus not having it. I lay in a gray area. Thankfully, for once I was not overachieving as I lay on the perfect side of this gray area.

If anyone could avoid radiation, it would be me. This was based on the fact that the cancerous tumor I had was small (considered a T1 in cancer staging). I had only one lymph node that was cancerous (considered an N1 in cancer staging). It was fully encapsulated, which meant that the cancer had not broken out of the node; the larger insitu tumor had yet to fully bloom into cancer and they were able to remove all of it with clear margins. Lastly, even though the breast tissue that had been removed was loaded with cancer cells, they had removed everything. Did this make radiation a moot point?

Without radiation therapy, there is only a one-in-ten chance of recurrence at the same site over an eight—to ten-year period. I wish I'd asked the doctor: "What happens in the eleventh year and beyond?"

Because my lymph nodes had been removed, placing my immune system at risk, having radiation greatly increased the chances of getting lymphedema by twenty-five percent (See Chapter 67 on lymphedema). When radiation treatments include the chest area, the lungs or the heart can also be affected, depending on the side being radiated. For me, the right lung was the issue. One early change is a decrease in the levels of surfactant, a substance that assists in keeping air passages open and fully expanding. Being a smoker, and with emphysema and COPD (Coronary Obstructive Pulmonary Disease) in my family, this was not an issue to be taken lightly.

While the symptoms could be treated with steroids, I had several concerns. Once you have had radiation therapy, it can never be used again in the same area. Radiation could greatly hinder the pectoral deltoid. There would be a ten to fifteen percent chance of radiation pneumonia and skin problems. And after radiation, cosmetic surgery issues would become more complicated. The time may not be right for me and radiation, but it may be a good insurance policy to hang on to, to be used down the road.

At this point in time, I was leaning towards *not* having radiation therapy. Based on the above information, I had decided to proceed as follows: 1) There was no rush to make a decision, as radiation would follow chemotherapy one month after I had completed the total chemo series; 2) I wanted to hear what the radiation oncologist had to say at the University of Chicago about why she/he felt so strongly that I consider radiation, if for no other reason than to be totally informed about the subject, personally experience the other side of a medical sales presentation, and to get this other position fairly represented in the book; 3) I wanted to confer once again with Dr. Connolly; 4) I needed to do a bit more research on not only radiation but also on the potential concerns with reconstructive surgery that radiation presented, and the future quality of life.

This subject would be revisited in the near future.

When I was a kid, I loved playing Monopoly. I still do. I considered myself a land baron and would buy every piece of property I could afford, and would place houses and hotels on each one as quickly as possible. Being a kind but very smart landlord, I was willing to provide temporary bridge loans to those who landed on my property but were unable to afford the rent or the mortgage.

OK, so the bridge loan bit is a joke . . . But had I known about bridge loans back then, believe me—I would have offered it as a solution.

Holding a "get out of jail free" card was always a good thing to have, just like owning real estate. It probably always will be.

Yesterday, I sent Dr. Lucy Chen via email, eleven follow-up questions that had come out of our meeting on Monday. The single most exciting news was that I had received a "get out of jail free" card from the oncologists; I did not need to schedule my colonoscopy (normally due at age fifty) until well after this drama had ended. The chemo should kill anything that lingered in my body. I could delay the bootie-roto-rooter test this year and wait until after I had gotten over the boobie issue. Who would have thought that chemo could have a benefit like this?

It's all about timing!

Chapter 35

I Have Never Shopped For a Rug
Like This Before (Part 1)

Flashback to nine months ago.

My high school friends—The Magnificent Seven, as we call ourselves—went with Carol to get her wig, which was also known among those who lived the experience as a "cranial prosthesis." We were all like little girls playing in Mommy's closet. We tried on virtually everything in the boutique. We had a blast, as we desperately tried to make this an event that wouldn't be too dramatic or maudlin for Carol.

It was difficult, if not impossible, to find anything close to my hair color. I didn't like the way I looked as a redhead or brunette. The browns that they had were too mousy-looking on me. Blonde wasn't working, either. Then off to the side, I noticed this thing called a hair ring. It was stuffed into a dusty corner on one of the stylist's shelves, perhaps with the knowledge that there wouldn't be many people needing or wanting its color combination.

It was my color exactly.

I put the ring on. It gave me fuller bangs and a few longer pieces of hair along the sides and around to the back. Kind of like a painless version of the latest hair extension craze. I would need to wear a hat to cover my head if I were bald, but the ring would be the "hair" surrounding it.

We were all shocked at what a very good match it was. I quickly took it off.

"It's nice to know that someone with my color hair is out there and had enough hair to donate," I said. "But I hope and I pray that I'll never need it."

"Don't worry, guys," Carol said. "Cancer strikes one out of seven women. I'm taking the hit for all of us. You are all safe."

The stylist in the room with us, a two-time breast cancer survivor, made a poignant correction as she interjected, "Girls, I need to tell you that that statistic changed some time ago. It's no longer a matter of '*if* you will get cancer'; it's a matter of 'when' and 'what kind.'"

That stopped all of us in our tracks. The joking around quickly stopped. The reality had chilled us to the core.

Nine months had passed since that visit to the wig salon with Carol and the girls. Having been forewarned by Carol that I couldn't simply walk into the place and buy a wig, and fully knowing that my hair color would make it impossible to just whip it out of an inventory, stored away in Box No. 11 on the seventh shelf up—I dropped by for a solo visit ahead of time.

It hadn't even registered with me that heads have different sizes, and that the wig needed to be fit to a specific shape and size. There were so many new things to get up to speed on that had not been a part of my world before.

I stopped by on March 4th and selected what I hoped to be the right base color. Having been involved with printers and inks and color matching all of my life, I had acquired a keen ability to recognize a true color match. But even the owner, a skilled colorist, said that I would be "a challenge." I'd heard that one before.

The colorist used the hair ring I had played around with six months ago, to match dyes for the wig I had selected. When the Mag 7 would be together on March 15th for my appointment, and we would all be going through this same damn drill for the second time in less than a year, at least we would have something close to my color to start with. I hoped.

Chapter 36

I Have Never Shopped For a Rug
Like This Before (Part 2)

Saturday, March 15th

My girlfriends and I arrived at the boutique for my 11:00 AM appointment.

The boutique was appropriately called "Naturally Yours." Having been there before, we knew the inventory, the way things were set up, some of the salespeople and yes of course, we had even gotten to know the owner. This was a shopping Mecca for women facing breast surgery, chemo, radiation, reconstructive surgery and life after it all calmed down.

The goal for the day was to make sure that the color they ended up mixing and applying matched my hair. I was silently praying that my selection eleven days ago was spot-on, so we could simply proceed with the fit for my head and order the wig to be later styled by Toni, my hairstylist. Then we could continue with our plans and head on to the Mexican restaurant for lunch and margaritas!

Naturally Yours is quite a place. There were bathing suits and bras with hidden pockets for a falsie (the politically correct term is "prosthesis.") They also had jewelry, hats and specially designed shirts. There were all kinds of things for the girl who appreciated accessorizing. They had baseball caps with ponytails that hung out of the hole in back, in every color imaginable but mine. There were other hats with wisps of bangs that were visible below the visor and some included a short or long hairstyle sewn into the back and sides. They had an extensive selection of dressier hats. Really cute caps with ties and scarves to wear during the day and tight-fitting cotton caps that reminded me of a swim cap or something that a fashion-forward doctor would wear during surgery. I was told that these were a big help at night so your head wouldn't get too cold. I was also told that after chemo, the little "buzz" of hair that would be left on your head would slowly fall into the cap during the night and you would simply have to turn the cap inside out in the morning and watch as your last bits of hair fluttered into the garbage can.

Even writing about this inevitable event bothered me and made me anxious. My hair was so much a part of how I saw myself, and I was only twenty days away from the Big Shave. I knew that this would be another devastating loss, and one that I had to experience, but it was happening too quickly; way too soon after my first loss last month, which made it all the more agonizing.

The shedding would continue until chemo really kicked in between the second and third treatment. I would begin to resemble Michael Jordan, Yul Brenner, my dad, my brother Bob or my cousin Steve with those amazingly shiny, smooth and very sexy bare heads. But they were male bald heads and that was normal. Men without hair are more easily accepted in the world than a woman without hair.

At the boutique, there were hats that were so uniquely constructed that not even a windy day in Chicago would allow them to fly away. Unfortunately, hats were the one accessory that I had never been able to get into because—hell, they would totally screw up my hair! Now I'd been given the chance to widen my horizons. I loved to accessorize, and getting "hat hair" would no longer be a concern or an excuse. And I had a drawer full of scarves. I could easily tie a scarf fashionably around my neck, on my handbag, on my coat or as an accent on a pair of pants. Now I needed to learn how to tie a turban.

Naturally Yours was unable to find a color that matched mine as soon as I had hoped. But they found one that they felt would provide them with the base colors they needed to work with. They would keep the hair ring and frost various colors as close to it as possible on the wig. This was a challenge when you had seven colors of hair all mixed together on one head, like mine.

They gave me the hair ring as a gift, probably because its color was no longer available. Or because they had not been able to sell it and I was the first person to even want it.

I selected a wig made of real hair. If they messed up the color, we would just need to start all over again. Much like when you mess up coloring on your own hair.

I also bought a wig made of synthetic hair. The stylist put it on my head. I guess it looked . . . OK. But have you ever tried something on that looked nice when you were in the store but once you got home and you tried it on again, you thought, "What was I thinking?" I would need to return to the boutique to get lessons on how to work with this thing, and really decide if I would ever wear it. And if I *did* keep it, I would need to have it trimmed so I would look more like myself.

Wearing a wig may be uncomfortable for some people in the summer months. Depending on where I needed to go, who I would be seeing, and their comfort level with being seen with a woman who was either oddly bald or obviously sick (because who would wear a cap, decorated with scarves or beautiful pins during summer?), I would usually go *au naturel*. The only woman I could think of who looked amazing when bald was Iman, the model married to David Bowie. She had proudly shown the world that bald could be beautiful on a woman. But her features are so classically beautiful and striking that she would have looked fabulous in any hairstyle or hair color.

I kept pushing at the two bumps on either side of my head that both Shere and Mom also have, and I wondered . . . twenty more days . . .

Chapter 37

Alright, Enough Already!

After years of bitching at me for smoking, and of him walking around with his shirt covering his mouth and nose like kids often do when they catch a whiff of cigarette smoke—the tide had finally turned in Larry's favor.

Last Tuesday, after his continual complaints to anyone who would listen (which included an e-mail campaign to my girlfriends); I went to a general medical doctor so I could get a script to stop smoking, and also to finally set up a relationship with a doctor who was a generalist. I decided it was time to have a GP.

I prayed that stopping this habit wouldn't be too brutal. I had a great deal of self-control when I traveled, when I was with a customer or when I was unable to smoke for whatever "posted" reason—especially when I was traveling internationally, as there is very little one can do while thirty thousand feet in the air above an ocean for seven hours or longer. I didn't have nicotine fits or any real symptoms of withdrawal during these long periods of time, as long as I knew that there was nothing that I could do to satisfy my desire. But once I was in an area where smoking was allowed, smoking was the first thing on my mind.

I was addicted. There was absolutely no doubt about it. But I felt more confident about quitting than I'd ever had before.

When I pictured myself walking out of a chemo treatment and lighting up a cigarette, it just seemed wrong. I imagined this five-hour poison cocktail that would slowly drip into one of my veins and snake through my body, then being followed by a different poison *chaser* taken through my lungs.

Although while getting this non-smoking pill fully loaded in my system in these first few weeks, I would probably still be found puffing away from time to time. The pill would allow me to smoke in the beginning and then I would be gradually weaned off.

Bob arranged the appointment with an MD, and simply told me where to be, at what time to be there and whom to ask for. The plan was for us to go together, as he had found a male doctor for himself and a female doctor for me, both at the same practice. But he was sick with the flu and was afraid to get me sick before chemo started. So we arrived separately. He was going to try this stop-smoking gig along with me.

Since I had left my parents house, many, many years ago, I'd only had the need for a gynecologist and a dentist. Since turning forty, I'd added a mammogram radiologist and a yearly eye exam doctor to get a baseline for the future. I'd never really needed a regular MD before.

I have a wonderful relationship with Dr. Ahkter, my gynecologist. I foolishly hoped that she, the dentist, the eye doctor and the mammogram tech were all that I would ever need. I could count more than a dozen people I had referred to Dr. Ahkter who were now her patients—and I don't give out referrals unless I am one hundred percent personally convinced of the person's abilities. Dr. Ahkter had started her practice the same year that Bob and I started our business, and I was one of her first patients. She had my complete medical history and had handled all prescription drugs that I needed over the last twenty-four years, which hadn't been much. She maintained a complete file on me that included blood tests, cholesterol tests and the sundry other tests required by insurance companies who insured an executive's life. For our annual visit and examination, I was diligent about bringing copies of everything that had happened to me during the year that she didn't know about.

Throughout the twenty-four years that we have known each other, Dr. Ahkter had referred me to other specialists that I'd needed; like a mammogram radiologist, and someone to give me the eventual roto-rooter colonoscopy. She had been on me to stop smoking for years. Several years ago, she gave me a prescription for a pill to stop smoking, which I never used. When I asked her to give me a prescription last week, she couldn't do it. Things were getting harder now with insurance companies and government agencies. They were looking ever so closely at what doctors were prescribing. If a drug was prescribed outside of the normally prescribed drug base generally provided by that medical discipline, then it could be and often would be questioned. I quickly found this out when Dr. Ahkter was unable to prescribe that pill to stop smoking. I knew her hands must have been tied in triple knots.

Other than the normal, simple routine tests that we all need to get as we grow older, and due to my general good health and my fear of all things medical, I'd usually determine the nature and cause of any of my problems and would take care of them myself. In many cases, I'd simply put on my big-girl panties and deal with it. These problems were generally very minor. Most of the time, I decided that a self-diagnosis would be adequate. I was really quite good at pushing out of my mind the thought that only a fool would represent herself in a court of law, or determine her own medical treatment.

I'd survived something I'd been told was major, but in no way did it threaten my life. It was a self-diagnosed bout with kidney stones. It happened on two occasions, five years apart, and lasted for precisely three days. The pain was so profoundly intense that I actually wanted to die.

It arrived like clockwork every fifteen minutes, which provided me with fourteen minutes—ample time to look up symptoms on the Internet, check e-mails and voicemail messages, return a few phone calls, cross-reference the symptoms to be sure they could not be associated with multiple problems, and drink a lot of water before throwing—no, hurling—myself on the floor and writhing in intense spasmodic pain. After five to seven minutes of agony, I would have those fifteen minutes of relief!

I sweated it out without medical advice. All I did was to delay relief by not seeing a doctor, which in retrospect was really stupid.

Now, I had an MD and a script to stop smoking which I would start on March 13th. Additionally, I would start working out with a trainer that Larry had hired for me on Tuesday. She has had experience working with breast cancer patients.

Here I come—soon to be bald *and* buff!

I have an extraordinary collection of very special, vintage, slim-lined, incredibly well-designed cigarette cases. I'd used the same embossed, silver, slim-lined case for the last thirty years and had used the others on rare occasions. These others were all carefully wrapped in tissue paper and placed in thin profile boxes that were yet again contained in a larger box that was neatly labeled and sat in a regal position in my closet. This box happened to be right next to the one with all of my sexy Victoria's Secret bras that were being stored for hopeful future use. I decided that some of these cigarette cases could be used for business cards or placed in an evening bag holding money or credit cards.

I couldn't bear to give them up just yet.

With all of the changes happening all at once in my life, I'd decided that this was *enough!* Any and all suggestions for improvement were welcome but would not even be considered until this time next year.

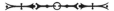

Dr. Song's Corner

Smoking is an extremely difficult addiction to kick—but for the purposes of surgery, an extremely important one. Tar, nicotine and carbon monoxide found in cigarettes have profound effects on wound healing. Most plastic surgeons will not operate electively on smokers. Patients should at the very least quit at least one month prior to surgery and during the six weeks after surgery, to help to mitigate against the deleterious effects smoking has on the natural healing and recovery process.

Chapter 38

The Mugascan

A Mugascan is a medical investigation of sorts.

It reminded me of a movie from the sixties, where a team of doctors and scientists shrank themselves and the vessel they would travel in. They were then somehow injected into a man's vein so that they could travel throughout the body to scope out something or other. I can't remember what they were searching for or what the name of the movie was. But it was a weird movie, like my Mugascan was.

This particular diagnostic test would measure the strength of my heart muscles, as the chemo drugs I would start on Monday were especially hard on the heart. A baseline was needed so that the oncology team would be provided with a starting point as to where my heart stood prior to chemo; regarding overall strength, the number of beats per minute, as well as how my heart reacted during the injection of these meds—so that changes could be easily recognized as I continued down the path of chemo treatments. Pictures of my heart would be taken with a special camera, following the injection of a radioactive material.

When I arrived at the Nuclear Medicine Department, Dr. Javid Ali, a nuclear cardiologist, injected a catheter into a vein in my arm. He was an amazingly gentle and compassionate man and he recognized and acknowledged my fear. He took his time and explained everything. To ease my concerns, he told me a few white lies about exactly how much fluid would need to be pushed into my veins.

It hurt like hell.

Larry and the doctor kept me well distracted with all kinds of conversation that I vaguely heard through the fog that was suddenly filling my head. I worked hard to concentrate on anything other than why I had to be there. Their conversation was useless dribble. What a bitch I can be.

Attached to the catheter was a thin rubber line that ran to a *very* large syringe-like pump filled with saline solution. From there, Dr. Ali used a needle to push a radioactive tracer into the catheter in my arm, along with the saline solution from the pump. Not only did it sting but I felt a major pressure and flush of warmth as the fluids were pushed. The material traveled through the bloodstream and directly to my heart. Larry said he couldn't believe how fast and how hard the cardiologist actually needed to push on the pump to alleviate any issues with its delivery.

I was asked to sit on a chair with my chest up against an X-ray monitoring screen, whilst a series of pictures were taken. It took approximately thirty minutes to complete the scan from start to finish. We were able to watch on the screen as the radioactive material entered my left lung and then my heart and how they both reacted. It was freaky and weird, very surreal. Dr. Ali said that everything looked fine to him.

I was now radioactive for the second time and for another day this year.

I would be called tomorrow if the results showed that I was unable to start chemo on Monday as planned. No word from them meant it would be a go.

Chapter 39

What Exactly Is a Skin-Sparing Mastectomy?

I had an artist for a surgeon and he offered me more than just a life-saving mastectomy. He offered me a chance to keep my original breast skin; and therefore, have a huge head start and a familiar foundation for reconstruction.

At first, while in the hospital and still drugged by my friend the morphine drip, and then at home with the Oxyconton and Oxycodone drugs, I hated they way my breast looked. It wasn't me. I struggled with the emotional and physical terror of what had happened in only six weeks' time and how it would affect the rest of my life. I was unbalanced and I felt ugly and disfigured. I had no nipple and I had a scar that ran about five or six inches horizontally. Weeks ago when Dr. Shere had first changed the dressing, I had cried like a baby and thrown up at the sight of myself.

It was still very hard to look at.

It had now been four weeks since surgery and Dickie the Drain was out. The hard, constricting, Barbarella/Madonna-like protrusion was gone. The part that looked like a horse had stepped on my upper chest was slowly filling back in; the tissue had somehow magically rearranged itself to make it look closer to me. The landscape of my back as I knew it and that Larry loves—had returned. I had been practicing a range of motion exercises and because of that, my mobility had also returned. But I was still numb on a small section of my back and couldn't feel much in the pit of my arm, on my breast or around it. My upper underarm felt as though it were constantly asleep.

It hurt a great deal if I moved the wrong way or stretched too much. The other morning, I had woken up feeling absolutely great, like I usually do; and like I usually do, I wiggled around and stretched my arms, legs and my back, uttering a loud and freeing moan. Ordinarily this was a wonderful feeling, getting out those kinks left from sleep, and starting my day peacefully in an acrobatic series of positions that I had performed for years upon waking up (while horizontal and still in bed).

That day, it had taken me ten minutes to recover from over-stretching my right arm. I had forgotten that I had new restrictions in my life, at least for a little while. I lay there flat on my back in bed with tears streaming down my face from the searing pain.

I couldn't move.

I knew that some of this would pass. Eventually, feeling would return to everything but the breast area and potentially in my underarm, as those nerve endings were gone forever and therefore no longer attached to what was necessary to maintain feeling.

I clung to the fact that I was alive. I would never have known about these two tumors (as deeply set as they were) or the cancer-ridden breast tissue that was just waiting to colonize into something detectable, had I not been a diligent and compliant patient.

My message is: don't mess with your health another day. Have the tests taken when the tests are due. Stay on top of your life's maintenance. Most people take care of their cars better than they take care of themselves. Making yourself a priority will give you the time required to have and explore options. You have to catch things early to have the largest set of options available.

A skin-sparing mastectomy is simply (funny word to use: *simply*; everything having to do with breast cancer is never simple) the removal of the nipple from which not only babies are fed but men seem to gravitate towards and women admittedly love as well. A nipple is considered breast tissue; with many breast cancers, all tissue must go. Under your nipple, if you were to look at a textbook drawing, all the important things are attached: lobules, ducts, tissue etc. Breasts—those life-sustaining and pleasure-giving beautiful pieces of skin—can also develop cancer. And all roads lead directly to your nipple.

After that little morsel had been removed and sent off to pathology, never to be used as intended again, they made a horizontal slice right on the center line of what used to be my nipple. My incision was about five to six inches long. Through this horizontal incision, they peeled back the skin with surgical scissors, anchoring it in several places and making sure that it stayed out of the way.

Next, they removed all the surrounding breast tissue, ducts, lobules, and of course, the tumor—the cancer.

During a mammogram, the technician will pull skin down from just under your collarbone, under your arm and as far into your back as she can pull forward. Breast tissue is way up there, just below the collarbone, as it is under your armpit and sneaks a little into your back. This requires that a large surface area of tissue be removed.

Dr. Connolly needed to reach inside of me to remove the axillary lymph nodes on the right side under my arm and next to my breast. Lymph nodes are aligned in a string. You'd think they could just pull them out like a string of pearls. But our bodies are more complicated than that. Nodes are encased in a Jell-O-like substance and are not easily identified by the surgeon. The resulting mass of Jell-O that the surgeon removes is sent to the pathologist and she/he painstakingly locates each node under a high-powered microscope, slices it into a zillion wafer-thin slices and tests its cancer quotient. As soon as I interview the doctor, I would find out in more accurate terms just how he was able to remove all of what he had removed through a five—to six-inch slit, *and* reach into my armpit for nodes!

It amazed me, intrigued me and yes, continued to absolutely gross me out. But I still had to know. I had read the surgical report; the things that I understood were gruesome in their detail, but I wanted to hear it in layman's terms so that it could be described in layman's terms in this book, but also in the doctor's words and sensitive to the correct description of medicine.

I had lunch with a friend on Friday. I was asked if I ever felt like my breast was still there. That phantom stuff again. Right after surgery and especially that first night, I was certain that I had *felt* my breast and my nipple—it had felt so much like they were still a part of me—and I'd wondered if the doctors had really done what they had planned to do. It wasn't until the next morning when the bandages were being changed and I had taken that first drive-by look that I'd realized that the mission had indeed been accomplished.

The next week after surgery, I would be talking to Shere or Larry or anyone else for that matter and out of the blue, I would feel my nipple brush against my pajamas. I felt it, I swear to God—and it had felt like it needed to be scratched. It had driven me absolutely crazy because I knew that I'd never be able to satisfy that itch. It was a cruel reminder of what was now truly gone. Just the thought of satisfying the itch on righty's remains, had scared me as well; not knowing what I might have been moving around or pulling at in the process. Some part of my brain had not yet recognized what had happened and it was still firing off on those nerves that had once been attached to the spinal cord. But it was getting a false signal.

Thankfully, that phantom feeling had finally stopped.

For about a year before my diagnosis, I had had an insatiable itch that would bother me under my armpit. It would come and go, had no pattern to it and occasionally, weeks would pass before it would recur. But it was something that I did take particular notice of. That was the first itch that I could never seem to satisfy. It felt as if it were deep within my armpit, and the only thing I'd found to provide relief was to grab onto a chunk of skin within that area, and pinch or put pressure on it. Maybe I was cutting off the blood supply, I wasn't sure, but it was maddening. Whenever I'd meet a woman who had had or was currently fighting breast cancer, I would ask if they'd had the same experience. The frightening thing was that more than half of the women I'd asked had said that they had. If this should happen to you, *run*—don't walk—to your doctor and have it checked out immediately.

I was now left with my original breast skin minus a nipple. All the nasty cancerous tissue inside had left this part of my body. It was my skin, only it had collapsed and was patiently waiting for the next step to normal, which wouldn't occur for many, many months.

I hoped that this would be the perfect "canvas" for the reconstruction surgeon. I looked forward to the results of that part of the process. I could only hope that the reconstruction surgeon has art in their background, like Dr. Connolly does.

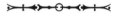

Dr. Song's Corner

Previously, it was the standard practice to not only remove the breast tissue, nipple and areola; but also the skin. But several landmark studies have shown that given the same stage of tumor, a skin sparing mastectomy (leaving all the breast skin behind and removing the contents) has no difference in survival from a regular mastectomy. Of course, the more skin you save, the better the reconstructive scar pattern can be—as the skin that will remain is your own. This is, of course, more important in an immediate reconstruction and a bit less so in a delayed reconstruction because the skin after radiation and healing will have contracted to a lesser or greater degree.

As for itching, this has been a common symptom with breast cancer patients we have seen. Let me be very clear: itching occurs all the time and there are many reasons for itching—some related to external sources (e.g., poison ivy, a new soap or lotion, or a new bra) and some internal sources or a drug reaction (i.e., allergic response), so please don't fly off the deep end if your breast or nipple itches. However, if the itching persists for any length of time or it is accompanied by nipple discharge, skin changes, dimpling or a new mass, don't ignore this. Seek your doctor's attention.

The thought behind itching is that there are deep sensory nerves in the breast; if the itching is in fact due to breast cancer, it is postulated that the sensory nerve fibers deep within one's breast are being irritated and cause itching. This is just a theory, but I've noticed complaints of itching deep within a breast (often, a patient states, "an itch I can't scratch") in several patients who are eventually found to have breast cancer.

As far as the method to remove axillary lymph nodes, some surgical oncologists (the very talented ones) will do a sentinel node biopsy through the mastectomy incision. It takes more skill and understanding, but this is possible. Of course, it also improves the eventual aesthetic outcome as no new scars are placed on the breast. The downside is that if the patient is smaller breasted and has a tighter skin envelope, or the tumor is low and the axilla is high, the access can be really tough. In my opinion, all surgeons should at least try to do this.

Chapter 40

Chemo, the New Cocktail for Me &
My Introduction to Red Death

Monday, March 24th, 8:30 AM

Shere arrived on Sunday night. She wanted to be here for my first chemo treatment. She seems to know when I need her most, even though I tried very hard to convince her that I would be fine and that she should stay home. Bob was on kid duty with the boys that week, as Lisa was a chaperone with both girls and their friends on spring vacation. Larry was here, of course. I was absolutely terrified of what was coming up and I was very grateful that they were there with me.

It's rather ironic but for all of these years, I had never allowed the nurse at the gynecologist's office to take blood—and it was a simple finger prick. I was afraid of needles and lancets or whatever it was that they used. One day, I asked them what they were testing for and I was told that it was a test for anemia. I laughed, saying that it was virtually impossible with my schedule for me to be anemic. If I were anemic, it obviously wasn't slowing me down a bit.

I now faced more than just a finger prick once a year. Anemia was suddenly an important issue that I must be careful about, as well as low blood counts, changes in my bone marrow, and changes in my heart's function. Blood must be drawn and needles and catheters would be plunged into my arm every two weeks for months. The next four months were going to be quite a period of adjustment and growth for me. I would probably still pass on the gynecologist's finger stick.

My blood work today, unlike others I'd spoken to who were able to get by on a finger stick test prior to chemo, amounted to two huge, full vials. They did a complete blood chemistry test and now knew everything there was to know about my blood, down to the last red blood cell in my bone marrow. They provided an entire printed page of medical mumbo jumbo about my blood that I would soon research and decipher. The good news was that an hour later, after the results had come in and I had passed the blood tests, I was told that last week's Mugascan had proven that my heart was healthy and totally ready for the onslaught.

I was ready for chemo.

We met with Dr. Nanda briefly and then we were introduced to Nurse Brigit Gallus, who explained every drug that they would use. Brigit asked me to sign a document noting that we had had this discussion. We talked about the risks and the side effects and what I needed to do if something occurred and lasted for more than twenty-four hours. It was a lot of information to absorb but they included a nice little package of printed materials for future reference.

My biggest concern would now be infections or getting a cold or virus, as my immune system would quickly begin to weaken.

I imagined that I must display my medical fears right at the surface. Maybe it was just a change in my eyes or body language that tipped everyone off; or could this team have my records marked with big, red letters stating that I am a medical chicken? They seemed to know, without asking, that I was terrified. I didn't even need to mention it. It had to be based on the fact that they had been down this road countless times with other people and were hoping that based on that, they might deliver a better experience.

Brigit took things slowly and told me what she would be doing before she did it. Larry decided that it would be a good idea to cover my eyes with his hand while the IV catheter for chemo was set being up. He has a big hand. He called it "the shield." I was squeezing the crap out of Shere's hand and nearly drawing blood from her while I simultaneously tensed up the muscles throughout my body. I had firmly anchored myself to the chair, braced for the inevitable.

The nurse implored, "Suzanne, please, you need to relax. Breathe through your nose."

I was as tight as a drum and could easily have bounced that needle off my arm and right into the stratosphere. My darling Larry decided that he would assist with the nurse's request. While he maintained a full "shield" with most of his palm to spare me from a vision of all the needles and other gross things, he had somehow placed two of his fingers over my mouth, using the same hand. I was forced to breathe through my nose.

I swear to God, we had fun even while having to deal with this. We were laughing our butts off, Brigit included, by the time the needles were in, securely anchored down and attached to all the tubes and pumps that were ready to deliver the healing poison to me.

The first four chemo treatments would consist of the following schedule every two weeks: blood work (two vials!); blood spinning tests that would determine my ability to continue with a treatment on that day; four oral drugs to combat nausea; inserting into my arm an IV catheter that is attached to a bag of saline solution that would slowly drip into my vein; three very large pumps of a drug called Doxorubicin (also known as Red Death due to its color and its amazing poisonous strength), a large pump of saline, three large pumps of a drug called Cyclophosphamide, and finally another large pump of saline.

I was keeping a watchful eye on the Red Death drug, as it could easily leak out of the catheter and burn the surrounding skin so badly that it would require a skin graft and render that vein pretty much useless for future chemo treatments. This was part of the reason why they pushed saline first, followed by the delivery of the drug to see if a leak will occur in your vein; before introducing the caustic drug treatments. I had no problems at all in that regard, as Nurse Brigit had done a fabulous job.

This was encouraging because if my veins had been too weak to accept the assault, the other option would have been the placement of a port. That would have required yet another surgery to have it placed in my chest, through which all chemo treatments would be delivered; and then another surgery to have it removed later. It appeared that my veins would be able to handle the onslaught of four months of chemotherapy treatments.

Dr. Nanda gave me a prescription for three things. An anti-nausea medicine, which I would need to take twice a day for three days after chemo. If that didn't work, she had prescribed another one that they call a "rescue drug." This drug was very strong and should work immediately. She wanted to be notified immediately about any sickness or unexplainable physical changes that I couldn't control within twenty-four hours. I would feel fatigued at the end of the week and there were myriad other side effects that I may or may not experience. I will detail those if and when they occur. The doctor, the nurse and Shere warned me that these drugs were cumulative; I may feel OK for a few weeks and then—*boom*. Stuff could start to happen.

Here was my latest challenge: I could go back to the hospital the day after each chemo treatment for a bone marrow shot, which was designed to stimulate white blood cell production in between treatments—or Larry or I could do it.

I laughed hysterically at the thought of *me* giving myself a shot. I would have to fashion the needle on the wall somehow, and then back into it. But that would leave as a challenge to that solution, the issue of plunging or pushing the drugs into my system. I could never do it.

I was hoping that my insurance plan would cover the purchase of the shot from Walgreen's, our local pharmacy. Larry would give me the shot. That would save a great deal of time and anxiety; at least I wouldn't need to travel an hour each way, park the car, sign up to see the doctor or nurse and then finally get the shot, only to reverse that entire process while making my way back home—a three-hour event at best. Doing it ourselves was, of course, the most cost-effective way for the patient, the hospital and the insurance company. But insurance companies often look at things very differently.

Larry was excited about this new task. He asked Shere to send him veterinary doctor needles so he could practice. But he wanted to practice on *me,* prior to wasting any medicine. Hadn't this man ever seen the television show ER or one of those medical programs where they teach an intern how to give a shot using a peach or an orange? Here's the deal: he had one shot at giving me the shot. The potential remained that we just might need to find another option.

We were at the hospital for five and a half hours and had been home for twenty hours.

Tuesday morning after chemo, I felt great. I had slept well. I had eaten three meals the day before, which didn't happen often. I wasn't feeling sick or tired and my hair was still firmly anchored on my head. Things were going well with this first treatment.

Chapter 41

Getting the Shot from Larry

One of the nurses called on Tuesday to see how I was doing after the first chemo treatment and to make sure that I was able to get the Neulasta shot from Walgreen's. She also wanted to know if Larry was still comfortable with giving me the shot.

She asked me how much I was charged for the shots. I found this a rather odd question and asked her why she was interested. She said that each shot generally cost $2000, and that they had always been interested in what the final cost was to a patient who had insurance, as opposed to the patient who didn't. With the insurance plan I was on, the shot had cost me $15. What in the world do people without insurance *do?* It was a terrifying thought. These days, most of us are at risk in keeping our jobs and therefore, our medical insurance!

After dinner, I read the huge instruction leaflet that accompanied the drug and pre-loaded syringe. It took about ten minutes to go through what I felt was important to know. I happily skipped past the bullshit that I knew I would never understand nor have the time to question, challenge or change. I passed the leaflet to Larry; he wanted to read it as well. Forty-five minutes later and after having read the document on both sides three times, he finally proceeded to get everything ready.

You'd have thought we were doing a biopsy in the kitchen. He sterilized everything, including me. Then he needed to read the document just one more time. I was now hanging out without any pants on and getting more nervous by the minute. We had decided that the shot would go into my thigh. I was trying to decide if I could flee the premises and still maintain our relationship.

Pop. In it went. Nice and smooth and easy and not a drop of blood in the plunger or the needle. Doctors Shere and Kurt and Army Medic Dad would have been proud. I felt a little sting at the first prick of the needle, then again as the drug went in. But it wasn't bad at all. I'm not sure if Larry or I was more relieved once it was over. I sensed, though, that this one had been harder for Larry. He immediately fell asleep on the couch while I just sat there amazed that it had even happened.

Chapter 42

The First Few Days after Chemo

Monday after chemo, I had a late lunch with Larry and Shere. Feeling completely like myself, I went shopping with Shere and ended the day with a huge Italian dinner with the family. Tuesday morning, Shere left for New Jersey. I worked all day in the office at home. Wednesday, I felt pretty good and decided to venture downtown to shop at my favorite haunts.

At 3:00 PM, driving home from the city, I started to feel subtle changes.

I was attempting to stay tuned in to these changes so that I could accurately describe how chemo was affecting me. I know that each person's experience is different, but I had also learned that much of it is the same. There are so many potential symptoms with treatment, and you might not hear about all of them from the medical professionals. Maybe, after reading my book, someone would find comfort in the fact that what they are experiencing is normal, or they would find relief in knowing that they had dodged a particular bullet.

I felt tired and less focused, kind of in a slight fog; like the feeling you get when you're coming down with a cold and it feels as though the top half of your head has gone missing. As soon as I arrived home, I fell asleep waiting for Larry to get off work.

We had a funeral to go to that night. It was an uncomfortable drive to the funeral home. I was experiencing small changes all over my body, from top to bottom, firing off one after the other. None that hurt or were frightening, but they did give me great pause. I didn't know what to expect next.

At the funeral home, after about ten minutes of standing with our friends in a room that felt devoid of air, I had to sit down. I was unable to regulate my body temperature and I kept swinging between hot and chilled. A light mist of moisture broke out on my face, chest and arms. My legs were cramped. Was it the crowded room? I wasn't claustrophobic. Was it too hot? Was it the funeral home, the sadness of place? I had never met the man who was lost to all of these people. Was I simply affected by the grief of my friends? Was I having a reaction to chemo? I just didn't know.

We stayed through the ceremony.

Thursday morning, I woke up at 5:30 AM after a restless night. I took my anti-nausea medicine and within half an hour, threw it up. Pretty effective. Had it already started? I thought I had a few more weeks before symptoms like these would begin. I decided to stay close to home, just in case.

Nine hours after I had thrown up, I thought: *Maybe it was a fluke.*

I'd been constipated for three days and because I had always been very regular in this regard, it concerned me. The pains in my tummy were agonizing. I took Ducolax and milk of magnesia, hoping for some relief. The thought of eating was a bit worrisome. How much could you push through one end before it must exit through the other? Relief in that area seemed to be the goal of the day. I laughed at the thought. Making a *bowel movement* the goal of the day? Where had the Suzanne that everyone knew, fled to? She should have been traipsing around Europe, having the time of her life trying to figure out Tezza's three F's for life.

The glands on each side of my head, near my ears, had been slightly swollen the night before. I only noticed this when I put cream on my face and neck. Today they were just a tad tender. My fingers were swollen and that slight fog in my head was still present. My lower back and my legs hurt but not constantly;

every once in a while, I would feel a tightening of the muscles. For about three hours last night, my body had ached the way it would with the flu.

Then it suddenly stopped.

Just like that!

I imagined that the drugs were slowly infiltrating all of the little nether regions of my body and that this was the cause of the changes that came and went so quickly. It was an interesting experience, as I never knew what the next hour would bring.

Today, I took it easy; having thrown up so early in treatment, albeit just once, completely freaked me out. I hadn't expected this to happen until after the second or third treatment, when the drug would be more prevalent in my system.

Friday morning, I felt pretty damn good. I had taken a nice, long, hot Jacuzzi bath for about half an hour the night before and it had helped my aching muscles calm down. Larry had tucked me into bed and I must have fallen asleep within minutes. It was now well past thirty hours since I had thrown up, so I chalked up that experience to being a fluke.

My body wasn't programmed to readily accept pills at 5:30 in the morning. I made sure there were crackers on the nightstand now, to put something in my stomach before taking any pills. It seemed to help.

Milk of magnesia had become such a familiar taste to me in those days that I could swig it right out of the bottle. Not very classy, but certainly easier and faster than measuring a proper dose with a proper dispensing tool so early in the morning or so late at night. It hadn't worked yet. I knew I was getting enough of a dose as sometimes I'd go for a second swig just for good measure.

One of the many nicknames that Larry had honored me with over the years was "Pebbles," the little girl character in the *Flintstones* cartoon, because I would occasionally wear my hair up in a high ponytail. That nickname now held a double meaning. Never before had that moniker been more appropriate.

Chapter 43

Doing What I Always Do: Reaching Through the Sky and Dreaming Big—Really Big

Several people have suggested that I write a book and spin breast cancer into something hopeful and move it as far of left field as possible. Textbooks were too clinically detached and often shrouded with fear and mystery.

I loved the idea of writing a book. My family, surely exhausted after so many years of hearing that one day "I will write a great novel" would finally never need to hear those words again. I knew for a fact that Larry was tired of hearing about it. Although he was absolutely convinced that we would need to collaborate if the book had any chance at all of becoming a bestseller, he felt that he had far better experiences from which to draw upon.

He can be so naïve.

Since I was a kid, I had dreamed of writing a novel and then getting it published. But I had always imagined that it would be a racy novel or some intricately woven and wildly fabricated mystery; not a true-life memoir. I had written many articles and had been interviewed, written about and published in many magazines relating to business. But they were never books that I had written. The closest I had come to being published was a printed page in a college textbook that talked about the business that Bob and I had built. It included a decent picture of us, at least. It is still in use at colleges all over the United States, so there was some exposure to be proud of. But it wasn't a book that *I* had written.

On my e-mail distribution list, there are four people who are published authors. I own autographed, first edition copies of their books. Michelangelo Capua has four books in print and one in the works; Bill Podijil with one book published and one in the works; and Ron Harper and Katherine Harper, both published. Having your manuscript read is rare enough but being published is even rarer.

"I am a published author"—this was simply one of the most amazing accomplishments and most exciting grouping of words that I felt could ever be said by anyone. Then one of my friends, quite a writer herself, suggested that I might find a wider audience by starting an Internet blog. I liked that idea, too. I liked the immediacy, the ease, the worldwide reach and the simplicity.

I've given this book-versus-blog idea considerable thought and have decided to do what I always do and reach through the sky and plunge headfirst into the unknown. Ease and simplicity be damned! I was ready to step out of my comfort zone once again, throw it back into high gear and work my ass off. I would attempt to write something compelling enough to be published and helpful enough to be purchased. It would meld the patient experience with the medical realities, including some of the best medical opinions I could find.

I had decided that should I be fortunate enough to find a well-known corporate sponsor and get published, one hundred percent of the profits would flow through the Zaccone Family Foundation and immediately be applied for use at the Breast Cancer Center at the University of Chicago. Once the Center was set up with some major item, we would buy another of whatever that item was and place it in another city or another country; and then keep on going.

Dr. Connolly and Dr. Song (whom you will meet in a future chapter) are also accomplished speakers. They would be able to train the doctors in these cities and countries on the use of this new equipment or technique. Chicago could pay it forward, and the book and the foundation could pay the way.

This was the fastest method I could think of to get to the *people* part of the drama: immediately affecting people who were alive today. Maybe we could reduce the number of "in memory of" stories that we all know too well. It would have an immediate impact on the quality of the experience for so many women and their caregivers, and those people who may not be as blessed as I was with the love and support that make facing the scary stuff so much easier.

I cautioned Dr. Connolly not to get too excited because this was still a dream yet to be realized. But it was a dream that was being dreamt by a very motivated dreamer. We had time to figure out how to use the money—that's always the easy part—but first we needed to find a sponsor and get published.

I definitely got Dr. Connolly's attention when I suggested that there must be some piece of equipment that he wished he had, some amazing research project that needed funding to be fully realized, something that would make his job easier, more accurate or thorough, more technologically advanced or better yet, less brutal or painful for the patient. I reminded him that when he goes into the Amazon to work with doctors without Borders and he wishes he had that second nurse, this book might fund that nurse's trip. I have friends in high places that have friends in high places who work in some pretty high places—and the collective energy of an amazing support group that would propel me forward.

I could always fall back on the blog!

Chapter 44

The Big Shave (Part 1)

It's the Monday before the Big Shave Party.

I began to doubt my ability to go through with it. I'd never loved my hair more than I had these last few weeks. Ironically, I had not had a bad hair day either; a cruel twist of things. Maybe I was just allowing what would normally be considered a bad hair day to slide on through, considering the future. Two options screamed at me: face it head on or get sentimental.

It was a loud, cold, crushing wave that slammed against my skull—my *naked* skull—throwing me off balance. With Option 1, I could feel the cool swoosh of air as I imagined that first swipe of the razor, that point where there was absolutely no turning back. With Option 2, I imagined the horror of waking up with random chunks of my hair lying on the pillow each day, or a soft veil of hair waiting to be swept away by the first breeze. (By the way, those in the business do not refer to someone losing their hair as someone with hair that is "falling out." It's called "releasing." But why pussyfoot around? Your damn hair *will* fall out.)

This shave party, being entirely my idea, was supposed to help me "take control" of the reality of my situation. Lately it had begun to feel like the situation was out of control. The options felt more like something being forced upon me with little or slim chances of skimming through it unfazed—or should I say *unshaved*? It should have been easier because it was inevitable: do it now or wake up to it tomorrow, or the next day.

If only I wasn't so vain . . .

Since the first chemo treatment exactly one week ago, I'd been collecting hair that I had found flying around the bathroom floor, in my hair brush after styling with the blow-dryer, or skimming on top of the drain in the shower. I had put all that hair in a Ziploc baggie. Shedding hair was normal for me, but these days I'd been keeping a very close eye on its loss factor. So far it wasn't falling out any faster than normal . . . I think. I'd never really measured it in this way before so I was really just guessing. The hair I had saved was virtually useless. This only made it harder to face the razor in six short days.

My girlfriend Debbie Donult (one of the Mag 7) and my parents flew in on Thursday to help us get ready for the big bash, hang out for Chemo No. 2 and lend their support. Debbie was the only one in our group of seven who lived out of the area. We were all thrilled that she was home.

I'd always thought that bald men were sexy. I suddenly had a new fascination with bald heads everywhere I went; especially with the shape, contour and sheen of Bob's and Dad's heads. I must have been identifying with the vision of my future. Here was another one of those odd moments: I'd gone from hoping to borrow Mom's shoes, bag and dress—to hoping for a nicely shaped head like Dad's and Bob's.

It's Saturday, late in the afternoon on the day of the Big Shave Party. Everything was as organized and prepared as it would ever be and we were ready for our guests. I had a Cosmo martini in hand and after a few bold and determined sips, I hopped in the shower and washed my hair for the last time. I hoped that I could blow-dry it into something that looked like the healthy, vibrant and lively hair that it was.

It would be my hair's final presentation. It's closing night after such a long rehearsal and an even longer run.

It had to be perfect.

Chapter 45

The Big Shave Party (Part 2)
What a Difference a Day Makes—
24 Little Hours

My life has always been energized by music. I can't resist using songs to occasionally define events. Hence, this chapter's title.

My shower experience was largely uneventful until the end. I'd been through the usual routine, and the last thing I always took care of was rinsing out my hair. I used my fingers as a comb to rinse out the hair conditioner. I ended up with two huge gobs of hair, one in each hand. I gently pulled them off my fingers, opened the shower door and placed them on the ledge. No tears. I went through this activity four times until it appeared that everything that was ready to fall out had fallen out.

It was bad. I didn't need a Ziploc bag comparison to be sure.

I put on my bathrobe, collected the hair from the shower's ledge, and placed it on a Kleenex to dry. Then I couldn't resist—out came the Ziploc bag and the hot and burning tears finally fell. There was more hair after this shower than in the Ziploc baggie, which contained hair from ten days' worth of showers. It was a sign. It was time to let go. My hair was certainly taking the cue, as it was letting go at a dizzying pace.

I walked downstairs to where Debbie and Larry continued to put a few finishing touches on things. I showed them the hair on the Kleenex and the Ziploc bag. I was shaking. We sat on a large leather ottoman and held onto each other, crying.

Last week, Larry had told me that he thought I had completely lost my mind to want to do this in such a public way. But it wasn't my mind that I was losing; it was my hair. I must admit that I was beginning to question my sanity as well. Larry had dubbed this event as "Cirque de Suzanne."

I was blessed that I always had the freedom to do it my way. Yet, I thank Larry for his continual support, for standing by my radical choices, even though he didn't always agree with them. He recognized that this entire experience had been a major change in my life plan, in *our* life plan, and he allowed me to feel the full swing of emotions that I'd known I would have to experience. A big part of that experience would be tonight but he would be there to help me finally take some control back.

We had decided very early on that neither of us wanted to cook. We wanted to be as free of the machinations of a party as we could, even though we were the hosts. The guests we had invited were people with whom we felt comfortable enough to not stress out over making sure they had something to eat or drink or whether they were having a good time. They would naturally have a good time and were close enough to us to know that they could make themselves at home in our home. We had food flowing across one long marble countertop in the kitchen. The bar area between the kitchen and the family room was complete with two of the foxiest bartenders in the area, Larry and Tom Matas. We had changed the cuisine from Italian to Mexican food. Beverages consisted of margaritas, of course, but we could not resist allowing the quirkiness of our personalities to come through—so we also had red and white wines, beer and Larmos (Cosmos), as well as various deserts like fresh homemade cannolis and Italian cookies, flan, chocolate and fruit. The variety represented us well. It brought together a diverse, eclectic, unique and special combination of food, spirits and friends.

We had forty-eight confirmed attendees on the list. Three couples and seven people in total called, as one or both of them were sick and did not want to infect me. I wanted them there but I thanked them for their kind consideration. My resistance was low and I had to be very careful about exposure to just about everything for the next three months.

People arrived throughout the evening, as several had had previous plans earlier in the evening. Things got wild. I lost count of how many cosmos I'd had because after only a few sips, my glass would be magically refilled. We were trying to decide if we should call them "Chemopolitans" instead of "Larmopolitans" for the next few months.

I was unable to spend much quality time with anyone, but judging from the laughter and the photographic evidence, it was a good party. The last person left at 1:30 AM. We were in bed by 3:00 AM.

Karen White came over the following afternoon and helped us finish off the food, clean up and veg out on the couch and watch movies. We were all very crispy. Larry said even his hair hurt.

My girlfriend Sophia Dilberakis had offered to act as the official photographer of the event. Sophia has been a professional writer for the past thirty years, has owned and operated her own Public Relations agency for the past decade and has also dabbled in photography. She is a well-known and respected packaging professional and had served with me and on her own on the Boards of various associations for the industry.

A few chapters back, I mentioned the lyrics to a song called "Living out the String" by Marc Cohn. A few years back, Sophia had written the biography for and was the manager of the major rock and pop guitarist Shane Fontayne, who had performed and recorded with just about every major artist under the sun (including Marc Cohn, Bruce Springsteen, Sting, Rod Stewart, Joe Cocker, Paul Simon, Shania Twain and John Waite). Sophia is a very dynamic woman and it did not surprise me for a moment when I learned that she was introduced to Shane by Grammy Award-winning trumpet player Chris Botti, who is also a close friend of hers. Things moved quickly from there. When they met Sophia, I was certain that they immediately loved her, just as I did. As such, she was asked to handle a lot of concert photography. When she volunteered to be the "tour photographer" for the head-shaving party, how could I resist? I've seen a sneak preview of her photos and they are spectacular!

There were several others who decided to do the Big Shave: Dad, Bob and Vince DiTrolio. They are all nuts; especially Vince, because he allowed me and Carol to shave his head.

I've never had short hair in my life. I have very clear, detailed, early childhood memories; my hair was longer when I was four years old than it was now. I couldn't do it yet. I couldn't do the Big Shave. But I managed to cut a lot off.

The story of my hair would find at least one more chapter, as it was falling out—pardon me, *releasing*—quite quickly.

Larry loved the shorter style. But I wasn't so sure.

Chapter 46

The Second Chemo Treatment:
Going Chemotose

Monday

As usual, we started out in the department that draws blood, one of my least favorite medical activities. They pulled out two tubes of blood for testing and approval.

I passed.

We could keep to the schedule.

I was a bit worried because of the *porre* I'd had over the weekend. (A "porre" is the Portuguese term for "a drink" or "a party." If the translation is inaccurate, I have six Brazilian friends who will correct me.)

The nurse who drew my blood was someone I hadn't worked with before. She noticed that I entered her domain like a walking dead boob, looking mighty scared. I hadn't mastered the art of hiding that emotion very well, as I've had little experience in being so very scared. I was accompanied by two people and I was holding their hands and squeezing the hell out of them. One of them was as big as a bodyguard (Larry) and the other was wearing a pink cancer camouflage baseball hat (Debbie). I was certain that the nurse had selected the easiest possible vein to get her job done quickly so she could send me and the entourage on our way.

We had a different nurse for this second chemo treatment. Her name is Lor Lawson. So much for the patient-nurse bonding experience, I guess. Since the nurse who had drawn blood had taken the easiest vein available, this left the chemo nurse with the not-so-easy ones. It was a lesson for the next treatment. Remind the nurse drawing blood not to use my better veins.

The chemo nurse had real work to do, pushing all the chemo drugs through. We needed a solid vein that would last several hours. She had to stick me quite a few times before we hit a vein that was stable enough. It was absolute torture. When she did find one, it kept wiggling around in an attempt to avoid the needle. The poor vein was as scared as I was, and was hiding out. I prayed that the nurse would make contact, as the option would be another surgery where a port is placed in my chest to deliver future treatments.

The thought of surgery must have been enough to pop that vein right back to the surface. Contact was made. The nurse had blood in the needle so we knew she had hit a solid one that would be able to withstand the push and volume of drugs. The delivery of today's Red Death, which was also known as the Red Devil, stung a bit. Dr. Nanda was there talking to us about how I would handle the treatments once at home. My reaction to the sting brought the nurse over. Lor immediately checked out a few things to make sure that the liquid Red Devil wasn't leaking outside of my vein. A leak could result in a nasty burn.

Lor was as amazing as Brigit. I hoped we could work with either of them for the next chemo.

After chemo, we had lunch. Then Debbie and I went shopping.

Tuesday

Debbie and I went to the wig place to get those hairy beauties cut down and ready for Toni's final touches of magic. The wig made of real hair came in as long as "Thing" (a tiny, four-foot tall creature with long hair that completely covered its eyes, ears, nose, mouth and entire body) on the comedy *Munster's*

Show. That was the perfect description for this wig before it was cut. Part of the cost of the wig was to thin it out and reduce the volume to something manageable, then cut it in a style that you were happy with and would fit your naked head. They would adjust it as your hair grew back.

Amy (the stylist) and Jan (the owner of the shop) strongly suggested that I shave off my hair completely so I could better fit the wig. I still couldn't do it. I had a Board meeting on Friday at the DiTrolio Flexographic Institute. I'm President of the Board; I would like to explain what was happening to me—with my own hair, and not have to worry about making some wig look decent that morning. It just seemed like too much pressure too soon for such a new and all-too-important opening day: me wearing a wig—in public. Shit!

Vince DiTrolio, the owner of the Institute, was at the Big Shave Party with his wife Cynthia and had actually asked me to shave his head, which I did. No one else on the Board knew. I was hoping that I could hold onto most of my hair for three more days and then the rest would be up to Toni to make this faux hair look like mine. We had a start.

Larry had woken up sick and was throwing up violently early in the morning. He didn't have a fever. We had thought it might be food poisoning; but no one else had gotten sick. Maybe it was a case of eating too much or having too sweet of a dessert at dinner and going to bed too soon on all of that. We teased him about feeling sympathy symptoms for me. It's possible. My dad's right breast had been hurting him for months and it wouldn't stop bothering him, even now after surgery had taken mine away; he still suffered.

Larry finally came home from work at around 2:00 PM. We stayed far away from each other, just in case he *did* have something.

I took Debbie to the airport, marveling all the way about how fast the last five days had flown by. I would miss her.

The issues that came up that day were—

I pooped like a champ, as I now knew the drill and had helped Mother Nature with Ducolax the day before chemo. I still had chemo head where I felt as if the top of my head had gone missing. I was losing hair fast in a scary way. The crown of my head was very tender, as were the glands on the sides of my jaw line under my ears. My eyes got tired easily but my mind was buzzing around and wouldn't allow me to rest. The inside of my nose went from dry and tender to drippy and tender. The cartilage was definitely being hit as well. It all continued to amaze me.

I tended to bump into things more than usual, which was *a lot*. Another nickname that Larry had given me years ago was "Bruizanne." Moving around as quickly as I used to, I was always bumping into or off of some corner, a table or object as I attempted to cut a second or two off my—-well, whatever it was that I'd been doing at that moment. Bruises were common. I needed to be extra careful now so I wouldn't look like an abused woman who laughed a lot. My left arm already looked like I was in the beginning stages of IV drug abuse. The only other symptom was that I was getting tired late in the afternoons. I fought the urge to sleep in the afternoons so I could sleep at night and keep to some sort of schedule.

It was Shot Night. Larry went through his drill, this time with more confidence. Now *I* was anxious. After taking the shot out of the refrigerator, we had to wait for half an hour to bring it to room temperature before it could be administered. I did what all Zaccone women do when they had to wait for something to happen: I started cleaning things. Everything and anything that looked remotely smudged or out of order was taken care of while I worked myself into a frothy mental lather just thinking about another damn needle stick coming my way.

Larry wore an industrial mask, in case he was carrying some germ or virus. He maintained the thought that the hospital mask was not as good as his personally selected and perfectly fit-to-size mask. He was probably right.

I was sitting on a chair with my leg up on another chair in the kitchen. It was a straight shot in with the needle and he was done.

He quickly moved around to rub out the knots in my neck and back. I love this. I'd turn into a piece of clay every time I felt him kneading those muscles. He has big, strong hands and knows just where to dig in my neck and back to turn me into mush.

That night, it was all too much. I was now mentally shot. I had worked myself into this *state*—it wasn't because of chemo or the shot. I felt as if I was going to be sick. I stood up to run to the bathroom and couldn't make it more than five steps. I had to lie down on the kitchen floor. That was all that I needed to do: get horizontal and stretched out flat on my back, breathing deep and lung-filling breaths. I was fine. What a roller-coaster ride this was becoming.

Wednesday

I woke up at 6:00 AM and immediately took the anti-nausea medicine. I began to get some office work accomplished. I soon felt a bit sick but I fought that battle and won. Mom was coming over that night so we could play dress-up with the wigs, hats and scarves just like when I was little, only we had never had need for the wig part back then.

After the first chemo treatment, it had taken until Thursday for me to feel any major combination of effects all at once. This second treatment had shortened that time frame by one day. I could actually *feel* this helpful little poison in my body; it was accumulating and moving around at a much quicker pace, saturating each and every cell and turning it upside down or inside out.

By 4:00 PM, I was wiped out. Mom came over to play with the wigs, hats and scarves and to teach me some tricks that her friend Heloisa Jennings had shown her. I was so weak I could barely assemble a meaningful thought or response. I couldn't keep my eyes open. My body was exhausted yet my mind was racing with all the things that I should have been doing but couldn't muster up the strength to do. These were things that no one could help me with: paying bills, working on the lake house insurance claim, GSI projects, et cetera. I'd never felt this before. This funky, cloudy, weird and difficult-to-describe combination of things that fired off then subsided; or fired off then stayed around for a while, draining my energy.

Mom and I were on the couch talking and it scared me to see the pain in her eyes as she sat with me, helpless and unable to pull her baby away from the fire. It tore me up. Her eyes spilled over with volumes of concern, love and fear.

I was certain that this was harder for my parents, Larry, Bob and Shere than it was for me. I *had* to do this—there was no other option—and with a lot of the experience, no one could make it better. In many ways, this was pretty much a personal journey but it was adversely affecting those whom I loved. It seemed unfair to drag them along this potholed and bumpy road with me.

I was up all night, completely restless. I was tired but unable to sleep. The aching I had experienced from Chemo No. 1 was back. I finally lost the battle and gave up at around 1:30 AM and allowed myself to throw up. My offering to the Chemo Spirit had obviously not been enough. The hungry bastard wanted more.

For the next four hours, I went from the porcelain goddess to lying on the floor in an effort to calm down and cool off. Then I would slip into the tub to soak in the Jacuzzi and warm myself in an attempt to stop the shivers. I would drag myself to bed to try and relax my muscles, and then the pattern would repeat. Larry laid his head on my chest at one point and was alarmed at the rate at which my heart was beating. He helped me set up camp in the bathroom and he sat there as helpless as Mom had been this afternoon.

I needed to get my heart rate under control so I could avoid another Mugascan or any delay in treatment. Larry gave me a pill that Dr. Nanda had ordered in case the anti-nausea medicine that I was already taking every eight hours wouldn't be enough. She called it the "emergency rescue pill" and was very clear about my using it and not trying to be a hero and waiting until things got really bad. It took fifteen minutes before the pill was offered back up to the Chemo Spirit via the porcelain goddess.

Was there an emergency pill for the emergency pill?

Thursday

I was still wiped out but doing much better. I woke up after two hours of sleep and created a whole new hairstyle without using anything but my hands. It's as though my fingers had retractable thinning shears; as I ran them through my hair, I removed a layer or two. So far, hair still fully covered my head. But I could tell that it wouldn't be long before I'd have a very different photo to share.

Chapter 47

Learning and Teaching Lessons while Allowing the Boat to Take Its Course

Lately it had been difficult to distinguish between a chemo or cancer-related ache, pain or symptom—and an ache, pain or symptom that would have occurred anyway. I'd always been very much in tune with my body and aware of its changes. But I was also known as one to pass over symptoms as just a part of life. Right or wrong, I would assess the situation then quickly get over it and move on.

For example, I had taken Christa and John—two of my godchildren—to Europe a few years ago. Debbie and her daughter Kelly had joined us. I'd broken my foot when Donna Cannizzo and I were at a trade show, the day before I'd left on the trip. I'd thought it was just sprained. Additionally, the airline had lost my luggage and I would not see it again until the night before we would leave for home.

Very early in the trip, I had had a decision to make and a lesson to teach; and both had to be handled in the right way. My choices had been to respond as I'd wanted to, from deep within the pit of my tummy by bitching and moaning and getting absolutely nowhere. Or I could respond as I'd known I had to and would: by showing the kids that attitude, and how you chose to respond to life's challenges, are everything. I had taken the high road: I laughed my way through Europe while walking around with a broken foot for nine days, and had the time of my life wearing the few things I always carry on the plane just in case, in sundry combinations.

Every time I started to feel cross or sorry for myself, God would send me a strong, immediate and physical message. Debbie and the kids may remember me mentioning this whenever it happened: a horribly crippled man would cross our path, or an obviously hungry and homeless person with only one leg would be sitting in the street and looking directly at me. Witnessing this kind of pain slaps you back to your blessings mighty quick and forces you to face the fact that things could always be so much worse.

Generally, I didn't give in to physical limitations or challenges. I've had two self-diagnosed bouts with searing pain from kidney stones that arrived and eased off every fifteen minutes for three very long days. I faced them, dealt with them, then pushed on and never gave them much thought.

Until now.

Since cancer, I've been in a heightened state of awareness. As the government would say or as that scary hospital voice would cry out in an emergency: *"Code red! Code red!"* Everything that happened or changed, twitched, tingled, pulsed, started or stopped was up for review and question. I wondered how many of these things would have even registered on my personal Richter scale just a few months ago.

My scalp was tender and tingled most of the day. I could feel hair actually releasing from my scalp as I typed. I could almost hear it breaking off. I was now wearing what looked like a surgeon's cap, only a great deal cuter and peppered with a mélange of colors that I liked. My newly acquired collection of caps and scarves matched most of my outfits. In case I decided to venture out into the world, I would at least look . . . *eccentric chic.*

The bottoms of my toes and feet had been very sore for the past seventy-two hours, but only when I walked on them or touched them. Was it because of the strappy, high-heeled sandals that I had worn on Friday? Maybe my feet weren't ready yet for summer shoes? Or had the poison finally reached the bottom of me?

I called Carol. She clearly remembered this happening to her, as well. She told me that slathering cocoa butter on my feet and taking Vitamin B6 would help.

I would need to bring this up with the doctor during the next visit. I had been told to tell them about everything I experienced and everything I put into my body outside of food and their prescriptions. I didn't even want to use eye drops to soothe my tired, stinging eyes without their approval; one of the symptoms they had warned me to be careful of was a change in eye focus. Should I be concerned that the eye drops may cause a reaction? Could there be a contraindication to the ingredients in the eye drops versus the ingredients in chemo, the Neulasta shot or the anti-nausea medicine? Better safe than sorry, so I would wait and talk to them next week about Vitamin B6. As far as the cocoa butter went, I ran out and bought some that day. It helped a lot.

Many people asked me why I hadn't shaved off all of my hair, as I'd thought I would be strong enough to do at the Big Shave Party. Why struggle with waking up each morning and combing out enough hair to provide to Mattel Corporation for a dozen Barbie dolls?

Well, I had decided to look at this experience as a journalistic, medical experiment. Now I knew what I looked like in several shorter hairstyles. In fact, since Tony had cut it, I was on my *ninth* hairstyle due to all of the hair loss. I was carefully documenting what had been lost after chemo treatments. Lately, I had been taking pictures of the actual daily hair loss since Chemo No. 2, when all hell had broken loose.

I was beginning to look sick. The reflection in the mirror was of me—in that drawn, balding, hollow and gray cancer-like look.

This may be morbid, but someone going through the first stages of chemo may want to know what to expect if they decide to go shorter in style but not totally bald. She may wonder how long her hair might hang on; she can use what she reads here as a gauge of sorts. She, too, may have a Board meeting or a family gathering or an event at which she'd prefer to have her own hair and not have to wear a wig, scarf or hat that announces to the world so loudly and clearly that she is sick. These things are worn differently when you have hair from when you don't. Trust me.

It may have sounded or appeared as though I was running from the truth or delaying the inevitable. Don't think for a moment that I don't know that. But somehow, through writing this book, things have changed. I needed to experience this for more than just myself. This experience should be available to anyone who may have to go through it tomorrow and needs to check in with a friend and make a decision based on the stuff they don't tell you at the doctor's office because the doctors didn't learn about it in medical school. Medical caregivers couldn't possibly tell you *everything* when it comes to cancer; there are just too many mutations and possible side effects. Resources like this can be helpful.

This had become a journalistic, research-filled, fact-finding, rule-busting medical experiment that I felt compelled to fully document. It had also become mixed in with a healthy dose of vanity when it came to the hair part. I feel confident that there are others out there just like me. Documenting the experience in this way would allow me to act almost as if I were an intimate observer chronicling the war for the folks back home. Brutally truthful in content and close enough to the front lines to be graphic in detail.

I had been learning Portuguese through email with Heloisa: *"Deixa o barco correr!"* (Let the boat take its course!)

With such a strong and determined captain and crew, I could let the boat run its course for a while without me.

Bon voyage!

Chapter 48

Hair Today But Gone Tomorrow—
or Tony, the Trucker and Tits

It had been twenty-five days since the first chemo treatment. It was the first day that I absolutely would not want to go out without something covering my head. When you are a woman, thinning hair tends to make you look sick or very, very old.

I'd noticed an interesting pattern to what went first. My hair was thinning around the area that framed my face. It was slowly moving through the center, top and the crown area. Looking at me from the front or on either side would bring about a second glance. In some areas, the hair was so thin you could see my scalp. I still had masses of hair on the back of my head and tufts on top and on the sides. Amazing, but I was losing hair in exactly the same pattern that most men lose theirs. I'd even tried the "comb-over," which looked as pitiful on me as it did on any man who tried to fool the world and failed miserably. If I wore a baseball cap, you would never suspect a thing. I was never a baseball-cap girl but I was finding comfort in knowing that I had several brand-new caps to fall back on when needed.

Suzanne's simple solution:

> Ice packs (the homemade kind, not the ice packs you receive from the doctor or dentist) work fabulously on a tingly scalp and issues relating to nausea. Fill

a large Ziploc bag with ice halfway up then fold in half. Insert that bag into another large Ziploc bag to prevent leakage. You may need to put a cloth or a cap on your head if it gets too cold.

You can also place a runner's ring (those rings of gel-filled fabric that retain cold water) around your head and pin closed or attach with Velcro straps.

A frozen bag of peas also works equally well for visits to the porcelain goddess.

It was an emotional Tuesday.

I was with Tony Scavo, my stylist who works at the Marianne Strokirk Salon in Chicago, as she whipped Wig No. 1 into shape.

Tony is an artist with hair. She knows precisely what to do for each client and their type of hair. She cut the wig into a style that would have been absolutely adorable had it been placed on any head but mine. On me, it looked like a mop. It felt strange, confining, and looked totally phony. Like I was trying to be someone I was not. I couldn't carry it off. At the shave party, we had taken some hilarious pictures of the wig being worn by some of my girlfriends, Bob and a few other crazy men. Other than the guys with mustaches, everyone had looked pretty good. *They* could pull it off.

I left one of the wigs and the hair ring with Tony so she could work on them at her convenience. I left, smiling, with the other wig on. It wasn't her fault that I looked like a clown in a cranial prosthesis.

I cried as soon as I got into the car and didn't stop until sometime after I got home. Once I had reached the highway, I whipped the wig off my head and put on my surgeon's cap. A trucker who had been next to my car had seen the whole drama unfold and had almost lost control of his rig. I'd been too embarrassed to enjoy the full hilarity of that situation as I normally would have—you know, hang around at the same speed and look him in the eyes and smile while sharing a side-by-side vehicular moment. I had sped away, tears streaming down my face the way they had a few weeks ago just after surgery.

I was not a person who cried easily about things relating to myself.

Ask Larry.

In so many ways, I'm a changed woman these days.

Ask *me*.

Chapter 49

Larry & the Three Bald Zaccones at Chemo No. 3

Shere arrived on Sunday afternoon. After dinner with Larry, Bob and Lisa, Shere and I went up to the bathroom to shave off the rest of my hair. It was driving me crazy, as it looked so straggly and thin. It made me look sickly even when I wasn't feeling that way a good part of the time.

Shere wanted to do the honors. We took pictures with the man-style "comb-over," making it ever more chic by adding a barrette. We took a few pictures of what was left of my hair from the front, the back and the sides; twenty-eight days after the first chemo treatment. Then we took a picture of the final result: bald.

My crazy and adorable sister had been insisting for months that she would be shaving her hair off in a sisterly show of solidarity. I had tried for months to persuade her that her support was felt each and every day; she didn't need to do this. She was a total lunatic to even consider it. The woman is a respected doctor of veterinary medicine with a thriving clinic; she has a handsome husband with whom she had four kids; she is also a Soccer Mom and a part-time cab driver to those kids and their friends. She neither needed to explain her baldness one hundred times a day, nor deserved to suffer the looks that bald women invariably get when they are out. We experienced that together on Monday afternoon before she went home. It was uncomfortable and eye-opening and something that everyone should experience just once, to be reminded of what people with afflictions feel every moment of each day.

I had asked my family to campaign against my sister's idea. What the hell had I been thinking? I had forgotten that she was just like the rest of our family; she would get something into her head and—"Damn the torpedoes, *full steam ahead!*"—there would be no changing her mind.

My first mistake was to leave her alone in the bathroom with the shaver. I had walked into the bedroom for a micro-second when I heard a buzzing sound from the bathroom.

"Just testing out the speeds available," she yelled, "so I don't hurt you . . ."

Yeah, *right.*

I walked into the bathroom and there she stood with a strip of hair three inches wide down the middle of her head GONE, her beautiful brown hair on the floor around her.

I burst out laughing.

We rolled around on the floor, laughing hard. Larry was too terrified to come up the stairs. Knowing full well what we were up to, he chose to remain in the relative safety of the living room, splayed out on the couch, waiting for the big reveal. Shere and I enjoyed a few preparatory drinks to ready ourselves properly. It took us a while to do both of our heads; we were laughing too hard. Bob was left with a great deal of fix-it work on Shere's head, as I had left a slight Mohawk on the top and had done a pretty bad job around her ears. We decided to leave mine the way it was; chemo would take care of the flaws in a few more days.

Larry took a picture of the three of us, bald Zaccone's, at chemo on Monday.

Monday

Things went well with this chemo treatment.

I had downed gallons of water before any needles came my way, something I had forgotten to do for Chemo No. 2. My blood was probably a tad too far on the martini side of life for that treatment, since it was just after the party. And like I said, my veins had gone into hiding.

This time, I used the relaxing techniques that Karl Zimmer, Yolanda Simonsis and Sophia Dilberakis had convinced me to try. It all worked together like a well-tuned instrument. The blood test needle and the needles for chemo that Elia Martinez, Nurse No. 3 wielded went in without any trouble. They still hurt, but it was not a brutal experience like it normally was for me. (No, I am not, and will never get used to needles.)

I now hoped that we would get Brigit, Lor or Elia for the rest of the treatments. It wasn't possible to "book" a nurse, so it might not happen.

Tuesday

Larry was out of town on business until Wednesday night. Shere went home in the morning, so Bob briefly "booby-sat" Bruizanne with an afternoon check. I loved his visits. He would bring me a healthy and cold protein-infused smoothie after he worked out.

Tomorrow, I would have meetings at work. Larry would be home in the evening. We had planned to take care of the after-chemo shot then. We would see what the old body had in store for me during this round. The shot, we were fairly certain, was what had taken me over the top, as far as the start of any major symptoms.

I asked Larry to drive the long way home from his seminar; told him to take his employees, who were with him, out for a nice, long dinner.

I was beginning to like this bald look. It definitely wasn't something I would have chosen to keep forever but I thought I could do it for the time that I needed to. It felt awesome to the touch, like soft little stubs.

The workout trainer came over to the house for the first time today.

Picture this:

Me. Bald. Buff. And eventually, with *both* boobs!

Chapter 50

In the Beginning

In the beginning, whenever I felt sleepy, I used to fight it off.

Now, I tried to remember to keep the matches away and the lighters well-hidden so that cancer wouldn't find them and burn the house down while I slept. I allowed my body to become a battlefield where the drugs battled with the disease. Chemo was working on a strategy, determining the best way to mutate and render the enemy useless without killing off too much of me. I prayed that a strong, centered, mind and body connection could overcome most of it and leave as much of me intact as possible.

Treatment No. 3 was not as bad as Treatment No. 2. I didn't visit the porcelain goddess once, and there were very few body pains. My eyes were extremely dry but were overproducing tears that seemed to constantly seep out of the outer edges, never reaching the places where they were most needed. It was an uncomfortable combination. My tear ducts seemed to be in overdrive but my eyes felt as scorched and dry as any desert on the map. I was trying very hard not to wipe the tears away, as the skin around my eye area was very tender and could become quickly and easily damaged if constantly pulled on. The doctor suggested faux tears.

I was now involved with more faux stuff than ever before in my life.

I used to be a night person. Not anymore. These days bedtime arrived at around 11:00 PM, I woke up at around 5:30

in the morning and ended up exhausted at around 2:00 or 2:30 in the afternoon. I took *naps*. Hard to believe but true: speed-racing Suzanne slept away each afternoon.

Food continued to taste bland, which made eating a major chore. I was hungry but nothing seemed to satisfy me. Much of it made me choke as I attempted to get it down. Soup, water and smoothies were about the only things that I could easily tolerate. It felt as if my throat had become smaller and food couldn't travel through it freely.

The inside of my mouth now exfoliated. I could peel off a layer whenever the mood struck. The sides and undersurface of my tongue were sore, as if I'd been sucking on a sour candy the entire day. The doctor prescribed a special mouthwash to help with this odd symptom. It's a very thick, cherry-flavored rinse that rendered your mouth numb in about two minutes after using it.

Aside from faux things, I was also collecting things that made you go numb. Lovely!

I didn't have thrush or mouth sores; I hoped that I would never have to experience those symptoms but it was possible that I would.

My nose continued to move between dry and tender, to drippy and tender and I was certain that the consumption of Kleenex in the Midwest had recently topped all records. Occasionally, if I stood up too quickly, I became super dizzy. I could usually make it a few steps and then—*bang*. Wherever I was at that moment, I needed to sit down. This had frequently meant the floor, as the dizzies kind of hung on for a while. It was an interesting experience but could be troublesome if out in public. I kept reminding myself that people often *paid* for this feeling.

Yesterday, Larry and I had an appointment in the city. He dropped me off at the front door and then went to find parking space. After our appointment, I learned that we were five blocks away from the car. Normally, that would have been a breeze. A nice walk on a beautiful day with a handsome man. But I was unable to walk. I was shocked and a bit scared. I knew without a doubt that I couldn't make the short distance. I started to cry. It was difficult for me to believe that I felt completely unable to walk five damn blocks in my favorite city in the world, in the safety and on the arm of Larry. I was crushed. Absolutely crushed. I couldn't allow cancer to win another round. I had to fight it head-on.

While I was wrestling with myself, Larry hailed a cab, which magically appeared from around the corner. The poor driver had to know that something was wrong with me. I was shaking, white as a ghost, bald as an eagle and silent tears dripped down my face while I concentrated on breathing techniques, trying desperately to pull it all back together. The driver was kind and thoughtful and carried on a friendly and pleasant conversation with Larry. It was clear that they were both overcompensating for what was obviously a tough moment in our day.

I had yet another opportunity to witness one more profoundly touching and very human moment: the kindness of a stranger in silent understanding.

As I prayed for all cancer cells to leave my body, Larry continued to hope that there was nothing that a nice meal and a little exercise couldn't cure. He made sure that I ate and kept well-hydrated, as those issues had never been consistently important enough to me. Now they needed to be.

Larry had the trainer coming to the house regularly.

I took vitamins religiously. For someone who rarely took a pill for anything—not even a headache—I now seemed to be taking an overabundance of them. I felt as if I needed a spreadsheet to keep track of everything.

I'd never once doubted Larry's love through all of this; although I'd been amazed at the depths to which he had shown it. Occasionally, it turned into "tough love," and as aggravating as this was to admit, he'd been spot-on with his advice just about every time. Lately, his loving care seemed to pour more freely and easily from each cell of his being. I would hug him and sink comfortably into the warmth of his body and the strength of his arms. Our tears would mix together and melt into our skin.

I was safe.

Chapter 51

The Week before Chemo No. 4

My scalp hadn't tingled in the last two weeks. Was the assault over or had chemo just stopped working? I still had some fuzzy hair left on my head and it seemed to have stopped falling out. It was sparse and felt much like a very short Army cut. Maybe I would be able to keep this bit of hair and get a head start on growing it all back. My doctor highly doubted that so I still had a chance at a Yul Brenner look.

My treasured long eyelashes and my eyebrows were slowly losing their hold. I'd always been a stickler for a clean eyebrow area. Even now, when I saw one that shouldn't have been where it was, I got out the tweezers and began the excavation process. Lately, that process had become quite funny. I simply went near the poor little hair with the tweezers, and it fell out on the spot. Preferring a smooth leg and underarm, I still shaved—just not as often. And a Brazilian wax has *nothing* over chemo!

My nails continued to grow long, strong and healthy. Thank God.

I was on the skinny side of my closet, as far as clothes were concerned. For some people, losing weight is an expected result of the chemotherapy treatment. I continued to pass all of the doctor's diagnostic tests so I wasn't all that concerned. Having clothes that fit me and were already in the house told me that at one time, I was *that* size.

Just for the record, Larry, Bob and Shere were getting alarmed. But then again, Larry, Bob and Shere were getting alarmed about a lot of things when it came to me lately. I felt I was doing quite well.

I fell asleep easily, although I did get up three or four times a night. I had taken an Ambien sleeping pill only once in the last three weeks. Ambien only seemed to work for about four hours and then I would be wide awake, watching stupid reruns on TV until I fell off again. My eyes were too dry for reading. I wondered if it was better to not take a sleeping pill at all, and just deal with the requisite two to three times a night that I woke up. The wakefulness only lasted for about thirty minutes and then I would fall off to sleep. I had energy most of the day, especially the week after chemo when I took care of *everything*. I met with the trainer as scheduled, no matter how many excuses I had ready and waiting (and holding on to for a rainy day).

Quitting smoking was a goal for another fiscal year. I couldn't do it. There were already too many pills to take to add another to the schedule. Frankly, I needed the calming affects that nicotine offered, now more than ever. I had reduced the number of cigarettes I smoked each day, in a big way. I was smoking probably half a pack a day and I only smoked in my car or in my office with both windows open. I would tackle this addiction, just not this year.

Many people have mentioned that they wished I didn't have to go through so much pain. I appreciate their thoughtfulness and support, but I have to be honest: pain wasn't really the best word. There *was* pain, yes—during those days after surgery, and while enduring the body pains after chemo and Larry's shot, when the symptoms took their cue to begin. And of course, there is pain for me anytime a needle is involved. But for a good part of it all, it really wasn't painful. A better grouping of words would be "totally annoying."

On the Mondays that I had chemo, I would have as normal a day as any bald woman would have once I had left the hospital. The same could be said for Tuesdays and Wednesdays. Wednesday night was typically when the weird stuff began to happen. It was a cornucopia of symptoms that started and stopped, and then started up again, and seemed to hang around for an entire day. Then the symptoms would taper off and leave me one by one. Aside from the constants (dry eyes, drippy to dry nose, the occasional dizzy spell, a sore mouth and tiring more easily than was normal for me), "pain" wasn't really a part of the equation. "Annoying" is really the best word for it. Completely annoying and draining.

Chemo No. 4 would be tomorrow. I was halfway through this part of the drama.

Chapter 52

Camp Chemo: the First Five-Star Camp of Its Kind

Monday

Chemo No. 4 was uneventful.

I dreaded having to do it all again, knowing what might be coming in seventy-two hours. While the entire drill had now become all-too-familiar and the fear of walking into a hospital was now somewhat palatable, I still hated the whole needle bit. As strong a mind that I believed I possessed, I was afraid that the needle continued to take me over the top. It was internalized. I didn't scream or make a scene but if you were a camera traveling through my mind, you'd have had one hell of a bumpy ride.

It looked like Elia (Chemo Nurse No. 3) would attempt to be my nurse throughout the balance of chemo. She has a very engaging personality and laughed easily, as all the others did. Elia, Lor and Brigit had told me that this was how it was with the Chemo Department. You rarely got the same nurse each time but Elia completely understood the benefits of the relationship so we would try to pair up again in two weeks.

She seemed to be the best technically when it came to me and my crappy veins. She found a vein where I swear I never knew I had one. She used that creepy band they all wrap way too tightly around your upper arm and then gently felt around with little taping movements and massaging techniques until she had found what she was looking for. I was too weak with fear to help the situation by making a real fist. I could only close my hand. The best they would ever get was my fake fist. Like I said, I was getting used to faux things.

There were obvious veins that could have been used, but they looked a little tired from previous stabs so her search took a little longer than usual. She eventually found her mark and the needle went right in.

Once in a while, life just comes at you without asking for your consent. You're going along doing your thing, teaching lessons, learning lessons, observing how others handle situations, trying to understand their plight, their fright, their excitement, or their intentions, deciding which battles to fight and which to walk away from, working on being a good friend, an engaged family member, a leader with guts and integrity, learning to be a better example at all of the above, making mistakes and hopefully correcting them, experiencing people, places, other ideas and cultures and figuring out which of those you will embrace, which you will change, which you can't and which you will totally discount. And then out of nowhere it all changes for you. It all changes because now you are studying *yourself* in a more critical way than you ever did before.

This was a good thing. This had been a very good thing. It had forced me to recognize and acknowledge so much, but the hardest issue for me had been learning that in many areas, I was completely powerless. How do you accept powerlessness? I started to write about how this feeling affected me. But then I realized that it made absolutely no difference who you are, what your background is, how you relate to your family and friends, what socio-economic place you hail from or have aspired to. Powerlessness is one of those universal elements of life that connects all of us. What is there to do?

It's a good idea to search for the good that is often so well-hidden or intertwined within the bad. Sometimes the bad just comes at you from somewhere, completely out of left field. It challenges you to discover it, spin it around and turn it into something manageable and fair. And if "manageable and fair" isn't possible, as in some scenarios, then at least comfort can be found in deciding that putting a positive spin on your world is a far better place to exist, no matter what the circumstance.

The silver lining I had found was being diagnosed and going through chemo in late winter and early spring.

It was Wednesday after Chemo No. 4. It had been four weeks since I had sung to the porcelain goddess. I'd recently discovered that a cold marble floor could be heaven on earth in between those spasmodic bouts. It provided an instant cool-down. I was not able to do a full body press, lying face down flat on my tummy as I craved to. Can you imagine the uneven rocking motion that would have been caused by having only one boob? It would have been an odd little balancing act, to say the least. Larry may be ambidextrous but I was still very, very flexible for an old girl. I knelt on the floor, sat on my heels, lowered my chest gently to my thighs, leaned forward all folded up like an origami flower and placed one cheek at a time on the cold marble floor, savoring the moment. Very Zen-like.

When I got nauseous, I fought it big time. Always have. It was always a fight to the end to see who would win the battle. The bummer was that there was little that could be done if you took your anti-nausea medicine and then threw it up. I hate throwing up. I tried to stave it off by taking deep breaths and swallowing constantly as those warning juices flooded my mouth, taunting me to give it up. I tried to remain as still and as cool in temperature as I possibly could. I'd remember that whenever the kids were sick I would place a cool cloth filled with ice cubes on the back of their neck. It seemed to help or at least distract them. Funny thing was, it worked for me, too.

When throwing up, should I stave off that feeling or was it best to just give in to it and let it all happen? It changed each time.

Another silver lining was in having a bidet right next to the porcelain goddess. I now used it for something other than what it was intended for. It doubled as a place where I could rinse out my mouth. We called the entire bathroom area "Camp Chemo." It was a very nice camp. Five-star for certain! I had an ideal setup, moving from the porcelain goddess to the bidet to clean out my mouth, then when possible slowly making it to the other side of the room to rinse with the water pick and mouthwash. A soft blanket and a pillow were ready with a Posturpedic wedge that Larry would place under my knees. A bottle of water, ice cubes and Shere's eye mask were nearby. The Jacuzzi, filled with hot water, was purring as I resumed my Zen-like position and waited.

Chapter 53

The Genetic Counselor and Chemo No. 5

I mentioned to Dr. Nanda, my chemo oncologist that I was interested in knowing if I had inherited a defective gene that could be identified through genetic testing and may be involved in the development of particular cancers such as colon, breast, ovarian and melanoma (skin cancer).

Knowledge is power.

I felt it was important to know if my family was at high risk of developing these cancers so that extra care could be taken during their mammograms and gynecology tests. My aunt had been diagnosed at age sixty-five, which is an age when breast cancer occurs most frequently. My diagnosis had been given earlier, at age fifty. I was concerned about what this might have meant for my sister and my four nieces.

My mother is an only child and my father had a sister who had given birth to three boys. We have a smaller gene pool of past women-related cancers. The test had to be given to a woman who currently has or has had breast cancer: me. I'd spoken to a Genetic Counselor the week before Chemo No. 5 and had answered questions so that a family history could be documented. I was told that I would need to provide two vials of blood for this test. I was assured that I could do that on the same day that I had chemo and had to give two other vials of blood for the chemo tests. The fact that it only involved one needle stick, made my decision easier. I was in.

The diagnostic tests were called BRCA1 and BRCA2. Results would be available in one month.

Through our discussions, I'd learned that these tests would also tell me what my chances were of developing breast cancer in my left breast, as well as my chances of developing ovarian cancer. Only a small percentage of people carried this gene; something like eight to ten percent. There was some comfort in that number. But those who carried alterations in the gene had up to an *eighty-five* percent chance of developing cancer in their lifetime.

Personally, I would have liked to know the chances of another cancer that chemo may not have eradicated, setting up shop somewhere else in my body. Larry and I were constantly being reminded by the doctors and nurses that chemo wasn't always effective in finding and killing off all the bad cells. The medical community was still playing around with the combinations, and the chemistry mixtures were considered an art and not a science. It had been only twenty years since the oncology community had had enough statistics to rely on from the few trials that had been completed.

It terrified me to contemplate another round of surgeries outside of the reconstruction surgery that I already faced. This surgery was intended to head off a new potential monster lurking within me. It would be a long month as I awaited these results.

I'm a multi-tasker. I wondered if Dr. Connolly, (my breast surgeon) would understand this about me and accommodate yet another out-of-the-ordinary request. During a routine surgical follow-up meeting in the same week that I met with the genetic counselor, Dr. Connolly and I came to an agreement. If I was found to be at high risk, and should the medical team and I decide that surgically removing "more things" was in my best future interest—he would arrange to take care of it all in one long-ass surgery. These types of duo-medical surgical disciplines could be done but needed to be scheduled well in advance. My get-out-of-jail-free card for the colonoscopy and annual Pap test would soon run out; I might ask them to just get everything done in one shot.

A year of medical nightmares had become my new personal limit.

Chemo No. 5 went well. It was a long day. This was a new treatment protocol. We arrived at 9:00 AM and left at 5:30 PM. They took four vials of blood; two would go to the genetic testing center and two would be for tests for my chemo reports. My blood stats were within their acceptable range, although I was getting low or moving off the charts in a few areas. Now Larry would be on me more than usual for the next two weeks, attempting to persuade or force-feed me or to do whatever he'd feel necessary to bring those levels back up.

I was passing the tests. I had not been denied treatment. I was feeling OK most of the time, so I wasn't all that concerned.

Going through chemo had compromised all kinds of things in my body chemistry. This time, I was less than inclined to attempt to beat the numbers. It was a race I was engaged in but was not obsessed with. As long as it didn't delay a treatment, I was happy.

Larry was on a personal mission to be certain that everything was perfect. He tracked and compared the numbers from week to week, often conferring with Dr. Shere for advice and affirmation of his plan. He is a good man to have on your team.

Nurse Elia was the chemo nurse today. We crossed our fingers that we would be in her care for the next three treatments, and be able to end it all on a familiar and celebratory note.

I must not have been hydrated enough, as it took two attempts to find a vein that was strong enough. This treatment would be delivered via an IV drip and would last much longer than the first four treatments, when they used nine syringe pushes. We needed a good strong vein that would handle the newest chemical assault.

The next four treatments were with a drug called Taxol. A fabulous little benefit to this drug was that they gave you two large syringes of Benadryl first, which would fend off the reactions to Taxol; hives, hot flashes, itching, nausea, breathing problems, accelerated heartbeats and a few other things that I could no longer remember as I was quickly drifting into the cosmos. I had taken half a Xanax before the first needle stick of the day; coupled with the Benadryl, I was on a medically approved and monitored high.

I was asleep throughout most of the treatment.

This was a marvelous respite for me and provided Larry and Shere with a long period of time to take pictures without my knowledge. They took photos of me completely passed out, wearing the little surgeon's cap to keep my head warm, and of me surrounded by half-eaten food and "get well" balloons.

Larry and Shere were major entertainment for the nursing staff and other patients receiving their treatment. I had worn a pair of Manolo Blahnik shoes with nice high heels and had taken them off to cuddle up with a warm blanket during treatment. My sister the veterinarian, who wears more practical shoes and has much smaller feet than mine, decided to strut her stuff around the large chemo room in my Manolo Blahniks. She cracked up anyone who was awake enough to see her.

Later, as the nurse freed me from all the needles and paraphernalia, she told me about their antics and said that they always looked forward to our visits for the comic relief in an otherwise sad environment.

There is a nurse named Victoria Frazier-Warmack who often sang while she did her paperwork. This was yet another soothing moment in our days as patients. We all listened closely to her as she serenaded us into a soothing and restful place. It made the whole drama a bit less scary. I loved her voice and the way she just let it out.

Once home, I was a literal glob of nothing. I continued to enjoy the effects of the Xanax-Benadryl combo. Shere made dinner and cleaned everything up as I struggled to stay alert. I finally gave in at around 8:30 PM and went to bed.

My darling little sister was on a mission of her own. She stayed with me for a short time and wanted to be sure that she had put everything in order before she left. She had found the laundry basket. I had noticed this and had hidden the basket before I'd gone to bed. She later found my hiding spot and washed, dried and folded the laundry, watered all my plants, emptied the dishwasher, emptied and recorded the output from my drain tube and woke herself up every four hours to deliver a pain pill to me.

I have always been used to and very comfortable with doing things for others. I found it very difficult to have things done for me. During this experience, I'd learned to release the guilt in accepting these outpourings of love that I continued to receive in person, by phone and through e-mail. The hard part was that I wasn't that sick for a long enough period of time where I couldn't have done things for myself. I had lowered the Type-A expectations that I'd always embraced and had accepted that I might not be on top of things as I normally was. And I was OK with that for the time being.

During the blood draws, while waiting to be called in, I sat next to a woman who told me that she had leukemia and had only two to five years left to live. She was fighting hard. Not only had she lost her hair but she had also lost all of her fingernails and toenails. On my other side was a man from Pakistan who had had a kidney transplant in Pakistan. He told me that I wouldn't know how good I had it in the U.S. until I went outside of it for health care. He was struggling now, as the kidney had not been a true match.

There I sat between two people who were obviously suffering from things that were greater than my own. The best thing for me to have done was to continue to soldier on and not allow myself to feel anything other than gratitude for all my silver linings. I hoped I would remember this after the Neulasta shot this week.

Tuesday afternoon

I was feeling pretty darn good. I was getting used to having drippy eyes and a constantly runny nose. These were issues that

I no longer counted and I was thoroughly enjoying the residual effects of the Benadryl.

After seeing that my white blood counts were within range, Larry and I agreed to hold off on the shot until the next evening. The doctor was OK with that. This would give me the day to rest, catch up on things around the house and take care of paperwork and phone calls from the office. Driving may not be such a hot idea today so I would wait until tomorrow to handle all of my running around. I had two days to eat as much as possible before the Neulasta shot shut down my throat.

People have asked me what that meant—to have my throat "shut down." After the shot, which was directed to the bone marrow and boosted my white blood cell count, my throat closed up to about one-third of its normal size. I could feel it as it happened. Eating felt like I had swallowed a pill that had caught in my throat and no matter how much water I drank, that pill was lodged and lodged good; and I could feel it slowly and agonizingly drag down my throat and pass my sternum. *That's* what it felt like to eat. It's when sustenance becomes liquid, as eating anything solid would have been too painful. It's also quite annoying, as my stomach would be literally growling for food but I'd be simply unable to eat. Quite a conundrum; and one that wasn't easily overcome.

Five down and three to go!

(Side note: Surprisingly, I still had the hair that Shere had not buzzed off a month ago. It wasn't much, and it surprised the doctors and nurses, but I could feel it on my head. It felt *good*. I reminded myself that it would be there in volume again one day.)

Larry gave me the shot on Wednesday night.

It's very early Thursday morning. I hadn't slept all night. There were aches and pains in my muscles, joints and bones. I began to feel my throat closing down at around 2:00 AM. The palms of my hands were sore and they stung when they were touched at any point where there was a crease. All of those little creases also hurt when they were placed in water. The same thing was happening with my feet, and I could peel layers of skin off of them even after having continually slathered cocoa butter on them for the past week. My nails were extremely sensitive. I'd had a few shakes and shivers but not as bad as earlier weeks. I'd thrown up only once. All of the symptoms I was experiencing were symptoms that were expected with this regimen.

Neuropathy, a nerve disease, was a concern for this treatment phase. Neuropathy is when your hands and feet are numb and tingle. If this occurs, the doctors must be alerted immediately.

I called the doctors about the stinging and soreness, hoping to catch whatever it was early on and find relief. The answer was pretty much "Take an Ibuprofen and deal with it, babe."

I couldn't seem to find a position that was comfortable. I was sick of being sick. I looked forward to a new day.

Chapter 54

Embrace the Suck

John, one of my godsons who is in the Army's 82nd Airborne Division and had left for Afghanistan in November of 2008, was home on a short leave. He took me, his sister Christa (my goddaughter) and her boyfriend Alex out to lunch. We caught up with each other for a few hours. He told me of an Army saying that seems to apply to a lot of things in life: "Embrace the suck." Essentially, this means that "the situation is bad, so deal with it because there is nothing you can do to change things but soldier on."

John's mission includes leaving everyone and everything he loves, and traveling halfway around the world to a place he's never been to. Although I hope to have inspired within him my love of travel, I doubt Afghanistan would occupy a top spot on his travel list. The place is ungodly hot, many of the people don't like you or trust you, and you never really know who does and who doesn't. You need to wear full body armor weighing up to fifty pounds which they call "Battle Rattle"—just to take a pee. You take care of these bodily functions in a portable toilet they call the "Blue Canoe." The hours are long when you are on duty and the hours you are off duty are boring or filled with other nasty work. All you really want to do is sleep. A long hot shower and a shave are not always possible so they use moist anti-bacterial wipes. And the food—well, anyone who attends business meetings where they serve buffet-style dinners would think that they were having the ultimate in high cuisine when compared to the slop our men and woman eat while fighting for our freedom. Oh, and in Afghanistan, you have to watch out for incoming fire at all times.

The living conditions aren't even close to what I would call acceptable. When you sleep with a bunch of other guys who snore, grunt and groan throughout the night—I guess you quickly learn to embrace the suck. Did I mention the sand mites, camel spiders and scorpions? It takes serious balls to carry out such a mission without crumbling. In the past five years, over eight hundred fifty thousand of our men and women have faced this challenge. I am in awe of each and every one of them.

"Your finely tuned negotiation skills would do little to keep you alive in this jungle we call the "sandbox," John said.

"I would have gone AWOL almost immediately," I agreed. (To be AWOL or Absent without Leave, is an illegal offense in the USA. It's not a decision to be taken lightly.)

I think about John a lot. He is like my own son. My love for him has no margins and the thought of him placing his life in jeopardy drives me absolutely crazy. I would double my time with chemo or make just about any deal to be certain he returns to us safe and in one piece—body, mind and soul.

Wednesday after the shot, my symptoms began to show up as expected. By Friday, I couldn't take it any longer. I tried hard to embrace the suck. For over two days, I lay awake in bed with continual body aches and bone and joint pains so severe that I just wanted to end it all. I was at my wit's end.

My whole body was firing off pain, and there was no relief for even a moment. If my upper body was hurting, my lower body might give me some rest. But once the pain had left my arms and elbows, it would move to my back, or my hips, settle in my thighs or knees, travel to my ankles, the backs of my legs, my toes, my feet or run a cycle—including several areas all at once.

I hadn't known I had muscles in my feet. They must be from the Louboutin and Manolo workouts. The only relief was when I was in a hot Jacuzzi bath, but I couldn't immerse my hands because they would sting so badly. Between the dehydrating baths (too many to count but at least they were available to me) and the pain and constant crying, I seriously doubted I could do three more rounds of Taxol. I checked the list of symptoms to expect; it clearly noted that what I was experiencing was to be expected. I decided not to call the doctor. I didn't want to hear, "Take an Ibuprofen and deal with it, babe" one more time. I'd tried Ibuprofen for two days and it wasn't working.

When Larry came home that evening, he had other ideas. He called the doctor. Dr. Nanda called us back within minutes after we paged her. Larry answered the phone and explained the situation. At one point he said, "Doc, there seems to be continual misfires in the synapse of her nerves and—"

She immediately asked to talk to me.

It hurt too much to laugh last night but tonight we had a few chuckles at Dr. Nanda's response to *Dr. Larry's* assessment. Larry has been hanging around Shere far too much, using and trading doctor-speak.

Dr. Nanda suggested that I take two Oxycodone pills, left over from surgery, and then she ordered a drug called Dexamethasone, which is some kind of steroid. Although these symptoms were expected, they could be controlled and the pain could be eased.

I had a sudden weird craving for a banana split. Off Larry went in search of a banana split and to pick up the drug *du 'jour*. I ate the banana split while sitting in a steaming hot tub.

The drugs finally kicked in and I had some relief. The pain subsided.

I slept.

Saturday morning, I woke up to the birds singing outside our open bedroom window, and listened to our resident owl, which I've yet to actually see, talking to the rising sun. It was time to get out of the house, breathe in fresh air and get groceries for Monday's barbecue. We would be celebrating the Memorial Day weekend to honor our troops—past and present—who are suffering or have suffered much more than I am or probably ever will. I was home, surrounded by loved ones, and I would come through this, eventually, and in one piece. Would they?

If you have cancer, you may have to experience this phenomenal assault of poisons. You may willingly ingest it, all in the hopes that it will make you better.

Here is another piece of advice: using toothpaste and mouthwash can be another very shocking part of this experience. So far, I have avoided getting thrush in my mouth but instead I've gotten a very sore mouth and tongue. Brushing my teeth, using mouthwash, eating spicy or salty foods and yes, even drinking a martini—all reduce me to tears. The burning sensation is incredible! I've gotta tell you, I'm my Daddy's girl in many ways but in this way especially—we love everything as hot as it comes.

But *this* is painful hot.

The doctor had prescribed something called Magic Mouthwash. It works but only temporarily. My girlfriend Carol suggested that I try Biotene, a toothpaste and mouthwash brand that she had used throughout her cancer journey. This is available over the counter at most drugstores. It has made every difference in my dental health regime. It doesn't sting and the ingredients help to alleviate the burn generally associated with the use of toothpastes and mouthwashes I would normally use. The pain relief lasts so much longer than if you use Magic Mouthwash.

I am embracing the suck! I am embracing the knowledge of those who came before me who have freely offered their sage advice to make my journey easier to live with.

It's Memorial Day weekend. I love you, John. Be safe and smart and careful. Share your college education, your amazing instincts, your leadership skills and your sensitivity. Come home more brilliant than you already are.

Chapter 55

A Medical Imbalance:
The Current Teams Plan for Radiation

Larry and I arrived at the University of Chicago for an appointment with the radiation oncologist who is on my team of surgeons, nurses and sundry "ologists." I walked in, convinced that it would be a cursory meeting. I would listen to what they had to say, ask the questions on my list then definitively proclaim that radiation was not for me.

It started out badly.

We were there for a consultation. I had made that clear when the appointment was made. I knew they were aware of this, as they had commented that they generally do not see patients until after chemo treatments have been completed; and they questioned my desire to discuss my situation this early. I was honest with them. I told them that through my research, I felt that I wasn't a strong enough candidate to find a benefit that overcame all of the risks. I wanted to hear the team's reasons why radiation was necessary. I told them that another radiation oncologist's opinion had concurred with my surgeon's belief and my feelings.

The 2:30 PM appointment began with the usual documents. I asked them why they weren't electronically connected to the other departments who have this same information. I was tired of having to write my whole damn history every time I saw a new medical discipline within the same hospital. They gave me an understanding smile that said, "Sorry, darling. There ain't much I can do."

I was quite put off by some of the questions. Why in the world would a radiation oncologist be concerned if I am or have ever been physically abused? When I got to those ridiculous questions—ridiculous for me, at least—I summarily ignored them.

We were then led into a room to meet with Nurse Sue, who pretty much asked the same questions that I had chosen to ignore but that she felt were necessary. She took down my weight and height, an area I'd already noted in the previous paperwork, and blood pressure. She didn't ask the "physical abuse" question. We had a few laughs; she seemed to understand the absurdity of some of these questions.

We met with the radiation fellow next. A fellow is an intern and a specialist of sorts with a vast knowledge of the medical discipline that he or she works in. The radiation fellow was professional, very nice and had a calming bedside/exam-table manner, even though I did not choose to sit on the exam table and instead selected a chair. I'm from the old-school; positioning during a meeting, and even in an exam room that was meant to be a consultation meeting room, is critical. The radiation fellow will definitely become a future star in the medical world but her purpose for being there with us was another time stall. She simply read aloud my history since diagnosis. It was clear that this was her first read on the background of my file and I guess we were supposed to be impressed with her reading abilities, as she offered very few answers to our questions. It was maddening. Then she said she would rather have Dr. Chmura get into the details. Larry and I looked at each other in amazement. What a flipping waste of time!

After the walk down memory lane, she handed me a smock to change into for a little exam.

I had had enough.

Recognizing that this seems to be the way things happen in our health care system, especially when at a teaching hospital, I told her nicely exactly why I wasn't going to change into the smock and kindly asked to see the doctor we were supposed to have the appointment with over one and a half hours ago.

"This was scheduled to be a consultation, darling," I said, "and our appointment with Dr. Chmura was over an hour ago. I'm tired of strangers poking around my body and what the hell does my *surgical site* have to do with a consultation that's supposed to tell me if I am even onboard with radiation?"

Many friends had warned me very early on in my cancer experience that you would get used to this "hurry up and wait" mentality and that even disrobing in front of countless groups of people would be no big deal. I had absolutely no problem with meeting any number of people involved in my health care, or disrobing in front of them. But if this drama was to be the case for a consultation, I should have been told to allow two to three hours for it and been given a reason why a physical was needed during a consult.

This radiation fellow handled everything with professionalism, respect and understanding. I was happy that she was on the team, but I was aggravated by the process. I continue to believe it is best to fight the process or the system not the individual, who carries it out.

We waited.

And we waited longer.

Unless there is a real medical emergency or something really important has happened, I absolutely hate it when a person's time is being abused to this extent. Had an emergency been the case, they should have said something. An emergency was not the case today. I told Larry they had fifteen minutes more and then I was leaving. He agreed that it was becoming ridiculous.

"But," he added, "I haven't come this far and taken off yet another afternoon of work not to hear what the good doctor has to say."

We were staying.

I did a slow but oh-so-controlled burn and walked out to the nurses' station and told them that we respected the department's protocol and the importance of taking time with each patient, but we had an appointment with the doctor for a consultation and *not* a full medical history review of the last five months. I told her that we would be leaving in ten minutes if he wasn't rustled up fast.

Bingo.

After I returned to the examining room, Dr. Steven Chmura appeared in mega-seconds. He looked like he was about twenty-five years old and was visibly uncomfortable having to enter a room with a somewhat perturbed patient about whom he had obviously been warned. The good doctor appeared a bit nervous, which made his explanation at the start of our meeting, all the more difficult for him. This immediately changed how we connected to him, in a positive way. Our attention, reactions and body language moved into a more sensitive pace and place. I felt the air shift in the room as Larry and I warmed to his obvious brilliance. Dr. Chmura must have felt it too; he became more comfortable, animated, and less clinical, and he displayed his sense of humor and freely showed his humanness.

This is one very smart man.

We learned that he is married to Dr. Lucy Chen, the chemo fellow upstairs who works with Dr. Rita Nanda. Dr. Chen is an up-and-coming shining star herself. Together, she and Dr. Chmura are one dynamic duo.

If only someone would correct these maddening scheduling issues! That's a big challenge for a doctor, as they never know how much time each patient will need and how many questions will uncover other questions. These doctors are constantly rushing from one room to another. It must be maddening for them when all they want to do is to practice medicine. It's maddening for *me* to wait for them to enter my room and practice.

Dr. Chmura began the story of why a person with my statistics, clear margins after surgery, a T1 tumor with only one node out of twenty-eight that were cancerous and a full round chemotherapy set complete—would possibly need radiation. We listened carefully as the story began with radiation activities during the 1920's.

When he got to the 1950's, I interrupted, "Please, get to the present and answer my questions."

And so he did.

Dr. Chmura's contention was that the numbers of nodes that have cancer are not always relevant. This was based on his extensive research and the resulting medical white-paper that would be released in the first quarter of 2009, along with several other radiation oncologists. Having just one cancerous node placed me on the higher end of the lower risk levels, simply because of lymphatic involvement. While surgery removed the tumor and the surrounding breast tissue that was found to be cancerous, and all margins were clear of cancer; cancer still had to learn to travel outside the tumor and burrow through my chest wall, muscle and ribs to end up in the lymphatic system. It also needed to repurpose itself and learn to live in a new location using a different blood source. God, that makes so much sense.

Dr. Chmura told us that chemotherapy had little effect on local control. If one tiny, microscopic cancer cell lived outside of those clear and negative margins near the tumor that was removed, only focused radiation on the specific area would kill them. I would be treated in radiation Levels 1 and 2, which is a rather large area that includes the surgical site, the axillary lymphatic system, just below my collarbone and under my arm. This treatment would focus on eighty percent of the affected area.

He told us that having radiation treatment after a full chemotherapy treatment has kept more women alive after ten years' time.

The treatment time, from start to finish, would last for half an hour. It would run for six weeks, from Monday through Friday. Thirty rounds.

Larry asked him if everyone on the team agreed with his opinion. Yes, he said. And he listed every one of them by field of expertise. I did not hear Dr. Connolly's name or his field of expertise ever mentioned.

I asked Dr. Chmura how this would delay reconstruction surgery. I was really disappointed with his answer. After I complete chemo and go through a resting period, I would start radiation. After radiation I would be required to wait another six months before reconstruction could begin. The area needs to heal, new nerve endings would need to find connections, blood movement would need to be improved and time must pass safely before the next surgery.

I asked him how the radiated skin took to reconstruction surgery. He admitted that it wouldn't be as aesthetically pleasing in comparison to skin that had not gone through radiation. Radiation could harden the skin, discolor it and change the landscape that the plastic surgeon has to manipulate.

Dr. Chmura presented quite a compelling argument. It was 5:30 PM. All of our questions had been asked and answered. It was time to leave the hospital. He walked us out of his department, along with the fellow. Larry and I felt that it was a very classy move.

We drove to our favorite Italian restaurant nearby and talked about the information we had been given. We drove home in complete silence, locked in our own thoughts, our heads spinning.

Some time had passed since that meeting with Dr. Chmura, and new questions had developed. If chemotherapy is not a sure-fire method to eliminate all cancer cells from a body and has been found ineffective for local control, then why is radiation done after chemotherapy in so many cases? Why don't they get those little buggers that are so close to the original source of cancer first, and then follow up with the chemo poison that would hopefully act as the clean-up crew? Is there an after-radiation test like with some cancers using the CA-125 blood test that will show if radiation was effective? Is the jury still out on this area of medicine? Many of my friends in similar and more precarious positions have not had radiation. Are they at risk? Am I simply another body needed for further research? And if I am, is it important that I agree to travel this road so that we acquire this important research for future generations?

Radiation treatment can also cause lymphedema, which leads me to another tricky medical issue to balance. Dr. Chmura told me that a woman who has had surgery, a full chemo regimen and a full radiation regimen will "probably live longer after ten years than others who have not completed all treatments." OK, but during that time, I am at greater risk for lymphedema if I have radiation—and it gets even worse. You must be diligent in wearing the compression sleeves for the rest of your life while flying and scuba diving, as lymphedema can occur years after surgery. If I pass the ten-year mark for cancer survival and if lymphedema came into my life, I could acquire something called lymphangiosarcoma, which is a tumor in the lymphatic system. The scary part is that the average time between mastectomy and the appearance of lymphangiosarcoma is about ten years. You may end up cancer-free in ten years but pick up this nasty little medical mystery right about the same time. After a patient develops this disease, the average survival time is a little over a year.

The cause of the disease lymphangiosarcoma is not known. It appears as a bluish-red bump at the affected area. First, a purple-red, slightly raised area in the skin of the arm or the leg appears. It looks like a bruise. Later, more tumors appear and the bumps grow larger. Death usually results from metastases to the lungs. This is a rare side affect but is entirely possible and must be understood and considered.

Dr. Chmura also said that generally any cancer that rears its ugly head after breast cancer, often travels to your bones, brain and liver. This is exactly what happened to Aunt Joan. I know it is unclear whether a mastectomy versus a lumpectomy would have made a difference in Aunt Joan's case, and we aren't sure if she even fully completed all chemo and radiation rounds, but it is important to be asking these questions.

What's a one-boobed girl to do?

Get a *third* opinion, of course!

I never would have imagined that there would be a third chapter devoted to radiation. This jury was still out.

Chapter 56

Chemo No. 6—With Withering Contempt, Half-Concealed Irritation and Feigned Amusement—I Move on to Weary Disdain I Am a Human Chia Pet

We tried to book a chemo seat by the window but my cache of frequent flyer miles didn't count at all. A window makes it easier to get a Wi-Fi signal; we can check our computers and PDA's while enjoying a view of the outside, where the world continues to pulse urgently, comfortingly. That wasn't possible today but I could see a tree outside a nearby window. As we waited for the show to begin, I considered launching myself through the window and down the white flowered branches to the street below, to escape what I knew was coming. The waiting was brutal. But nothing would happen until we got the all-clear from the blood tests.

Mom was with us today. I couldn't convince her that this would be the single most boring thing she could do all week. But she is a mom, and I sensed that she felt the need to share my experience.

The day went well. I followed the drill set forth by Dr. Shere and Larry. I had pounded water for two days prior to chemo. While the needles still hurt, it was one entry for each needle that had to enter my skin. Kurt, my brother-in-law had given me two rings that he had embedded with "special powers." I am not superstitious, but things went more easily whenever I wore the rings during chemo. I now remembered to wear one of them each time.

Mom's a trooper. She had been up since 4:00 AM and was not feeling well. I didn't find this out until the next day. To make matters worse for her, I was a total bitch on the way to chemo. I needed to get well within myself to prepare for what was coming. She tried very hard to distract me with conversation but I was having none of it. Once the needles were in and all the stuff was set up, I was back to the Suzanne everyone recognized—but until then, it was generally best to just let me ruminate.

Mom was with us from 7:45 AM until we finally got home at 5:00 PM. She went home and immediately crashed, only to wake up the next day and make homemade pasta, red sauce (Italians call it "gravy") and lasagna. She brought it over for a family dinner at our house with Bob, Lisa and the kids. My mother is an amazing woman. She did it all with half of her face swollen from an infection in her ear, which didn't show itself until after she was home that day after chemo. I'd gotten my stubborn streak from her. It had become easier for me to understand her need to be with me at chemo. It had absolutely killed me to see her looking unwell the night after chemo when we were having dinner together. I wanted to help her, even though there was nothing I could do. Mom and I are rarely sick and she had always been the healthy rock of Gibraltar in our family, invincible and always pushing through whatever confronted her. We teased her that she would outlive all of us. We lovingly call her the original Energizer bunny and continue to use the nickname we gave her as kids: "The Roadrunner." It hurt to see her in any pain.

Now I get it, Mom.

A Chia Pet is a clay sculpture that is usually in the shape of an animal or a person's head. It is soaked in water. Seeds are applied over its body and are watered each day. After a week or so, little green sprouts emerge from the clay mold where the seeds have grown; giving it a hair-like, grass-covered look. A

Chia Pet is one of those stupid novelty items that have been around for thirty plus years, successfully delivering huge amounts of revenue to its shareholders. (I know. It blows my mind, too.)

Surprisingly, my head still has hair. Well, maybe a better description would be "little hair sprouts all over the place," like a Chia Pet. The doctors were amazed that my hair was still hanging on. It was pretty cool, like a soldier's buzz cut.

Then last night after chemo, I saw Carol. It was our monthly night out with the Mag 7 girls. We went to see the movie *Sex & the City* at a place called Hollywood Boulevard. Ted Bulthaup, the President of our high school class, owns several of these theaters that serve alcohol and food and have high-backed comfortable chairs that swivel and adjust with a table in front of you. We arrived early and sat around in his office reminiscing. After a few drinks, we toured the back rooms where the stars hang out when they open their movies, and Ted showed us all of the equipment required to make the theater run. We were led into the theater through a private entrance and he allowed us to pick our seats before he let the masses in. Carol, who had recently ended her breast cancer battle, was there. She looked amazing. She had grown a beautiful short hairstyle that felt like the finest of cashmere. I have never felt a softer head of hair except on a baby. My new goal was now a cashmere head, not a prickly Chia-head.

I still hadn't worn any of the wigs out in the real world since I'd left the places I'd bought them at. They felt confining and hot and I was afraid that with one good whip of my head, the thing would sail off into the air. Or end up twisted around with hair falling over my eyes and nose. Even with the special tape that you can put on the front and back, the wigs still worried me. I had slowed down a bit but only by a few hundred miles an hour and only on some days, so the possibility of flipping my wig was all too real. When I tried to style it into something acceptable, I ended up looking like a little girl who had raided Mommy's closet and put some hairy thing on her head without a mirror or a clue. Obviously, there was a definite front and back with long hair and bangs to indicate which side was which. But I don't know . . . I just couldn't make it look right. I had given up for the moment.

I remembered being on holiday with Larry one year and seeing an elderly couple having breakfast. The woman's bra strap was hanging out and somehow it had gotten all twisted. The man had a trickle of melting glue running down his forehead. The glue was there to anchor his hairpiece. We ran into this couple several times. The man continued to sport his glue and his wife her disheveled look. Larry and I promised each other that we'd never allow something like that to go uncorrected in our relationship. But I could hardly expect Larry to go with me everywhere—the man *does* have a business to run!

At business meetings, I wore a hat. Once the meeting attendees had found out what was going on with me, I usually took off the hat. The last few days, I had even forgone the hat and just gone *au naturel*. The looks I got moved from a double take, a smile of understanding and the "What the hell were you thinking, lady?" look.

Larry actually found a place in the city that did the best job on yet another wig. The color was perfect and the cut worked. The problem was always *me*.

Twenty years ago, my sister-in-law had had a brain aneurism and of course had to have her head shaved for surgery. She is a confident woman and, like me, chose to go bald until her hair grew back. One day, while shopping, a woman had come up to us and gushed, "I just love your hair. Where did you get it styled?"

"Loyola University Hospital," my sister-in-law had replied coolly.

The woman had turned green and beat it out of there fast.

I had prepared my own quip but had never gotten the chance to use it. I would have said, "The University of Chicago Hospitals. They gave me some new, trendy chemo treatment and this was the result." Feel free to use it if you are asked about your hair stylist while going through your bald head drama.

Tuesday night, we decided once again to postpone the shot until the next evening. This would give me a much-needed day to catch up. So far, there had not been a symptom in sight. I had been tired last night after chemo and had kept falling in and out of it while watching the movie with the girls, but I'd slept very well.

Today and tomorrow would be full of business teleconference calls and catch-up work. I was very grateful for the distraction that work provided.

On Wednesday, at around noon, I began to get a spacey feeling in my head. By 2:30 PM, I was experiencing those dreaded little twinges in my muscles and bones that were associated with Taxol, the new drug they had given me. It started around my shoulders and then slowly and painfully moved downward.

I was trying out something new. Researching and experimenting are in my blood. I didn't want to take the pain pills and the steroids right away after chemo, as directed. I was interested in learning if my body would settle into the new chemo drug set on its own. Knowing that these last four treatments would be with Taxol and some other preparatory drugs, I wondered if the first reaction two weeks ago was just my body trying to figure out how to handle the latest assault from a new set of drugs. I decided not to take either of the pills prescribed. The thought of taking steroids did little for me because of their many known side effects. I wanted them to work when they were badly needed and not waste their intended effects by using them when I *thought* they might be needed. I preferred to save the use of pain pills for when I was *really* in pain. I had recalled the speed at which they had worked when I'd finally taken them for Chemo No. 5, so I was willing to ride the wave and see how I might react this time. I was glad I had done the experiment.

I ended up taking a steroid and a pain pill at 3:30 PM on Thursday. After four days the pain was getting pretty bad. I jumped into a hot Jacuzzi bath and soaked until the water cooled off. After getting out of the bathtub, I quickly fell into a deep and restful sleep. My throat was still tender and seemed smaller in diameter than was normal. Thankfully, it hadn't totally shut down like it had during the previous two months of drugs. I could eat.

After dinner last night, I struggled valiantly to stay up late enough so that I could take another steroid and a sleeping pill and hopefully sleep though the night. A deep and restful sleep had eluded me the past several nights. I woke up every few hours and all I could do was stare into the blackness, knowing that I wouldn't easily return to the safety and the escape of sleep. My sleep patterns changed quickly when I started these new chemo drugs. I gave it the best I had until I couldn't bear it any longer, gave in and got up.

Friday morning, I was pain-free and ready to move back into life. My experiment had allowed me to skip taking six steroids and six pain pills: a sixty percent reduction in drug intake. I was pretty sure that after today, it would be good to stop them both altogether.

The next week would be a free week: no chemo.

Chapter 57

Chemo No. 7, Shot No. 7 and the Land Of Oz

Monday

Seven is one of my lucky numbers. Chemo No. 7 went well.

Tomorrow, Larry would give me the last of seven shots.

Today's support system included Mom and Larry. Larry dropped us off in front of the hospital then went to park the car. We were whisked into the process surprisingly faster than any time before, so I had the "Mommy shield" for the blood test needle, as Larry wasn't able to make it in there fast enough. The two-tube blood test was the most painless of them all, so far. Beverly, the nurse for these tests, was very good at what she did; it barely hurt. She promised to be with us next time if we asked for her when we checked in.

Larry arrived in time to be the "shield" for chemo's needle sticks. Elia, the chemo nurse attempted to place the needle and catheter into an area of my arm that would provide me with the most unrestricted movement, as I had to be there for three to four long hours in order to take in the complete IV drip. The poor little buggers had decided to go back into hiding after Beverly had done her job. After three attempts, Elia finally decided to use a big vein right at the bend in the crook of my arm. This location was an uncomfortable place for all that stuff to be hanging around, tethered to the IV system for such a long period of time. I naturally wanted to bend my arm when

I moved. Whenever I forgot that the IV was there and bent my arm, it hurt like hell because the needle and the catheters were so large. I was in tears several times that day. A full day later, I could still see a red lump and the large hole that marked the point of entry.

They offered Benadryl in pill form or through my IV. They worked equally well. There was only one difference: when given through the IV, the Benadryl sped through my system like lightning and I ended up *really* high, *really* fast. *Pow!* Starting out at ground level, I slowly climbed a gentle slope, much like going up the side of a scary ride at an amusement park and then briskly moved to a higher and higher elevation where I became very relaxed and oh-so-sleepy—just hanging there suspended in the clouds. It was quite different from having a few strong Cosmopolitans. *This* cocktail was much gentler at the start but so much more intense later, and I could feel the build-up moment by moment, the force of it literally washing over me and pulling me under, completely overtaking me. It was mind-blowing.

If you are interested in knowing how your body reacts, like I am, and if you can fight the desire to sleep—you can actually mark time through critical thinking abilities, the changes in your attention span, and the overwhelming feeling of just wanting to sleep. It reminded me of Dorothy in the *Wizard of Oz* as she danced and sang her way to the Land of Oz through the poppy-seeded Opium fields. As I moved through these stages, I felt absolutely totaled. What a ride! It was truly the best part of my day. Too bad they don't give this to you for all the treatments, or bottle it for home use.

The combination of pills and liquid drugs that they had given me, made me pee a lot. Today, all of the pills were pushed through the IV catheter in liquid form. Together with Benadryl and Taxol, and all the water that I was required to push into my system to stay hydrated, I was in and out of that chair almost every forty-five minutes. Once I was all hooked up and until I left the hospital, I generally hit the bathroom a minimum of five times. Today, I made a new record. Most of the other patients must have decided that it was a good day to go into another zone and had opted for their Benadryl or equivalent to go through their IV, as the majority of people were knocked out cold and the chemo room was eerily quiet. I tried to stay awake. I wanted to fully experience and record my body's responses to the Benadryl before I became unable to fight it any longer. During the first two Benadryl experiences, I had just let it take me away. I'd fallen out rather quickly. Today, there was a different agenda. I checked my voicemail and e-mail several times, responded to them all, and had the usual meeting with Dr. Nanda. I went to the bathroom a lot. Reading a book was impossible; my eyes would not focus and concentration was fleeting. Having too much respect for writers not to give a book my complete attention, I quickly gave up.

When I needed to go to the bathroom, Mom would unplug the equipment from the electrical outlet and wrap the cords around the moveable IV system. I would grab hold of the IV pole and walk over to the bathroom, where I always seemed to meet up with or meet eyes with the same young man. He was probably in his late thirties or early forties, very thin, bald, no eyebrows or eyelashes, with a completely ash-white complexion and on the same need-to-pee schedule as I was. After meeting several times like this, we looked at each other more closely. Despite the age and gender difference, and the fact that I still had some eyebrows and eyelashes, it was like looking into a mirror. We both laughed. I told him that it was nice to hear him laugh and reminded him that the best time to laugh is *anytime* you can. He nodded his head and smiled but he didn't say a word. His silence spoke volumes.

What do you think of that as a title for this book? *The Best Time to Laugh Is Anytime You Can.* I'd had that on my list of potential titles for three months now, and after seeing this guy's face—looking so sad but resigned to the process, knowing intimately his sense of powerlessness and how absolutely tired of it all he is—those words seemed appropriate. The best time to laugh is anytime you can. It looked like he might not be laughing too much these days and I wanted to share the wealth.

His silence spoke volumes to me because most of the people that I'd met here were generally eager to engage in conversation. I was afraid to ask Elia what he was fighting and if he would be OK. I wasn't sure I wanted to hear the answer.

An hour earlier, while checking email, I had learned that the husband of someone I've known for over twenty-five years had died on Friday from his six-year fight with cancer. His had been a much larger battle than mine, on all counts. He had been in and out of chemo throughout these long years and had been very sick a good deal of the time, but he never complained and had been an amazing example of strength and grace to all who had known him. They had called him Chemosabe.

Ed Rose will be sorely missed.

Until this moment, I'd chosen to believe that he, and the many people like him, were truly winning. That God and the angels had recognized that each one of them had achieved notable victories in their lives and would be given this challenge—and if they handled it honorably, they would ultimately win. But Ed had left us and it was a cruel reminder that not much had changed. There was still a stark randomness with cancer. Ed's triumphs were temporary, his progress illusory. He had won many battles but the war had been ultimately proven useless. Or maybe it had been too late, with not enough of some critical "thing" or too much of something else. It's random. I could feel my heart weeping.

I decided it was time to allow the drugs to take me away. I curled up with a blanket and pillow, reclined the chair and drifted off to the Land of Oz to ask the Wizard for courage—for me and for Ellen, Chemosabe's amazing wife and my friend.

Chapter 58

When Everything Is Coming Your Way, You're in the Wrong Lane

The bone, muscle and joint pain that I seemed to get in combination with the shot after chemo, were fairly easy to handle until Friday at around noon.

After chemo on Monday, I'd felt the need to take only one steroid and one pain pill on Wednesday, which had given me great hope that I was assimilating the drugs—finally!—after the seventh flipping week, and that it would be fine to drive for a few hours to the lake house.

On Friday, I had an appointment to meet a real estate agent about renting a house near our lake house in Wisconsin for the Fourth of July weekend. On Christmas Day, our shower steamer had been broken in a freak accident and water had been pouring out for at least three weeks. It had pretty much ruined our award-winning, two-year-old lake house. It was still under construction. This would be the perfect opportunity to check on how things were progressing.

He showed me several rentals, none of which would work, as we always have at least ten adults who stay over for several days. Occasionally, others would stop by for the day, or a day or two and bunk wherever they could. These properties were far too small for our group. After seeing the last option, we parted. I was thoroughly disappointed. I went to see my house and waited to hear from this guy who was going back to his office to check all available rental inventories from other offices in the area. It was the perfect last-minute scenario. But planning anything in those days needed to be last minute, so I didn't get my hopes up.

Orren Pickell Builders, as always, was doing a great job. Everything looked magnificent and was moving forward nicely. As I walked through the house, I couldn't help seeing and feeling the many metaphors on the rebuilding of this house in comparison to the rebuilding of my body. This builder had built a remarkable house in the past; I was building the same house with just a few improvements. This time I needed to rely on them to make the right decisions in many areas, as I wouldn't be able to drop by every few days to take care of questions or problems. There were many times when we would talk on the phone while I was in bed or lying next to the porcelain goddess having just thrown up, and they were either in the conference room at their office or at my house, executing whatever it was that we were working on that day. It was another beautiful orchestration of efforts.

Halfway through the house, there were abrupt and unexpected changes in my body. My left knee started throbbing, and then stopped. I took the next set of stairs more slowly, as I was probably cramped from driving for so long. Then my shoulders chimed in, followed by my shins, back, ankles, hands and hip.

The circuit of pain was starting and I was trapped on the top floor of the house.

A warm layer of moisture erupted on my face, neck, chest and head. I had eaten breakfast and had drunk water during the entire trip, so hunger and hydration were quickly ruled out. There was no place to sit down that wasn't dusty. I walked outside. I didn't want to go to my brother's house next-door and let myself in. No one was there that day. I was sure that if I went there, I would get too comfortable and it would all be over. I had to get home. I called the real estate agent and left a message asking him to call me as soon as he had found something that would work for our group. Then I began the drive home.

As I drove through the many gorgeous tree-lined and hilly streets in the area, heading towards the highway for home, the pain increased to the point that tears had begun to stream down my face uncontrollably. I started to feel things that I hadn't experienced before. A huge rush of cold shot up through my head. I was keenly aware of my body's outside borderlines, but the center seemed . . . not even there. There was a cool buzzing at the edges of my body from head to toe, then the buzzing concentrated in my head. I felt a little light-headed. Then I started breathing again and regained some control.

Maybe I needed sugar. I made a Taco Bell drive-thru my next stop. Fountain Pepsi is the best flavor in the world! Maybe it was the sugar, or the cold liquid or my hopes that it would work—but it did.

I had about twenty minutes until I reached the highway. I tried to decide if this was a smart thing to do: continue driving when I felt so odd. I decided to continue driving; surely a very selfish and maybe even stupid decision to those who are reading this. I apologize for that. I wasn't going to tell this part of the story, but then I had decided to be honest so that others might reconsider at the onset not to venture off, alone in a car, too far from home when going through chemo.

I thought I had gotten the pattern down pat. I'd been convinced that Friday after chemo would be a good day to make this trip. I was wrong.

The pain wasn't in one specific area. It would come and go, attacking one part of me every two minutes or so continually chasing around my body. I was almost at the highway and, depending on traffic, an hour or so from home and the relief of a steroid and pain pill. I was unable to use cruise control because there was too much traffic and too many construction stops to have made it a safe option. I was also constantly looking for roadside stopping areas whenever I passed by a construction site, in case I needed to get off the road fast and chill out. Fortunately, the Illinois Tollway Authority had done a great job of setting up a place for cars to pull off the road. I'd been staying in the express lane, a single-file lane that moves faster than the local lanes with all its exits. And it had a decent-sized pull-off area available.

My tears, falling for so long, no longer contained any salt. Surprisingly, they didn't blind me. They were a soothing relief to the skin on my face and cooled me off as they dripped onto my chest.

I thought about calling Larry, Mom or Dad, Shere or Bob—so someone would know what was happening. But I didn't. All they could have done was worry and freak out until they knew I was safely home. Besides, I would have had to find my reading glasses to enter a password on my phone so I could turn the damn thing on and then dial. It was too much of a distraction in this traffic. I was almost home. I would simply wait.

My hands and feet were like blocks of ice. It felt strange to grasp the steering wheel and feel the gas and brake pedals. My fingernails hurt. My toes and the pads of my fingertips were becoming numb. I remembered that Larry had always reminded me to breathe through the pain when this happened. I tend to take a deep breath and push against it; taking short, shallow, staccato breaths. Now I breathed through the pain. It helped, and so did groaning like a woman delivering a baby. There I was—breathing hard, groaning and crying and trying to drive safely. What a mess!

I noticed my exit ahead and thankfully made each and every light towards home.

Home at last, I threw a steroid and a pain pill down my throat. I was now unable to move. I was stretched out on my bed and thankful to have arrived home safely without hurting a soul.

The phone rang.

It was Dad. I could barely speak. I couldn't formulate a logical sentence or at least one that was understandable. He thought it was a bad connection. He hung up and called back. On the second call, I hoped that I had gotten him to understand that I couldn't talk and that I was in too much pain. I hung up this time. Twenty minutes later, the doorbell rang. I was two floors up and ignored it.

It might be FedEx or UPS, I thought. That was their signal that a delivery had been made.

The phone rang again. It was Mom and Dad; they were at the front door. I asked them to use their keys. Mom filled my pitcher with ice water and fixed the bed around me. Dad lay down next to me, holding my hand and rubbing my back. That felt so good, so comforting. But having them see me in this state was harder than being in it. They were totally helpless and could not do anything to make it better. I couldn't see very well and that at least released me from seeing the pain that I knew would be evident in their eyes. I could feel it in their touch; that was hard enough. I convinced them that the pills were taking effect and that they should go home and not worry too much. Dad called Larry and they discussed whatever it was that they needed to discuss about me and then Mom and Dad quietly left. Larry appeared soon after.

Sleeping was a challenge. I was up and down every three hours. Maybe I should have taken the steroids and pain pills as directed but I stood by the method that I'd used, as I had greatly reduced the amount of drugs that would have been in my system. Besides, the pain would have occurred regardless. I should have been at or near home when it happened and not driving to and from another state. Making short trips around and about town with time in between driving is a good thing; you need to continue living and getting out in the world. But driving for several hours is not something I would recommend.

That is the lesson for this chapter.

My friend Yolanda Simonsis suggested that maybe the experience would have been less traumatic if I had simply let it happen and had taken the pain pills in advance of the pain, if I had allowed the Benadryl to take me away at the hospital, if I had gotten over my concern with steroids and had taken them as directed.

"So here's a devil's advocate question," she said. "Might your treatment experience or anyone else's be milder if you simply let the drugs do their part and choose not to experience all of the chemo drug effects in a wakened state?"

For most people, I think the answer would be "yes." It would be best to just let it happen and do everything as prescribed. I had done that for two sessions, and then had decided to try it another way so I could journal how my body had responded—which, of course, may not be how everyone will respond. But I hope this resonates with someone who might look at things the way I do, or experience them the way I did. It would at least provide them with a set of limits or a time line; a head start.

I went out with a bang when I needed to and stayed awake when I could. But on a more global level, I agree with them—and I need to emphasize that they give you this stuff for a reason. So take it as directed, unless you have a very good reason not to. Although I learned this lesson a bit late, being that the last chemo treatment would be on June 30th, I could at least find comfort in once again having done it *my* way: keeping steroids, pain pills and anxiety medicine to a minimum.

Each person walks their own journey. In order to live a more fulfilling life, we must share that journey so that others can make better choices for themselves.

Saturday morning, spotty pain coursed through the lower half of my body. But I could type and work on the book and catch up on e-mail. It was a good day to lie low and stay home.

Chapter 59

The Last Chemo, a Little Respite and Then Diving into the Next Step

We've all heard it said: pain, uncomfortable memories and trying times soften in their intensity with the passing of time. I found this to be true, as I tend to drop the negative stuff as fast as I possibly can and look for a way to re-frame it. I concentrate on spinning it towards the positive side of things.

Today would be the last of four very long months of chemotherapy. While the experience was still fresh enough to send little wiggly chills down my spine, I could already sense that those chills would fade very quickly.

I had decided a few weeks ago that the perfect end to this experience would be to have a celebratory, thank-you lunch for the entire Chemo department on the last day.

Moondance Diner, my long-time favorite, delivered platters of sandwiches. Everything was cut up into a quarter of the regular size to make it easier for those who were hooked up to IV's—and for the nurses scurrying around, taking care of us. Along with homemade potato chips and large platters of fresh fruit and brownies, we were all able to eat something that wasn't made at the hospital. Theresa Manuele, the owner of Moondance Diner, after finding out what was going on with me, decided that she wanted to split the bill and not charge me anything for the delivery to the hospital. This little luncheon was well-received by everyone who was at the hospital that day but especially by the nurses who were most definitely tired of hospital food. The mood of the department seemed to elevate a bit and conversations were started with people meeting over the area where the food was placed. It was a nice change in atmosphere.

Last night, my girlfriend Tomi had sent an email with a suggestion for this last treatment; a suggestion, like Yolanda's, that I am actually going to take.

"Tomorrow should be your last round of chemo," Tomi wrote. "How about, for research's sake, you take all the drugs the doctors recommend, at the time they recommend, to see just how much easier this whole process might be when you're not so stubborn? I can't help but believe that they've developed these protocols from experience and trial-and-error—they must have learned *something*—and they really don't want to torture you any more than necessary. We all hate seeing you suffer, especially when you don't have to. Good luck tomorrow. May you have your favorite nurse, may the needle not hurt, and may you sleep through it all."

I'd decided that I would take the steroids and pain pills in advance of the pain after chemo, as directed. But I'd never really suffered more than others did while going through the same treatment—and occasionally (quite often, actually), I had won the battle of the pain and had been able to override it without having to take any drugs. That having been said, I would take them this time. For research's sake.

Today's support system included Larry and Shere. When we checked in for blood work, I was told that Beverly was now working on the third floor. I was a bit disappointed. I'd wanted to see her and say good-bye. She was also the best blood-drawing technician that I had met. They shocked me by calling her and asking if she would come up to the chemo department to draw my blood. She came up to the sixth floor to take care of me. I was blown away that they would even consider calling her from another area of the hospital and that she would actually come up for a patient that she may never see again. The caretakers at this hospital were amazingly proficient, professional, knowledgeable and compassionate. Beverly's actions were a perfect demonstration of high-quality customer service, relationship building and what it means when people say that they are loyal to the brand.

Melody Perpich, the Genetic Counselor stopped by to discuss the results of my tests. She was smiling as she walked up to my chair. I tried to discern if that smile meant good news or if it was the first gentle emotion before she delivered the bad news. While only two percent of the population carried the breast cancer gene, I wondered if my odds were higher due to Aunt Joan's breast cancer and Grandma's uterine cancer.

I had a sudden sick thought that maybe God was going to let me experience all of it so that everything could be documented in this book.

This test was a hugely complicated decision and one that held implications far beyond one's own self. The results, if positive, would mean that I had to make a decision to remove my other breast and ovaries; my chances of cancer occurring in those areas would then be twenty to forty percent higher than the general population's. The suggested treatment for me would be to remove all of it.

This also presented an issue for my sister and four nieces, some of whom may have no desire to learn if they will get this disease and then in having to decide early on, how and if they will respond to that knowledge. But at least this knowledge would give them an early clue to the extra diligence that they must employ. If I carried the gene, they would need to be ever-so-careful and timely about mammograms and Pap smears. They already needed to alert their doctors of the fact that I had breast cancer, so that their ovaries and breasts would be checked thoroughly. While my diagnosis wouldn't mean that they would also suffer this disease, it would point to a heightened risk factor. A positive result would also present any number of problems with one's insurance company, not just now but also in the future if one should change carriers.

I had spent parts of the last five weeks contemplating both scenarios in vivid and colorful detail; and of course, usually ended up with the belief that I couldn't possibly have this gene. But then again . . . As such, this ambiguity had made me quite anxious while waiting for Melody to arrive. She started with the usual pleasantries that are expected from a doctor. Then she moved swiftly into the heart of the matter.

The results for the BRCA 1 sequencing, BRCA 1 full gene rearrangement, five site rearrangement panel, BRCA 2 sequencing and BRCA 2 full gene rearrangement—were all *negative*.

No mutation detected!

Women who have not had breast cancer have a two percent risk of developing breast or ovarian cancer. My risk was now at three to four percent. Melody cautioned me that my chances of developing these cancers had been significantly reduced but not completely ruled out. The possibility remained that my cancer risks would be increased due to other non-hereditary factors (i.e., environment), another hereditary cancer syndrome or a mutation in BRCA1 or BRCA2 that current technology couldn't detect. They were learning new things every day and I would be placed in a database to be kept up to date on any changes or improvements to testing or information.

Dr. Nanda made her usual visit with me while I was in the chemo chair. She reminded me that because I had not yet gone through a natural menopause, that estrogen would now be my enemy. Chemo would no doubt throw me into early chemical menopause, and it appeared that I was following protocol—I had not had a period in two months (yet another silver lining!). I would need to take a drug called Tamoxofin for about a year once I had completed chemotherapy. As soon as Dr. Nanda was convinced that I had completely stopped having periods (sometimes they stopped and then started up again), she would switch me to Femara, Aromasin or Arimidex; those drugs would have to be taken for another five years.

I now needed to make a decision about radiation. We would start the Tamoxifen drug therapy after radiation was completed. At that point, Dr. Nanda and I would review the after-chemo drugs' short—and long-term side effects and how best to handle them. If I decided to go ahead with radiation, it would provide me with plenty of time to research these drugs thoroughly. I know several people who had decided not to take Tamoxifen—and they are still alive—but I wanted to attack this disease with everything known to man. The Benadryl shot was starting to take hold and I was falling out fast, so I didn't push myself to learn *everything* today. I was sure I wouldn't remember much anyway.

I asked Dr. Nanda what tests would be given to prove that I was cancer-free. There were tests available (CA15-3 and CA27-29) but they weren't being given for early-stage breast cancers so I wouldn't qualify for either of them. Additionally, Dr. Nanda didn't agree with PET scans, as they can be harmful themselves. Because my cancer had been found early, she felt that we were attacking it from all angles with the combination of excellent surgical results, an aggressive chemotherapy treatment, and after-chemo drugs.

It was time to ask Dr. Nanda for her opinion regarding radiation therapy. She cautioned me that she was not familiar enough with the statistics or the side effects but that she certainly understood my concerns about having radiation, as I was floating in that gray area. She suggested that I go back to Dr. Chmura and thoroughly review with him the risk-versus-benefit factors, side effects, numbers and percentages. The last time I visited with Dr. Chmura, I hadn't even bothered to prepare questions, as I had been convinced that I wouldn't be having radiation. He had bowled me over unexpectedly with some very compelling reasons to have it, but I needed to get more information to make a fully informed decision.

The bottom line was: I needed to make a final decision very soon. Dr. Nanda and I both knew that. It was comforting to hear that she understood my dilemma. I had four to six weeks before radiation must begin, if I would have it at all. That decision had to be made quickly. I would make an appointment to meet with Dr. Chmura tomorrow.

Looking at it all from a different perspective, I saw myself balancing at the top of the apex. I had a wide-angle view of the past and shimmering glimpses of the future. The fears that I'd had after diagnosis, the terror over surgery, the physical and emotional changes during recovery, the roller-coaster ride called chemo, concern over the results of the genetic tests—all of these have been for the most part, the hardest parts for me. As I slid down the other side of that apex, I expected that I would go back to whatever would be "the new normal" for me. Before that happened, I would take a bit of time off from all things medical and use that time to put the lake house back in order.

I found a house to rent up at the lake in July. The Fourth of July holiday with our friends would go forward as planned. Watching the fireworks on the boat this year, and simply being with them, would be especially meaningful. We would toast the end of this chapter and my independence from the poisonous IV drip. At the same time, we would celebrate our country's independence. Most of August would be spent moving back all of our things from the many places where they were stored in Wisconsin and Illinois, hanging drapes and pictures, and making our house a home once again.

If I decide on radiation, then this schedule would change and my creative problem solving abilities would be put back into play again.

I finally understood Global Warming. These chemically induced hot flashes were *amazing*.

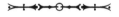

Dr. Song's Corner

Many women will find themselves in a situation similar to Suzanne's when faced with options/choices for cancer care. There are some wrong answers, like doing nothing when all of your doctors are recommending a certain treatment plan. Many suggestions are based on our collected data of patients with similar staging and biology of cancer. Like with Suzanne, it is recommended you seek sound information, challenge your doctors with questions and ultimately find a team of doctors that you trust.

Chapter 60

How to Keep It Moving

Every single person I have spoken to who has undergone chemotherapy, has suffered constipation—at one time or another, to one degree or another.

We know what causes this conundrum when life is normal but when being treated for cancer, any number of reasons can be added to the list. Some classes of chemotherapy drugs can affect the nerve supply to the bowel and slow down the natural movement and rhythm of the intestines. Additionally, these drugs affect appetite and physical activity that normally help to keep things moving. All these issues provide the perfect recipe for constipation.

Up to ninety percent of cancer patients experience cancer-related pain. Several drugs such as morphine, hydrocodone (Vicadin and Lortab) and Oxycodone (Percocet, OyyContin) frequently cause constipation. These drugs effectively relieve pain by binding to certain receptors in the brain and spinal cord, but they also bind to receptors found in the intestines—leading to constipation in about half of patients by disrupting contractions that help to keep everything moving down. Without these contractions, the drugs stay in the intestines longer. As the body absorbs water, these drugs cause everything in the intestines to become dry and hard.

This is one of the most common but debilitating side effects of people undergoing chemo treatments—and for those who, after surgeries, are also taking pain pills. Because constipation is almost guaranteed, you need to head it off by taking a softener; and in some cases, also taking something that increases contractions. Senokot and Senna Lax worked wonders for me. Ducolax—well, not so much. These wonder drugs increase intestinal contractions. Softeners like Colace help to retain water to soften it all up enough to be passed.

Nutrition plays a major role in this drama, too. Eating foods that are high in fiber (such as beans, peaches, squash, broccoli, carrots and whole grain bread) can minimize the problem. Fiber helps to hold water, making all that waste heavier and therefore able to move through the intestines more easily. This is the biggest challenge for cancer patients, as loss of appetite and constantly throwing up can quickly deplete your body of essential nutrients and proper hydration. You need to have something going in, to have something coming out.

Drinking water keeps your entire body hydrated.

Last but not least, exercising in some way every day not only helps you to stay in shape, but it also serves as a preventative measure for cancer patients who are at an increased risk of constipation. Physical activity keeps things moving, trust me.

There is no easy way out of this one. You will need to take the suggestions above and adjust them according to your body's needs. The best suggestion that I can give you is to head off all of this in advance when taking pain relieving drugs or having a chemo treatment by using softeners and drugs for constipation.

Chapter 61

Do Boneless, Skinless Chicken Cutlets Float?

Uncharacteristically, I kept putting off finding a bathing suit that would fit my new body landscape and the boneless, skinless chicken cutlet. I dragged it out for as long as I could and waited until Tuesday afternoon. We would be leaving on Wednesday morning to open the rental house and begin the holiday.

I headed back to the boutique that carried accoutrements for women with boob issues. I had become one of their frequent customers. I care enough to get and use the proper "stuff" when presenting myself to the world when I feel healthy and normal. The way I'd been—a bit off kilter in recent months—made doing it right even more critical.

Being a woman, I tried on *many* bathing suits before I finally found a few that I liked. Every maneuver that any woman has ever attempted in any dressing room in the world when trying on that dreaded piece of fabric, was deftly put into action. I put everything but water to the test.

It was hard to believe, but I found three suits that passed with flying colors.

I happily chatted with the girls at the desk as I paid my bill, and we shared a few laughs. We had become quite friendly over the past five months. Then I then went home to pack my new stuff.

Picture this . . .

It was the Fourth of July holiday. We were on the lake house property with our friends—Bob, Lisa, their kids, some of Bob and Lisa's college friends and *their* kids, Mom and Dad, and everyone else who owned a home in that little part of the world. Our group walked to the clubhouse pool. I was about to learn whether the boneless, skinless chicken cutlet (a.k.a. breast prosthesis) would float out of my bathing suit or stay put. Even after those rigorous dressing room tests and looking for bathing suits that had a little trap door built into the side to carefully keep the chicken cutlet anchored, I was still a bit uneasy about the trial run. Today would be the real test.

The girls were aware of my concerns and had agreed to run reconnaissance. Being backed up by the Mag 7 gave me a sense of security, as well as a bit of trepidation. I know these guys too well. I was afraid that if the chicken cutlet broke free, we would burst out laughing—hard enough to make it float away, traumatizing nearby children. Or, the little bugger might sink to the depths of the pool, and one of us would have to stop laughing long enough to dive for it. It was too soon to venture into the lake waters, as the chicken cutlet would surely be lost forever.

The others were aware that something was up. But I wasn't sure they got it just yet.

After spending some time in the hot sun, a few of us at a time would dive, walk, slide or slither into the water. I was quite happy to simply watch, safely sprawled out on a lounge chair, until the heat and the promise of a quick cool-off became too much to bear. Walking into the water, I did not feel any difference, shift or change.

Ahhhh . . .

I felt comfortable going a bit deeper.

I am happy to report that on that day, I didn't traumatize any children, ruin my reputation or harm a family's name. It was all quite uneventful—literally.

Five perfect days!

The weather was excellent. The people we annually share the holiday with were a fun group to be around, as always.

Insane amounts of food, mostly home-cooked meals were abundant and probably too many drinks were consumed. Best of all, new memories were made.

At the end of the weekend, as I reflected on how blessed I am, I realized that I'd made it through five consecutive days of social activity, which is the most activity I'd had in *seven* months. I was wiped out, very happy, totally content—and yes, boneless, skinless chicken cutlets really do float and they stay where they are supposed to be!

Life was good.

Chapter 62

Slash, Poison and Burn
& Focusing on the Long-Term

Just before leaving for the Fourth of July holiday, I had called the radiation oncologist's office at the University of Chicago and made an appointment with Dr. Chmura. I wanted a chance to get into the thick of the matter with him; this time while keeping an open mind. The doctor had already presented compelling reasons for me to consider radiation. Although his opinion differed from the opinion of the surgeon that I respect and trust, not carefully considering both sides would be unlike me. This time, I would be armed and ready with questions and research. Larry and Mom would be along on this mission; I would have the advantage of having two other sets of ears with me. Afterwards, we would go out to dinner with Dad, so no matter how it rolled at the hospital, we'd end the day eating well and having a spirited dinner conversation.

Since they had given me a four—to six-week period to rest after chemo, I planned to wait until August to continue my research on radiation and to make the final decision on further treatments. I looked at my calendar and realized that I was quickly running out of time. There is never a good time to plan for a medical procedure, as they say; but the planning becomes especially complicated when the medical procedure needs to be done every day for six weeks. It was going to be a challenge finding six consecutive, uninterrupted weeks. The best solution would be to figure it out by continuing with my research and radiation oncologist interviews, determine a plan of action and then get it done and over with.

Chemo ended last week, and I now needed to uncover the momentum that had been gathered and put aside for a rainy day. It seemed that the best use of my time would be to push forward; focusing on the big picture, and understanding and accepting the long-term benefits and consequences.

This decision would have everything to do with how the balance of the summer—and the rest of my life—might play out.

After careful consideration, exhaustive research, long talks with survivors who had had radiation and those who had decided against it, I decided to move forward with radiation therapy. When I walk into the next ten years of mammogram appointments, I want to be able to know that I had tried everything that was available to me to stem the chance of a local recurrence or a metastasis in another area of my body. After doing all of this, if it still happens . . . then it happens. I had done everything that I could.

My rationale included the fact that I had an invasive Grade 3 tumor. It had reached my lymphatic system. I also had a high-grade, stage 2B Ductal Carcinoma in Situ (DCIS) associated tumor that would most likely have grown into an invasive cancer. The surrounding breast tissue that was removed was also found to be cancerous. I was HER-2 negative, which closed off some of my treatment options and opened up others. My cancer is receptive to hormones—that means, I would need to take other drugs to ward off the beast. And lastly, having radiation reduced a local recurrence from fifteen percent down to five percent

I asked about the disease called lymphangiosarcoma (see previous chapter) that they suspect could be caused by radiation. It's so rare that they don't have viable numbers to present, which I verified with my own research.

I was very intrigued by Dr. Chmura's study, which was published in the first quarter of 2009 and speaks of the benefits of radiation therapy for women who have my specific type, brand, stage and grade of cancer.

My reasons not to have radiation revolved around vanity and time. Going to a hospital every day for six weeks really blows a schedule. But the most disappointing issue was that having radiation would delay reconstruction surgery by six to eight months (see previous chapter for the reasons). I would also need to accept that the radiated side of my skin may not be as smooth as the non-radiated side and some reconstruction options would not be possible for me after radiation. Fortunately, several of the reconstruction options that I had looked into were not options that I would have chosen to undergo anyway.

The various methods of reconstruction surgery blew me away and shocked my senses. It ain't just silicone implants anymore!

To use vanity or time as a rationale for not having radiation is a shorted-sighted view for someone who wants a long-term solution.

Yet, I had to consider the time factor. Without traffic, having daily radiation at the University of Chicago would be a three-hour round trip event. To plan for anything less than that is not a reasonable expectation in Chicago. Dr. Chmura understood this. When I told him I was ten minutes away from Hinsdale Hospital and five minutes away from La Grange Hospital—both of whom are affiliated with the University of Chicago—he asked how far away I lived from Edward Hospital. This hospital is about half an hour farther than the others I'd mentioned. Dr. Chmura looked me in the eye and said that if I wasn't going to come to the University of Chicago to work with him, he would rather have me work with Dr. Ann McCall at Edward Hospital.

When he looked me in the eyes, he was sending a very clear message. For him to refer me to a competitor and another hospital meant something, as it would have been so easy for him to answer the precise question that was posed. Which hospital was better—Hinsdale or LaGrange? Instead, he answered it more fully by stating what the best hospital in the area was and included a physician he knows and trusts for good measure.

When I called for an appointment with Dr. McCall, I found out that Dr. Chmura had already spoken to her and that they had set aside time for me next Friday. During this meeting, I intended for us to get to know each other, for me to be able to ask Dr. McCall a few questions specific to her treatment plan, go over long-term symptoms from her experience and then pull out our calendars. I'd already checked her out and liked what I had read.

One fact continued to move to the forefront of my mind, over and over again; the same fact that always tipped me over the side of going for all of what was being offered: the fact that I had even *one* lymph node that was found to be positive, meant that my cancer had learned to live outside of the host area and and had learned to thrive in my lymphatic system. Had one of those microscopic cancer cells moved to a lymph node(s) near my neck?

Chemo works throughout your bloodstream using different combinations of drug therapy to stop cancer cells from dividing, so they stop growing or die, which provides that whole body experience. But chemo does not reach the site of origination like surgery does and radiation will. Radiation is much more effective for local control.

I tried to focus on the long-term benefits, as most of the symptoms are short-term and don't sound all that nasty (i.e., flaking or peeling skin, darkened skin like when you tan, soreness or swelling, tiredness turning into exhaustion, puckering around the scar, shrinkage and shifting of the breast). The long-term symptoms are scary but very rare (i.e., rib fracture, heart injury, radiation pneumonitis, lymphedema and brachial plexopathy). It's still a crap shoot. There was just not enough long-standing data to provide reliable numbers or an understanding of who might experience what symptoms.

Equally disappointing is that there are no tests available to tell us if chemo or radiation was successful. If cancer returns, it didn't work; pretty clear cut. But if cancer doesn't come back, it cannot easily be attributed to a specific therapy. In other words, there is no way to find out if chemo or radiation was the savior, or if both had been necessary; just as there is no way to find out if skipping either of the two would make a difference. They just don't know. And because of that, I will attack it with everything that they *do* know, accept the risks and live a full life no matter how long it will be or what consequences I might encounter along the way.

The result is consistent with who I am: a long-term, big-picture thinker. A person who leaves no stone unturned but occasionally meets up with a creepy-crawler or two. I am OK with that. You should have seen what I had discovered while scuba diving in Australia with Terry Rowney and Peter. This six-inch centipede-like creature had snuck into my scuba boot one night and I'd met him the next morning after I'd put the boot on. It had bitten me and caused me to be flown off the Great Barrier Reef and returned to civilization in Sydney via a Medi-Vac helicopter and three planes. The medics had never seen anything like it before. I had never before seen a foot swell so quickly. Customs would not allow me to take a living "thing" out of the country, so Terry had kept it. He later had the taxidermist kill it and then had set it in clear resin for me to use as a paper weight: a true memento. The little bugger has one less pincher as he remains encased in his resin tomb!

Chapter 63

Hoping That This Will Extend My Expiration Date

I spoke with Dr. Connolly the day before I met with Dr. Ann McCall. Dr. Connolly and I reviewed his reasons for not wanting radiation for me and he suggested some things that I could ask Dr. McCall. I felt more comfortable after talking to him again, discussing my choice to go ahead with radiation and reviewing my ability to tolerate the potential symptoms. His major concern was to keep the radiation beams as far away as possible from my armpit. The risks of lymphedema are higher if radiation is used heavily in that area.

The Cancer Center at Edward Hospital is clean and modern, and the people that I was in contact with were all kind and helpful. The Center has an organized system set up that moves the patient swiftly from one event to the next and keeps them pretty much engaged with a human the entire time. It felt like there was progress being made because something was always happening and the time flew by rather quickly.

For over two hours, I went through all of that first-time-visit preliminary crap. It was another "consultation" appointment but this time a much stronger intent was behind it. I was on-board with the whole idea. I simply wanted to be sure that the doctor and I clicked and that I understood and agreed with her treatment plan. This visit did not include my usual entourage; it was a nice change to be one-on-one with the doctor.

As soon as Dr. McCall entered the room and before she had spoken her first words, I knew that we would work well together. She told me that she has had several conversations and exchanged emails with Dr. Chmura; she felt like she already knew me. She even asked about the book. The two doctors had collaborated on how best to treat my case. The plan seemed reasonable and they were open to altering it a bit to take into consideration the concerns that I had: lymphedema, heart and lung issues, and rib fractures down the road. I was still trying to figure out how to find six weeks of uninterrupted time; Dr. McCall told me that we could be flexible and that delaying radiation treatment by a few more weeks would not adversely affect the outcome.

On August 18th, I would be back at the hospital for what they call a "planning day." I would have CT scans so that Dr. McCall could easily identify the precise area of radiation and determine how she would steer as far away from my lungs and other organs as possible. Basically, the CT scan would define the treatment field. They hoped to be able to bend the radiation or stop at a specific layer so that the more sensitive areas and organs would be left alone. They would do a series of scans, and depending on what they would find and the extent of the treatment field that would be required, a mold of my body on that side might be required to assist me in keeping still so that the radiation beam would be delivered to the exact same area each and every day. I would also be marked with dots of semi-permanent ink the size of freckles. These marks would likely fade over time but are necessary for the six-week treatment period. Treatment would begin on August 25th.

Dr. McCall would steer clear of my intramammory lymph node chain, as there was no evidence that it would increase my survival rate or change recurrence rates. The areas that would be radiated were Level 1 and Level 2, my remaining lymph nodes, the chest wall and the lower two thirds of my armpit (I was hoping that the armpit percentage would be lessened after the tests). The equipment that would be used is called the Trilogy and the Varian 1X. I would see a radiation therapist every day and visit with Dr. McCall and a radiation nurse once a week.

At the end of our meeting, Dr. McCall hugged me before I could hug *her.*

There were only a few weeks left until I was to experience the tan of my life. I reminded myself that until then, I should "Live out the String."

Chapter 64

A New Twist to Cleavage
and the Tests before Radiation

It had been about six weeks since I'd last written. During that time we'd been on the annual Zaccone Family Vacation and had had a magnificent time. I had a chance to catch up with GSI projects, personal financial and legal issues, I worked on our Family Foundation, organized the final requirements before the lake house would be ready to move back into, reorganized closets and drawers at home and generally reveled in the freedom that I had from all things medical.

Before we left for vacation, I tried on just about everything prior to packing it to make sure that each outfit could be easily altered by a brooch, accessorized with a scarf or jacketed to hide my new landscape. The first night on vacation, as we dressed for dinner, I selected the one and only dress that I had not tried on back at home. No matter how I reconfigured my bra, the straps on the dress or the accessories—this dress could not be worn. It was far too revealing. I had a minor meltdown, and then I tearfully changed into another dress. I used to have a rather nice cleavage; now I had a rather nice "cleave edge." Yes, a "cleave" for the half still there that falls off the "edge" to nowhere, quite dramatically.

The Sunday before the pre-radiation tests started out badly. I burned the inside of my left hand while making breakfast and then was stung on the back of my left hand by a pissed-off bee as I watered the plants outside. Obviously, I had gotten too close for comfort to his hive. We'd been trying to get rid of this beehive for a while now. I was grateful that it wasn't my right hand, since I had to be careful about infections and any kind of trauma due to the removed lymph nodes in that arm. As my hand began to throb and swell and after Larry applied Neosporin all over the area, I decided I would do a little last-minute research on radiation. I headed for my sanctuary—my office (Larry calls it "the nest").

I've learned early on to be careful about what you read and choose to believe while surfing the Web, unless the information is coming from a highly accredited organization. On this day, I went to the American Cancer Society webpage. I happened upon an area of the site that noted personal stories. The one I read was about the challenges with reconstruction surgery after radiation. It was a story complete with pictures. It pushed me back over Niagara Falls, and tears poured for most of the day. Those tears reappeared on the way to the pre-radiation tests the following day.

The actual tests were a breeze. I lay quite comfortably inside of half of a horizontal tube while they decorated my chest with three little "X's," then covered them with very durable, clear tape that was supposed to stay on until my return the following week. There was an "X" smack in the middle of my chest in between what used to be my boobs, and one sat precisely under each arm on the same line. They were made with a Magic Marker type of pen. Swimming or baths for extended periods of time were out for six weeks and I needed to be careful not to pull off the tape while showering or drying off afterwards.

I was sent through the X-ray tube several times. Because I'm not at all claustrophobic, I simply closed my eyes and stayed as still as I could. I was able to breathe normally; I just couldn't move. I'm not sure if the equipment was highly sensitive and was able to detect moisture or if the radiation techs handling the tests were sensitive (they have a video camera trained on you at all times, as well as a microphone, so contact can be made instantly) but at one point, Becky Panayiotidef, a radiation tech returned from behind the safety of the glass partition that separated the radiation and X-Ray room from normalcy, and wiped the tears from my eyes. She asked me if they should stop, if I was scared, what was wrong. I explained that it was probably just a bit of the last eight months that had come crashing down on my head and not to worry, I was fine and we could continue. She wiped away a few more tears, gave me a handful of dry Kleenex, and instructed me not to move. We continued.

Dr. McCall came into the room, assuring me that I would not look like a circus freak at the end of radiation and that she would help me find the best surgeon alive for my reconstruction. I was feeling like nine miles of bad road and finding it hard to really believe her, even as I so desperately wanted to. I was trying to prepare myself for the possibility that I might be one of those who could have an unattractive outcome. Several of the pictures I had seen online yesterday were somewhat unsettling, and the memory was still fresh.

Today's tests would provide the doctors, nurses and radiation techs with an outline of the precise areas to be radiated so that they could leave as much of me untouched by the rays as possible.

I'd developed another after-chemo symptom. About a week ago, I'd gone for a manicure. Char, the manicurist, who is familiar with my fingernails, noticed that a horizontal line across many nails had shown up. The line was evident on about seven of my fingernails and it was at the exact same point across all of them. We agreed that it must be a mark that had been caused by a reaction to chemo and was finally showing itself as distinctly as a line on my forehead. I also mentioned to her that the nail of the forefinger on my right hand felt sore and a bit loose in the center. Upon closer inspection, she saw that although the nail was firmly anchored at the sides, it had in fact lifted from the nail bed in the center.

This was an incredibly uncomfortable feeling, as any pressure on my fingernail made me feel as if my nail would lift right off. It was bandaged up to provide some strength and security as I moved about my day. During the early days of chemo, while Shere and I were waiting to get my blood drawn for testing, we had begun a conversation with a woman who had not been given much time to live but was fighting like hell to beat the odds against her cancer. She had laughed at my concerns over my hair, as hers had been the same "style." She had shown me her hands, and there had not been a fingernail left on either of them. All of her nails had fallen off, completely fallen off. My heart ached then; it bled now. I checked my nails a zillion times a day. So far, it was just the one.

Next Wednesday, we'd start with a dry run. The treatment map would have been made and the dry run was scheduled for mid-morning to make sure that the map and the lines on my body would all line up, and that they could bend the rays away from healthy tissue and organs. Oddly enough, later on that same day, I had a six-month follow-up appointment with my surgeon; my hero. The one who felt that radiation was not necessary for me. Would he provide some newly discovered magical answer or another option to spare me from this next step? I doubted it.

The next day, I began the six-week journey through radiation. My appointment with Dr. Connolly went well. I was scheduled for a mammogram next month. It was just one more thing to ponder while I lay in radiation, acquiring the sunburn of my life.

I continued to experience occasional "numb fingers and toes syndrome" (mild neuropathy) but that came and went rather quickly. My eyebrows are really sparse, but I could see growth beginning. I no longer had any lower eyelashes, though I suppose I should be happy for the few that I did have on my upper lids. Once chemotherapy is complete, your hair, eyebrows and lashes should start to grow within six to twelve months. If they don't, then other causes are the issue, such as a low thyroid function. This should be brought up with your physician immediately.

I'd gained back some weight and food tasted much better these days. Every once in a while, I felt like I had drunk three shots of vodka in quick succession; a little off my game, kind of dizzy, a little high. My eyes were still very dry and then they would suddenly become watery, although each week I could feel a major shift as that symptom lessened. My nose was beginning to stop its constant running as hair slowly grew back to stem the flow, and the Kleenex Tissue Company was probably rallying the troops to determine their next biggest strategic outlet. My periods had stopped, at least for the past three months—so chemo had, in fact, thrown me into early menopause. The hair on my head was beginning to grow back and I could finally use my old toothpaste and mouthwash without burning the inside of my mouth. I'd shaved my legs and underarms only twice in the past five months. I would miss that benefit, big time.

I looked forward to when the chemo poison would leave my body completely, and to when I no longer woke up to a new physical surprise or side effect each day. They told me it would take about six months.

Life . . . well, it's still good.

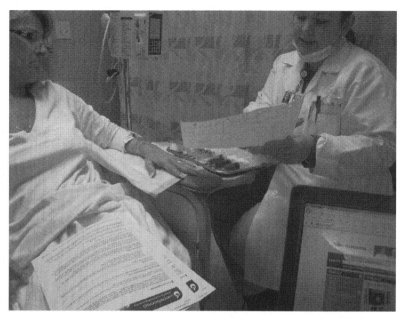

Brigit explains potential side effects of the eight syringes of poison

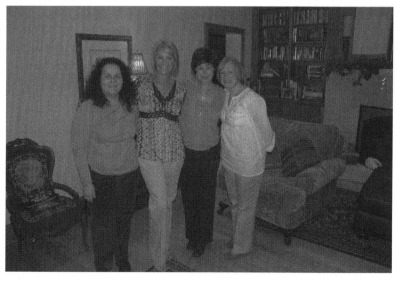

Cancer survivors: Sophia, Carol and Yolanda

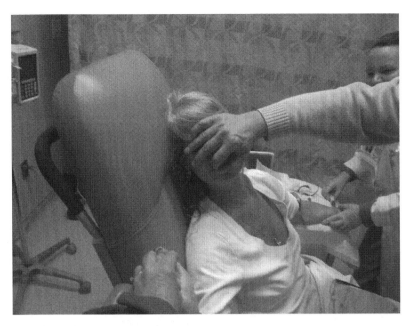

Chemo No. 1. "The Shield"

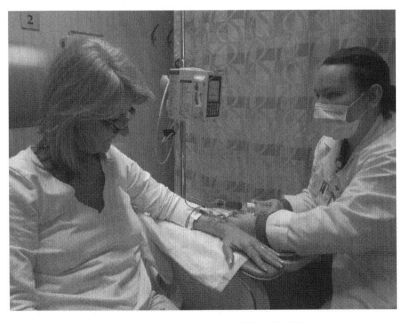

Chemo No. 1. With Brigit and The Red Death

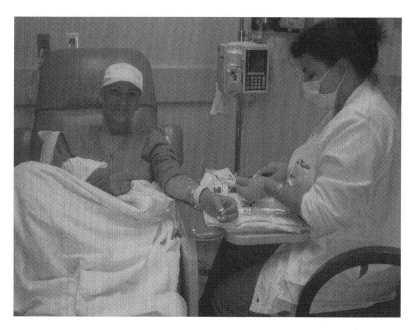

Chemo No. 4. Elia delivers the Red Death

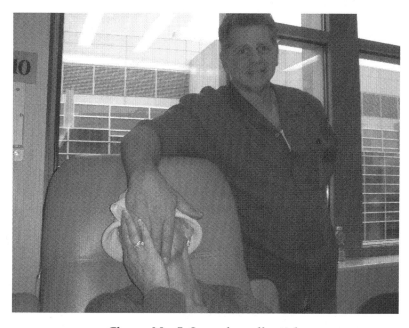

Chemo No. 5. Second needle stick

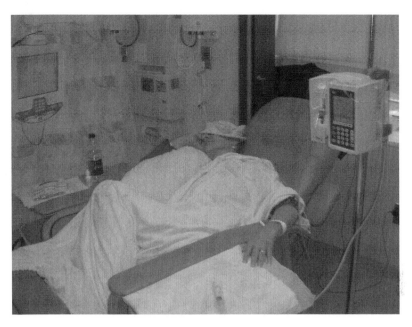

Chemo No. 5. Passed out

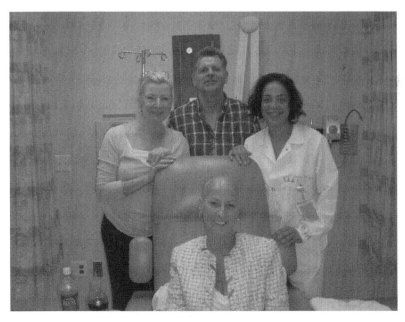

Chemo No. 6. With Mom, Larry and Lor

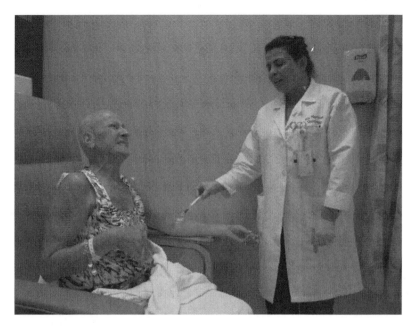

Chemo No. 8. The Burn Drug

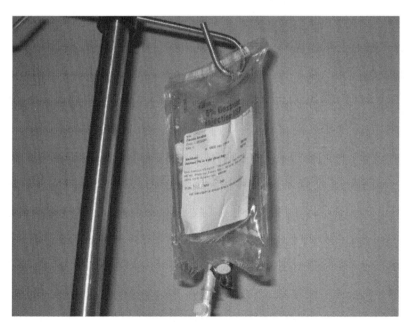

Chemo No. 8. The last dose

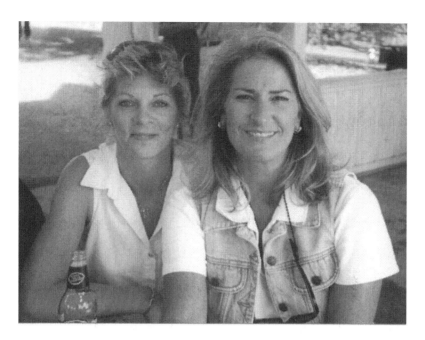

Connie, my BFF

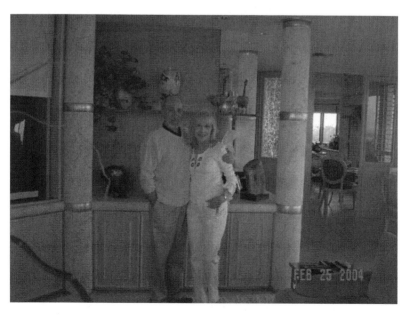

Dad and Aunt Joan

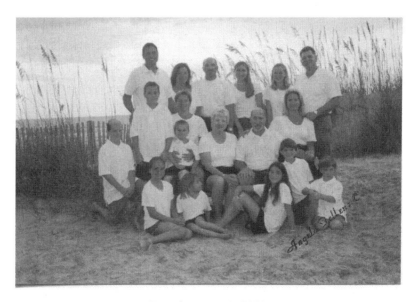

Dr. Shere's prescription

Family portrait 2003

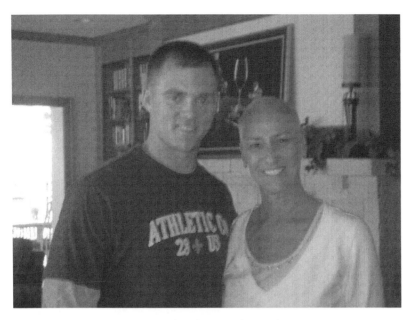

GI John embraces the suck

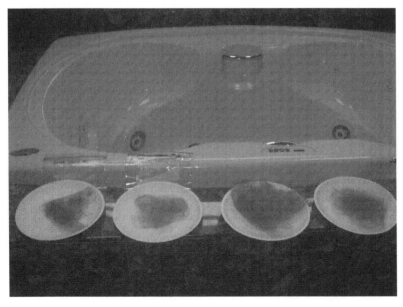

In order of the paper plates (L-R): Chemo No. 1, Chemo No. 2, during the shower before the Big Shave Party, after the shower

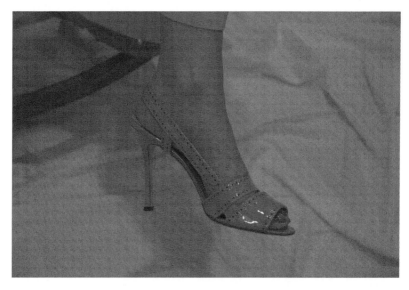

I've walked miles and miles in these slingbacks

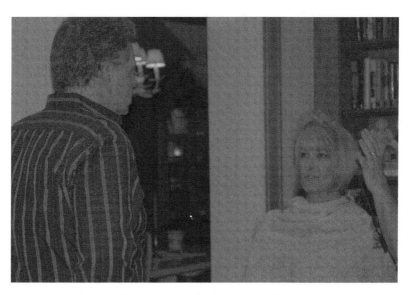

Larry checks out the new 'do

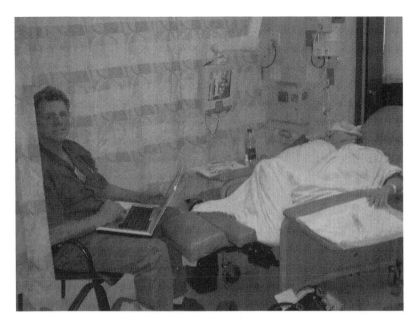

Larry works while I'm hanging there suspended in the clouds

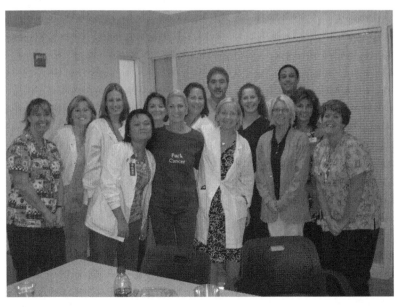

Last day of radiation. Fuck cancer! (Dr. McCall on my left,
in a black dress and white coat)

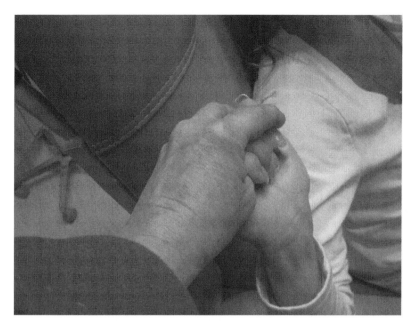

Me squeezing the crap out of Shere's hand

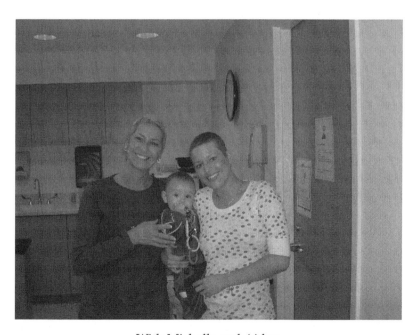

With Michelle and Aiden

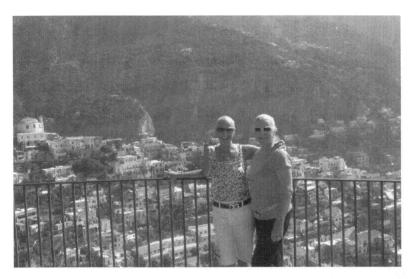

Mom and me in Sicily

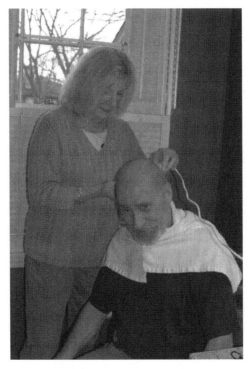

Mom shaves Dad at the Big Shave Party

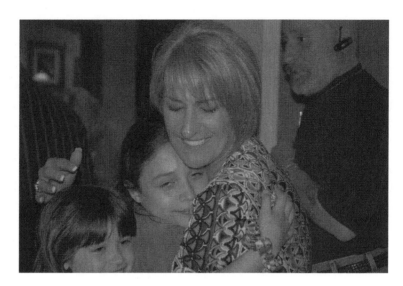

Olivia and Rachel approve the new haircut

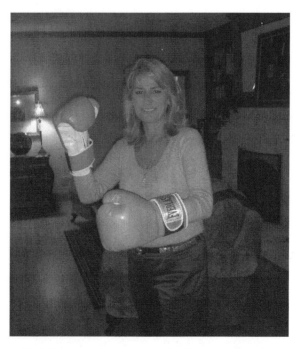

Pink boxing gloves given by Bruce and Anne
when I began my fight

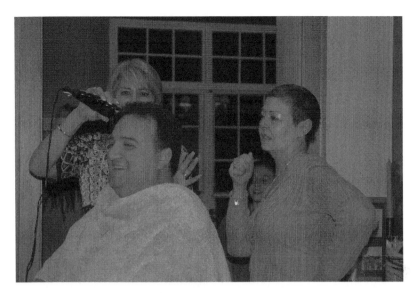

Shaving Vince

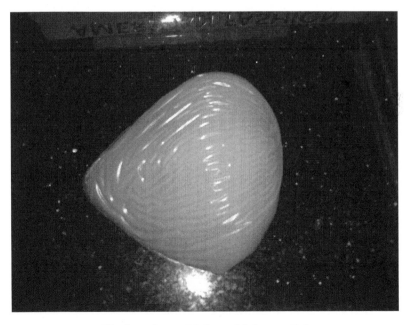

The boneless, skinless chicken cutlet

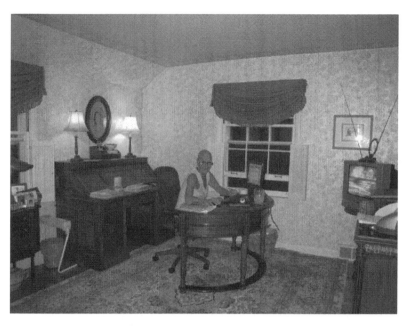

The day before my breast reconstruction surgery

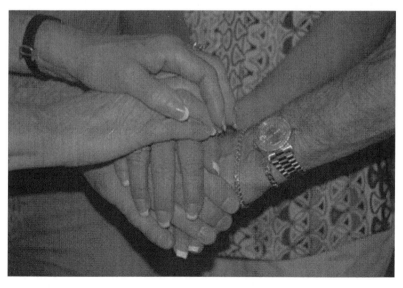

The family gets ready for the fight!

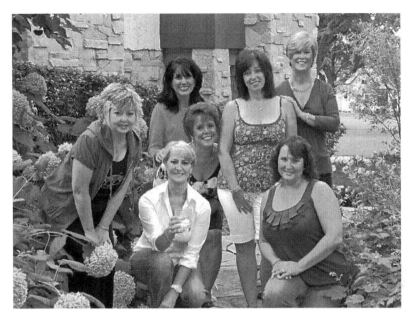

The Magnificent 7

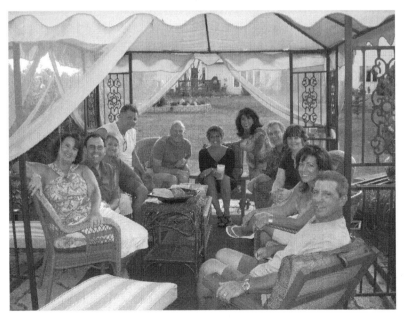

Mag 7 & their Men minus Deb and Jeff

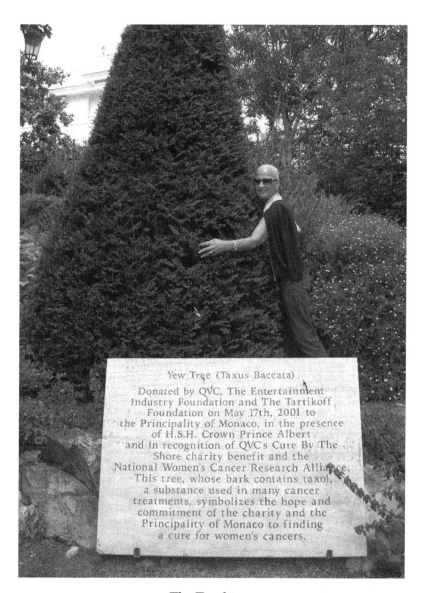

The text on the plaque reads:

Yew Tree (Taxus Baccata)
Donated by QVC, The Entertainment
Industry Foundation and The Tartikoff
Foundation on May 17th, 2001 to
the Principality of Monaco, in the presence
of H.S.H. Crown Prince Albert
and in recognition of QVC's Cure By The
Shore charity benefit and the
National Women's Cancer Research Alliance.
This tree, whose bark contains taxol,
a substance used in many cancer
treatments, symbolizes the hope and
commitment of the charity and the
Principality of Monaco to finding
a cure for women's cancers.

The Taxol tree

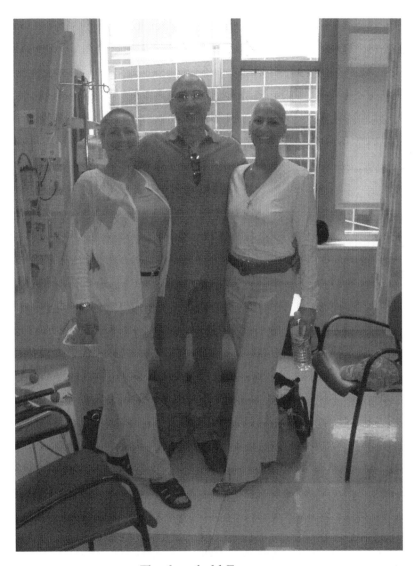

The three bald Zaccones

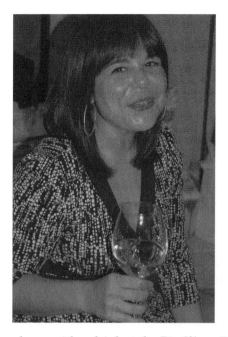

Tony relaxes with a drink at the Big Shave Party

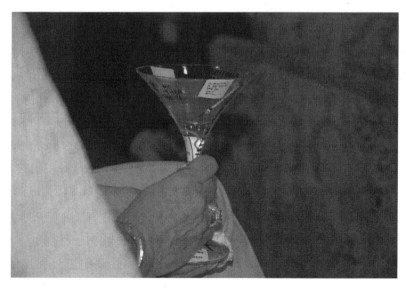

A martini a day keeps the doctor away!

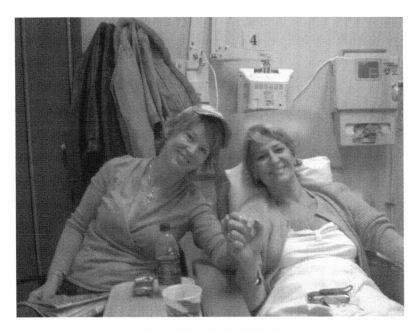

Chemo No. 3. With Debbie

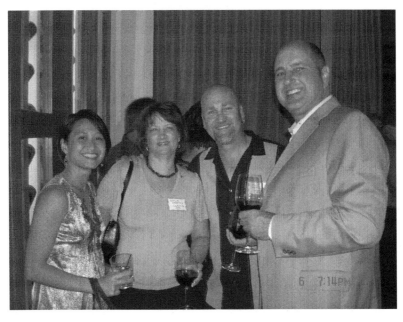

Hao, Leslie and my cousins Steve and Rick

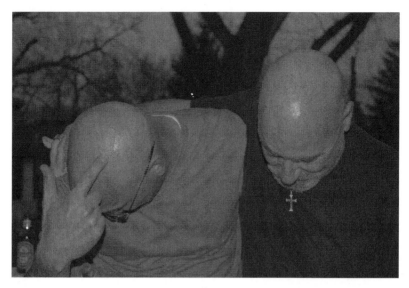

Hoping for a head that's as nicely shaped as Dad's or Bob's

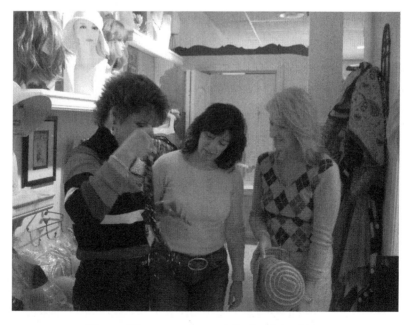

Karen, Donna and me at the boobie store

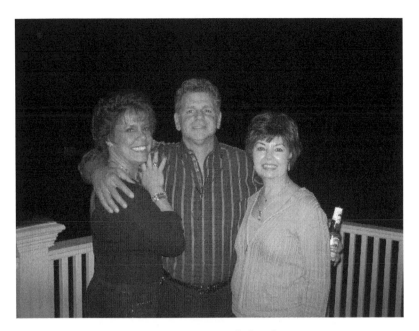

Karen, Larry and Carol

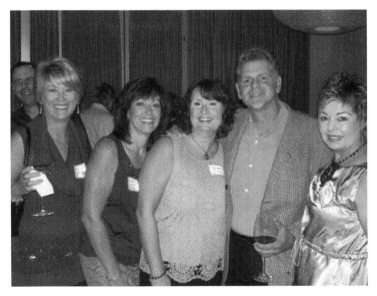

Larry and the girls

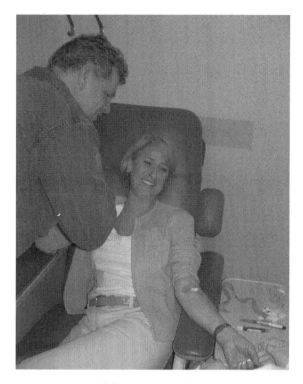

My crappy veins

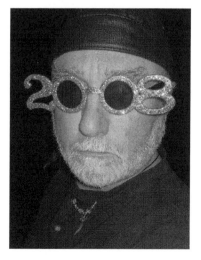

Jack bringing in 2008

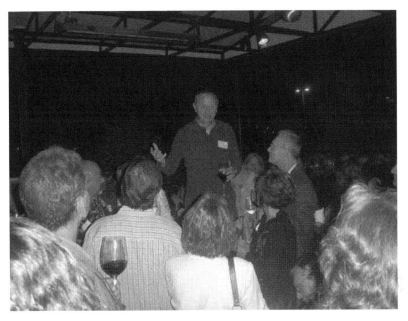

Terry's speech; Karl gets ready for his

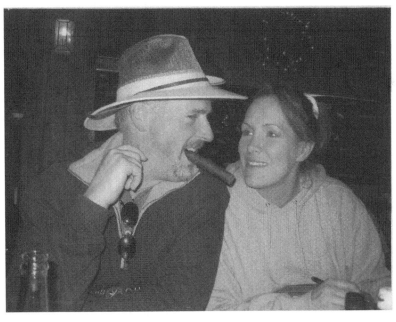

My cousin Bruce and his wife Anne

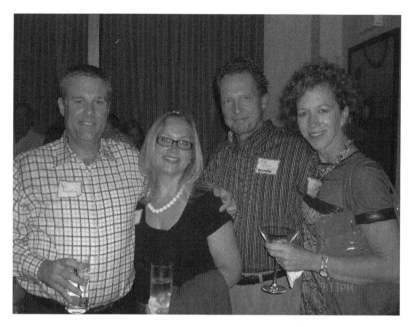

Bill, Kathleen, Mike and Cindy

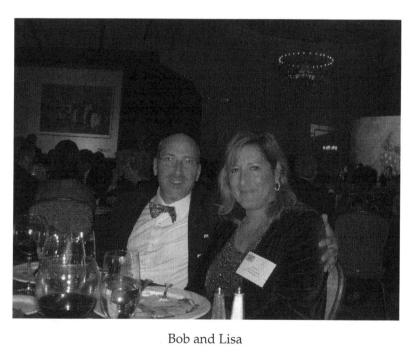

Bob and Lisa

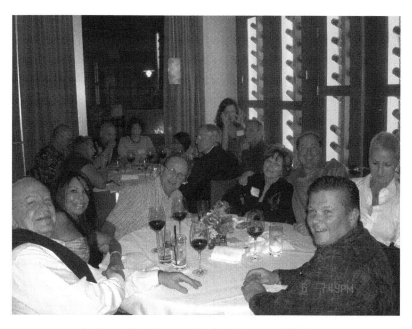

Jeffrey, Rita, Steve, Linda, Brian and Robert

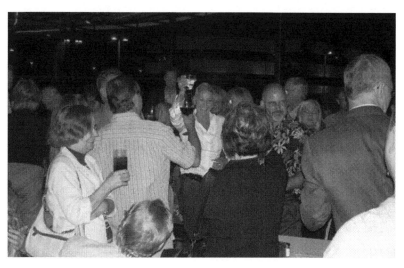

Accepting the toast from Terry and Karl

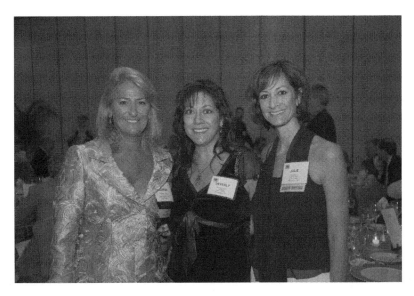

Beverly and Julie

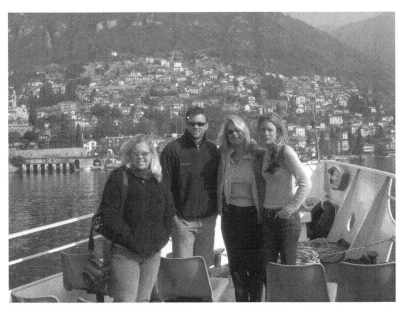

Christa, John, me and Kelly in front of
George Clooney's house in Italy

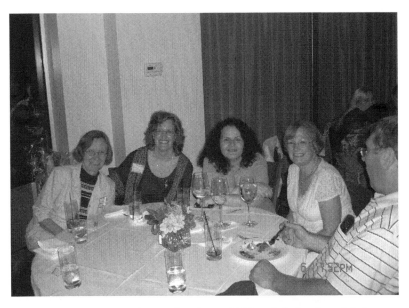

Jean, Jeanne, Sophia, Yolanda and Yolanda's husband Bob

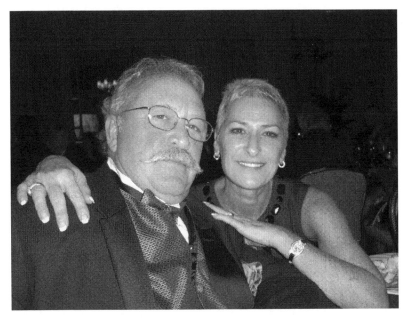

Paulie

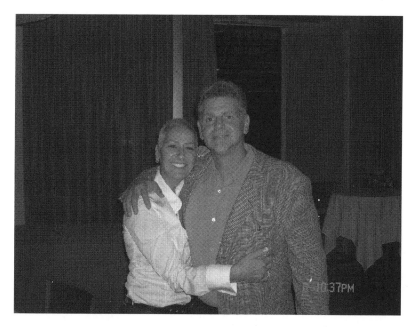

Larry and me

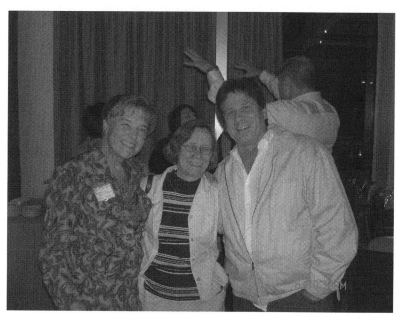

Katherine, Jean and David

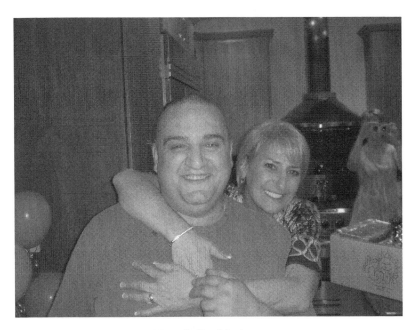

Vince's final haircut

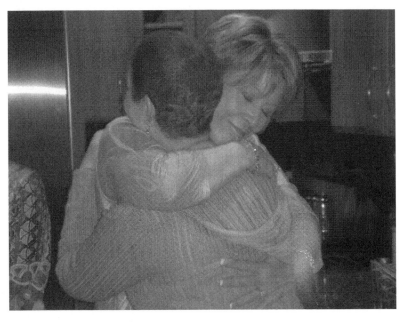

Debbie and Carol—can you feel the love?

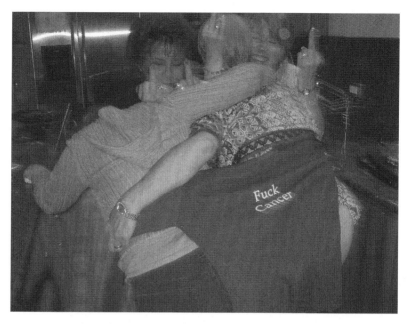

You can kiss my ass cancer!

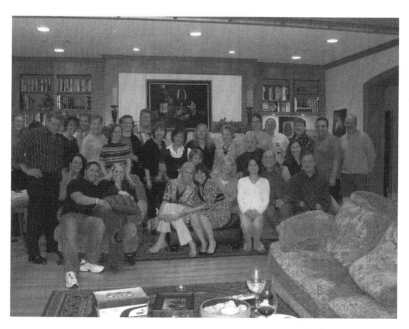

Some of the Big Shave Party attendees

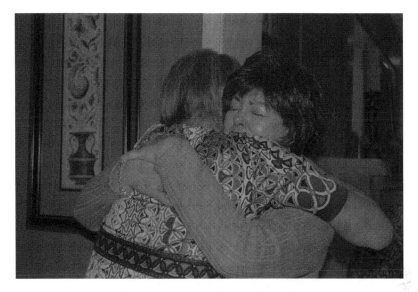

Carol crying over the shared experience

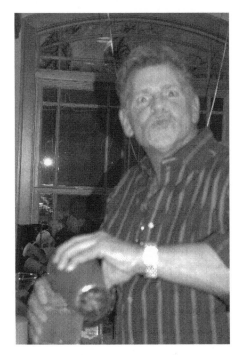

Making Larmos

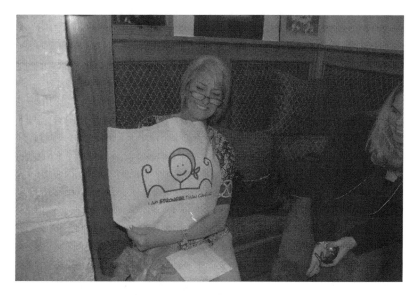

I am stronger than cancer.

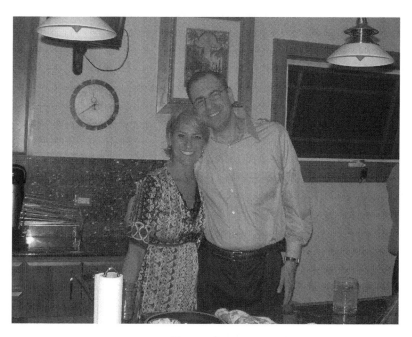

Tim and me

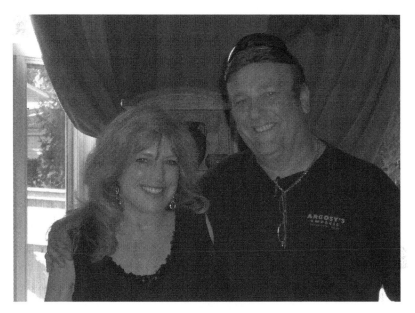

Cindy and Mark

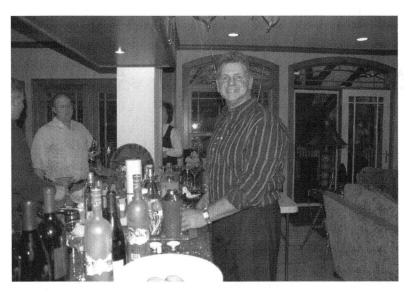

Larry at the bar for the party

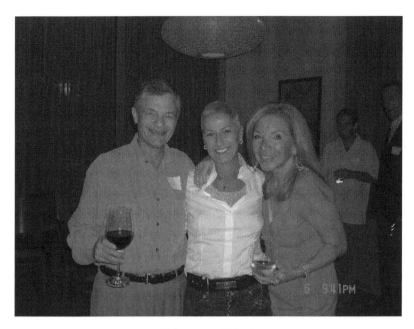

Ed, me and Toni

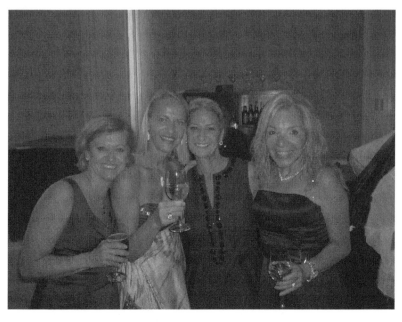

The Four Musketeers: Michelle, Karin , me and Toni

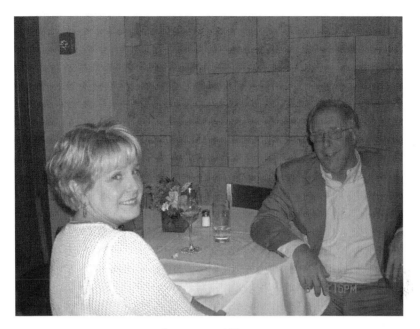

Jonette and Tom

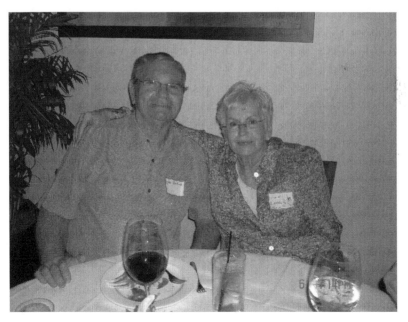

Larry's mom and dad

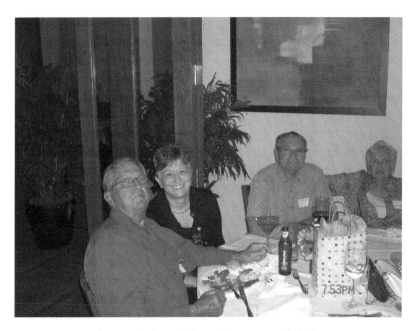

Leroy, Judy and Larry's mom and dad

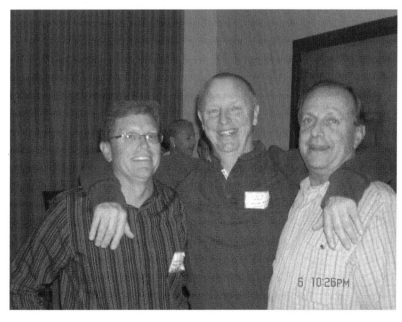

Mike, Terry and Steve

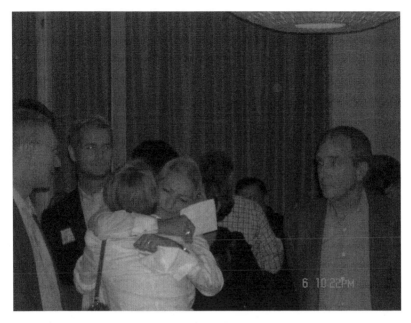

Minna and me

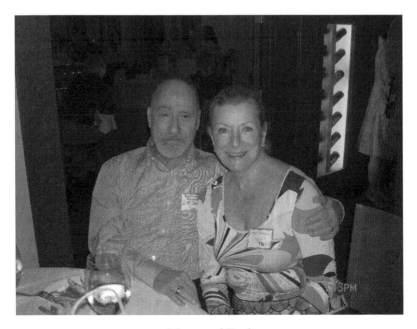

Mom and Dad

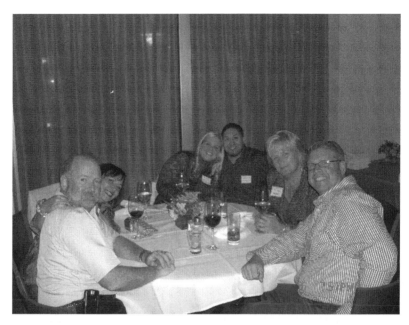

Phil, Marta, Christa, Alex, Claudia and Glenn

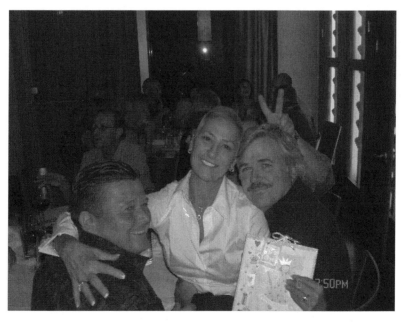

Robert and Randy

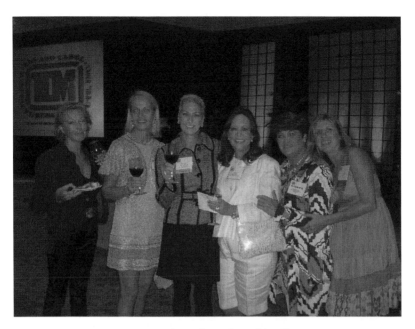

Some of my friends at TLMI

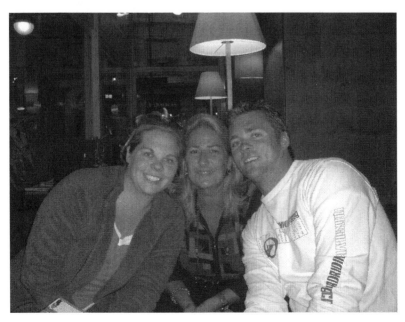

With Christa and John

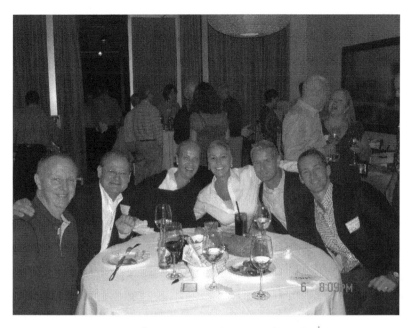

Terry, Ferd, Karin, me, Corey and Hudson

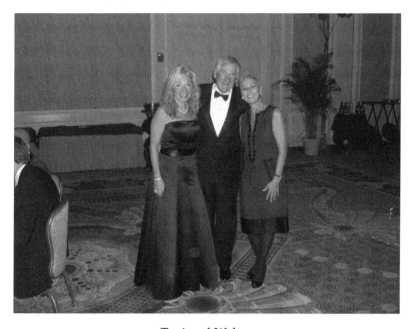

Toni and Walter

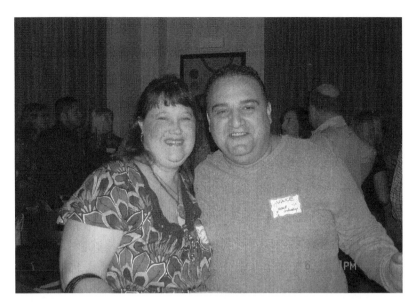

Vince and Cynthia

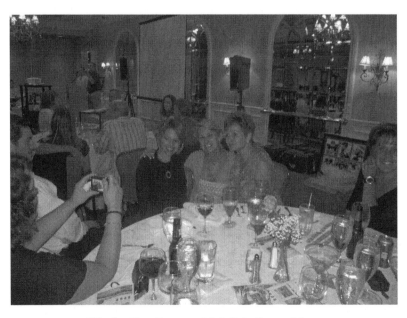

Windy City Event with Michelle and Jane
(Two of the Radiation Chick Gang)

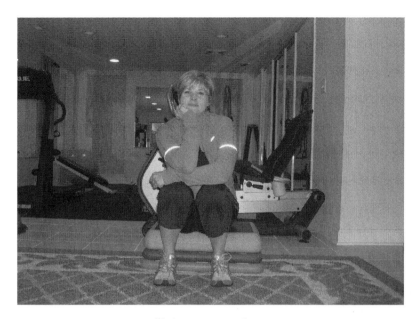

Tammy, my trainer

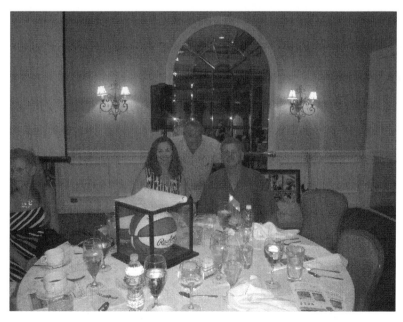

Tom, Marianne and Larry

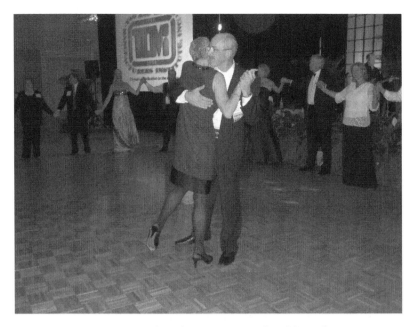

Dancing with Bob among a circle of friends

Coop, Linda, Judd, Tomi and Larry

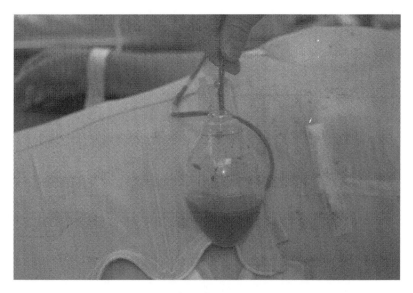

Dickie the Drain

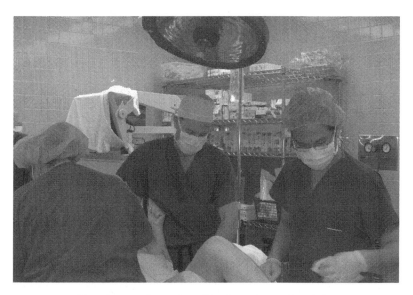

The doctors in action. Dr. Song is on the right

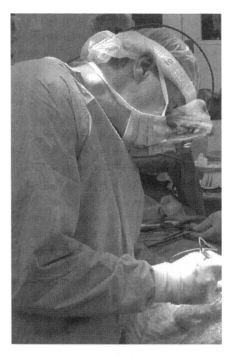

Dr. Connolly in Action

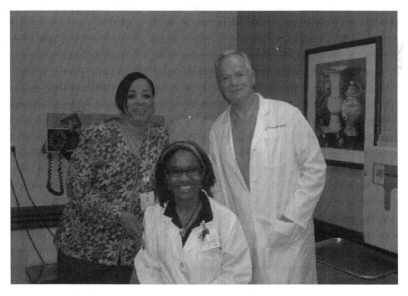

Reanetta Reed, Donna Christian, Dr. Mark Connolly

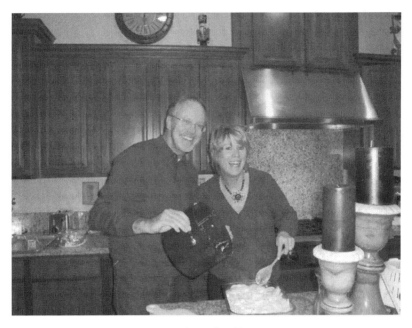

Deb and Jeff

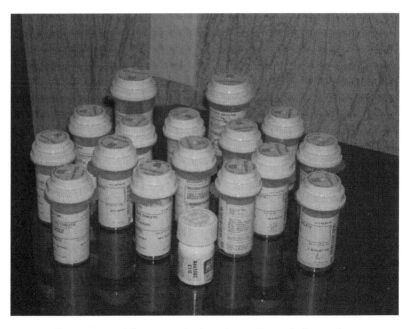

Just some of the prescription drugs I needed to take.

Chapter 65

From Strategic Planning to Strategic Plotting, All in One Day

For the past three days, our company had been engrossed in its annual Strategic Planning Sessions. I have always found this to be the perfect time to spend with our managers, reviewing their plans for the coming year after they have had similar discussions with their teams. On the second day of these meetings, I had to leave mid-morning to attend my Strategic "Plotting" Session for radiation at Edward Hospital.

As with all things medically related and never experienced before, I was anxious. Larry would meet me there, although I had tried to persuade him that it would be a waste of his time, as he would be allowed only in the waiting room. No one who didn't have to be there was allowed in the radiation area. For just a moment, I had forgotten the power of Larry's charm.

Upon arrival, I was whisked into the changing room, where they had mini gowns. What a cool idea. Instead of the long gowns that are usually provided and only get in the way, here was something that stopped where your pants started. A brilliantly simple design change that was a great deal more comfortable and much easier to manage. Jessica Keller, one of the radiation techs who had brought me into the changing room, was surprised at the ease and speed with which I took everything off from the waist up, put on the robe, and placed all my things in the locker and locked it before she had completed her introduction to their department. She didn't yet understand my motivation. In reality, I was simply trying to move things along so I could leave.

We walked down a short hallway and turned left into the radiation treatment room. It's a pretty scary place when you're the one being radiated. Machines protrude from the walls and ceiling and they move in several odd positions. It's cold. There are racks and racks of thick plastic molds that have been custom-designed for a patient to lie in, while the treatment is focused on one particular place on their body.

I saw a mask that reminded me of what Hannibal Lecter had worn in that movie with Jodie Foster. Evidently, the location of some cancers on the upper part of the body, mostly the neck and upper chest, require that the mask be worn and be anchored down to the table to restrict any and all movement. I've met someone who had to do that every day for six weeks. It was hard for her to be muzzled like that.

I found comfort in the well-designed system that they had worked out. I could already tell that this team would provide as good of an experience that could possibly be had, considering what must be done; but having a system in place that supports the end game so seamlessly and effortlessly is critical and oh-so-comforting for the patient. Anxiety grows while you wait around. They understand this and move you along as quickly as possible. So many parallels exist from this morning's Strategic Planning Session to this afternoon's Strategic Plotting Session, as far as the things that you must do differently in order to separate yourself from others: by going above and beyond what is expected in the personal and the product experience.

I was now on the same horizontal tube, and in the same position I had been in last week. My hands were above my head, clutching two poles that were there for me to hang on to. My arms fit nicely into the arm rests that seemed to be made just for me. My head was cocked to the left side to keep it from any errant rays, and to be sure that my spine was positioned properly according to the way they had strategically plotted my treatment plan. This kept my upper body in the same position each and every time. My legs were to be uncrossed. Above me was a three-panel pictorial of a beautiful scene that was there to distract you from what was happening. It was a nice attempt that fell short in the comfort department, at least from my experience. I was surrounded by tender, loving care so I could attempt to relax. I trusted this team but there were so many thoughts crashing through my head and they were louder than the equipment whirling around me. These people were amazingly efficient, honestly human and so in tune with my feelings. I felt comfortable allowing the experience to simply evolve without censorship. So I did. I allowed the experience to take me wherever it would take me.

Hillary Deeke, yet another radiation tech, sketched a green trail of ink on my chest that looked like an outline of some state on a map of the United States. A series of X-rays were taken and I could see the reflection of my upper body in the equipment that was coming around my left side where my head was tilted. The reflection was of a series of green lasers that crisscrossed my chest in strategic ways, zeroing in on the area that the doctors considered critical.

Tears were beginning to form. *Why* were my tears silently flowing again? It did not hurt a bit. I am not frightened by enclosed spaces, loud noises or odd machinery. I had laughed through much of chemo, once the needles were in; so why was I feeling such distress throughout radiation? Radiation was the easy part of the treatment plan, in comparison! I'd thought about this long and hard and could only come up with a few possibilities: chemo had literally pushed me into menopause and it had been way too early based on my family history. Maybe that was making me more emotional than normal. You know the age-old hormonal shift that is expected during menopause. All this was so new to me—and shit, I just didn't know. My heart was telling me that this was just a little piece of it, that there was more for me to consider that would be harder to reconcile.

While chemo was pretty much mandatory, radiation wasn't and here I was after all the research, the long discussions with others who have had radiation and those who have not, all those long months of soul-searching and trying hard to continue to react authentically, and I still needed to reconcile with the fact that I was willingly subjecting my body to this assault. And while the assault, for some, might be different or easier—for me, it continued to balance on that fine line between "Do I really need to do this or is it overkill?" and "Am I risking an end result that is less than what I had hoped for?"

I had yet to fully detach myself and walk forward worry-free from the results of radiation, so I continued to agonize over these questions, slowly making what should have been easy into a major event. Clinically, those in the know may reject these next thoughts, but I saw myself offering up my body to radiation rays that would, without question, affect my internal organs, those essential parts of me that I have not seen and really don't ever want to see. But then there are external results that I would see each and every day. Was I burning and hardening the skin that my surgeon had so skillfully left for me, along with the few minute senses that remained and continued to trigger a response even after surgery, when my nerves and sensory connections had been severed? Was I making a bad situation worse? Was I saving my life? Was I doing absolutely nothing but trying yet another medical invention that was yet to be fully understood?

Just before we were done with the tests, Larry arrived. We needed to drive separately today due to our schedules. How he had finagled his way into the treatment room, I've yet to discover; but it didn't surprise me. Suffice it to say, he had done it and even though he was out of arm's reach or my eyesight, simply knowing he was there was a comfort.

I was told that they wished to place tattoos on my chest to be sure that they would have the exact quadrants throughout these next six weeks. *Tattoos!* Radiation was supposed to be free from needles and all invasive procedures. They were willing to continue with the Sharpee markings but those wouldn't last through the six-week treatment plan and we would inevitably need to go through the entire planning phase all over again, several times.

I gritted my teeth, curled my toes and let them put four tattoos on my chest. I felt two of them (the bee sting was worse) and the other two were placed on the dead zone where feeling would always be a thing of the past. They dropped a dot of ink onto my skin and then inserted a needle into the first few layers to push the ink into the skin and create a mark. According to Dr. Connolly, these tattoos would be with me for life, although I must say that they seem to exist happily amongst the freckles on my chest and you'd never know their real purpose unless I told you.

Part 2 (the next day)

Today after the company's Strategic Planning meeting ended, I had an hour and a half before I needed to be at the hospital. The meeting room had been as cold as an igloo and I escaped as soon as I could. I longed to get to the warmth promised outside on a normal August day in Chicago. I decided to go home, check e-mail and take a quick catnap. That was a really bad idea.

I finally lifted my head from the warmth of the pillows and blankets at around 1:25 PM. I needed to be at the hospital at 1:45. Normally, this would be a thirty-minute drive; I was obviously going to have an issue today. Luckily, I had every light for at least seven miles, then the construction crap hit. I finally slid into the hospital at full tilt and wound my way around to the Cancer Center, thanking God that they had valet parking. I was two minutes late. The parking guy was familiar with me, saw my need to move fast, took my keys and promised to lock the doors (he knew my mantra when leaving my car). I pretty much catapulted through check-in, ended up in the changing room and afterwards spun quickly into the treatment room, somehow landing squarely on the radiation bed. *Whew!*

They placed a cold poultice, which intensified the rays, on my chest over the area to be radiated, and away we went. There was no time to get too worked up, but my psyche had had fifty years of training and it didn't take long for me to get into the reality of what was in front of me. It went quickly, probably no more than fifteen minutes, but I still had tears running down the sides of my face. I needed to get *that* in control. I am much stronger than what I was presenting to the world over these past few days. That is what I kept telling myself, at least.

Chapter 66

The New Chick Gang, a Caveat and a String

Arriving at the radiation changing room either before or after treatments and appointments, I saw the same women every day. We talked easily with each other, even as some of us remained strangers. Sometimes names weren't exchanged; sometimes they didn't need to be. We were serving our time for myriad reasons: breast cancer, brain cancer, Hodgkin's lymphoma. These were just a few of the cancers gracing this room. Larry always teased me about having too many groups of what he called "chick gangs," so he was not at all surprised when I came home with stories about the amazing women I'd met during this scheduled stop on my road to survival.

I met Michelle Rosch during my first week of radiation therapy. This year, after turning twenty-seven years old, she had been diagnosed with breast cancer during her eighth month of pregnancy. Her situation was so dire that her pregnancy needed to be induced a month early so that a bi-lateral mastectomy (both breasts removed) could be performed. She had the expanders for her implants placed during that surgery. Before chemo, she harvested as many eggs as possible so that she and her husband could continue their family one day. Her sister-in-law would carry their future babies. I was getting to know another fabulous example of an amazing family.

A month later, she began chemo and then went right into radiation therapy. She was scheduled for surgery in November to remove her ovaries and uterus, a complete hysterectomy, as she carries the BRCA gene for cancer and is at great risk for cancer there, as well. She was now going through full-blown menopause, complete with all the associated lovely physical responses, such as hot flashes—at *twenty-seven.*

I had to ask her: "How did you do it? How *do* you do it?" First having major mind-blowing surgery and chemo, now radiation, menopause and a *baby* during all of it! Of course, she had help from family and friends, but she said that her son Aiden and husband Michael had brought her through the hardest times. She fiercely lived on for them. And she was blessed with an incredibly beautiful and healthy boy who is always happy and smiling. He came with her every day. We all doted on him and Michelle let us look after him while she was having her treatments. He loved being the main attraction and he never failed to bring smiles to all of our faces, no matter where our minds had taken us that day. He symbolized a new chance for total health.

After nine months of this crap, Michelle and I had come to terms with showing our battle scars when the situation really called for it. It was especially easy to do this with someone in the sisterhood. Up went her shirt and she showed me her radiation area. She was about four weeks ahead of me with her treatments. Under her left arm, it looked as though she had been burned with an iron in some terrible torturous event. It was so red, dry, puckered, irritated and sore that it brought tears to my eyes.

Warnings and suggestions were given on what she had done wrong and how I might save myself from the same fate. "Moisturize, moisturize, moisturize." she'd say, "and then, moisturize again!" Michelle advised me to "lather on creams and lotions as thick as you possibly can and don't forget to reach up to your neck and your ears on the side being radiated."

She knew that she couldn't abandon the process and that she must cooperate and allow the medical people to do what they needed to do. Some may say she is courageous. Michelle saw it as a situation that she needed to see through to the end in order to be with her family. She shared her story without tears, anger or a cry for pity and she wore this adorable brown fabric head covering every day. I had a hard time believing that it was her radiation hat. It was probably the easiest and most comfortable thing to wear during her incredibly busy day.

Michelle wanted to know my situation—how long had it been since chemo ended?—as she was looking forward to getting a little hair back. Hers was coming in randomly, in just a few areas of her head. She couldn't go without those fabric head coverings or the specially designed hats that we "in the business" know all too well. I told her that it had been two months since my chemo ended. She quickly looked over at her husband, reminding him that in six weeks she would finally have a little hair.

Here before me sat this young family struck by such a horrible experience so early in their lives. I couldn't keep my eyes off of that familiar brown hat. I mentioned that I had a bunch of hats that I had bought and wondered if she would like a few, as I was done using them. An audible gasp meant I had hit a hot spot; she loved these things as much as I hated them. I only asked that she find someone who really needed them when she no longer did. For the record, I would not pass on any hat or head covering that was given to me. Those will remain with me as a special reminder of life, and how that piece of cloth kept me warm and allowed me to go out in public during those very early days.

The Zaccone Family Foundation's charter is to help people who have no other options, and while Michelle would not be a candidate for our help, I felt compelled to share what I had that she liked and I was no longer wearing. Michelle is one of those people who is easy to be around and I liked her instantly. Her attitude is so wonderfully honest and she consistently maintains an amazingly positive spirit for someone so young and experiencing such a loss. She was always helpful towards others paying it forward in her way. This disease needs young advocates like her. I was also confident that she would follow through on my request to pass on the hats when she was done; paying it forward.

Then there was Rose Maza, whose sister had died of Non-Hodgkin's lymphoma a few years ago. Rose was being treated for Hodgkin's lymphoma. She has three kids and is in her mid-thirties. Her oldest son pretends that everything is fine, while he silently worries about Mom, moving very carefully when he is around her. This is not normal for him. Her middle son cries a lot, like she does, and her five-year-old daughter keeps asking her what happened to her hair and when will it come back. Rose is terrified of dying. She continues to have bone pain, the chills, symptoms of neuropathy in her hands and feet and many sleepless nights that she spends on the computer—researching. Questioning everything that is happening to her versus what she is reading, and crying a lot. We hug every day. She must have her head bolted in place during radiation and her hands clamped down while she is situated in this uncomfortable form they had made for her to lie in. Rose was one of those who needed to wear Hannibal Lecter's mask. Her last treatment would be tomorrow, and we would all celebrate.

Jane Koulianos had found her breast cancer early on and they were able to treat her with surgery and chemotherapy. She was spared the issues with radiation altogether. Jane met Michelle and Aiden in chemo and they too formed an instant bond. Jane would arrive with Michelle when she could, and look after Aiden when Michelle went in for her radiation treatment. Jane, married with two children, holds the same fears that all of us do. We do not look forward to coming to radiation every day, but we do look forward to seeing each other.

The last chick of this gang is Ruth. Ruth went through a lumpectomy, chemo and radiation eighteen years ago before her cancer came back in the other breast earlier this year. She is in her early seventies and is a pistol. She reminded us that eighteen years ago, things had been prehistoric; we were encouraged by her words and our knowledge of how things have improved, but I know we all were silently wondering: *Will it come back for me, too?*

OK, but how does all of this relate to the chapter's title? Well, if you know of or learn of a woman in need of hats or fabric head coverings, send her my way. When I run out of those I've purchased, I will purchase more. The "caveat" is that the person has a true and honest need: *Do I buy a hat or buy food for my family?* And the "string" is that they pay it forward. We'll start small and generate a blazing movement that will hopefully grab the attention of many others.

Chapter 67

A Cord to the Right of Me, a Mammogram to the Left Here I Am Stuck in the Middle with One Boob

During each week of radiation I was to meet with one of the nurses, Sue or CeCe and then Dr. McCall. This meeting would take place every Wednesday after treatment. We would take care of the usual weight, temperature and blood pressure routine, a zillion questions would be asked and answered and then whichever nurse was available would take a look.

The first time we met, three days after I started treatments, Nurse Sue marveled at the excellent result obtained by the skills of Dr. Connolly, and she asked about my thoughts on reconstruction surgery. Once again, she was impressed by him. He had been quite clear when we talked about this subject months ago and I knew that I had to wait for at least six months after radiation before I could even consider reconstruction. Time must pass for all of radiations effects to end, and this time is crucially important to the final result. I certainly didn't want to have reconstruction early and end up with one boob higher than the other due to the shrinking and shifting possibilities with radiation. And I definitely wanted to reduce the number of surgeries to get to the final result.

Evidently, this was the time during early radiation treatment when nurses bear down and pull all of their energy in close, getting ready for a fight, a long discussion with a hysterical woman or one who just melts when they hear this news; many surgeons fail to go into these details with their patients. Some of the women I went through radiation with, had implants or expanders already set in their bodies and others planned to have their operation too soon after treatment. I worried about that for them. You kind of get close to these women. You see each other every day for six weeks for the same reason; how could you not get close? Many doctors feel that the trauma of waking up after surgery with one breast or no breasts and living with that for more than a year is far worse than the extra reconstruction surgery that may be required later, if they were to have to have radiation. I could relate. Not having to convince me that I must wait for the next step and since I answered just one question in a way that sent up her nurse alert, I was able to see the doctor earlier than scheduled.

One of the questions I was asked about was how my range of motion was progressing. I had been diligently working on that, beginning a few weeks after surgery, as I knew the problems ahead if I didn't. Tammy Hemmingway, my trainer, sets up her routines and exercises to target these areas, and even Dr. Connolly was impressed with my agility so early after surgery. It continued to improve each time that I saw him. But over the last few days, I'd noticed that when I reached up to squeegee off the water from the glass surrounding the shower, it hurt like a new pair of shoes. It was tight and I felt a sharp pull. I chalked it up to regular workouts and thought that I was probably developing some ultra cool-looking muscle that would look hot as hell in a bathing suit next year. Wrong. She asked me how much weight I was lifting. I told her that we move around from three-, five-, eight- and ten-pound weights with many repetitions. That wasn't it. Crap!

And then it came to me: moving the zillion and a half boxes into the lake house last week and occasionally adjusting the angle of some piece of furniture. Could that have been it? Nurse Sue confirmed that this was probably what moved things along, although the root cause was my having lymph nodes removed.

I had developed what is called a "cord" that runs along the inside of my right arm from deep inside my armpit down to just past my elbow.

A cord (a.k.a. axillary web syndrome) is a painful condition that has been identified as a complication of axillary lymph node dissection. Therefore, all women with breast cancer who have had lymph nodes removed must take heed. The syndrome often shows itself as a visible cord from the armpit area to—in some cases—all the way down to the hand, and is characterized by pain and what is called lymphedema or swelling in the soft tissue of the arm. Up to seventy percent of breast cancer survivors experience some symptoms of lymphedema, although many cases are mild. A cord is a lymphatic channel that becomes inactive once the lymph node has been removed. Occasionally, a lymphatic channel can become a scarred-down cord.

Everyone has lymphatic channels and lymph nodes. The channels are located throughout your body (even in your elbow) and are connected to the lymph nodes. You have somewhere between five hundred and six hundred lymph nodes. The channels are too numerous to count. The precise locations of each person's lymph channels are as varied as their fingerprints. They are very thin tubes that look and feel like fishing lines and are an important part of your circulatory system, as they carry lymphatic fluid to your lymph nodes. When your heart pumps with either increased exercise or movements, this very important filter helps pump blood and fluid throughout your system.

In my case, twenty-eight nodes were taken out of my body from under my armpit (axillary area). The lymph channels remain but are rendered useless and therefore can turn into post-op cords, eventually learning new pathways or simply dying away. When these small fishing line-like cords or channels scar down to the tissue and attach themselves, they become a painful cord.

Because many or most of my lymph nodes in that arm had been removed, the lymphatic fluid really had nowhere to travel through to get cleaned up and taken care of, so it moved around the arm until it was either absorbed by my body or redirected toward other fully operating lymph nodes in other areas of my body. Those other lymph channels and nodes would thankfully pick up the slack. Since the lymph channels in my arm are inactive, the cord becomes more prominent. It results in limited range of motion through my arm and chest wall. There has been some discussion amongst the medical profession as to whether the cord is made up of lymph tissue or nerve tissue; but in any case, the lymphatic system is incredibly complex from the initial vessels that pick up fluid to the lymph nodes that filter it.

The way to respond to this dilemma is through Occupational or Physical Therapy and intervention involving gentle stretching of the soft tissue which can be helpful in relieving the pain and increasing flexibility. After the cord is sufficiently stretched and the adhesions are released, the cord disappears over time. Heat is contraindicated and is only used as a last resort when all other treatment options have failed. Heat, as we all know, causes swelling and actually worsens the problem by flooding the area with more fluids than necessary. A fine balance must be maintained if and when heat would be applied, and it should only be applied for short periods of time under the strict observance of a professional; and the heat should be moist heat.

Wearing a compression sleeve can also aid in the reduction of fluid that goes into your initial lymphatic by reducing the space on the tissue to prevent excess fluid from accumulating. Some women need to wear a compression sleeve while working out, and any breast cancer patient who has had lymph nodes removed must wear a compression sleeve when flying. The reason for this is because while flying through the air strapped in an aluminum tube, you have decompression effects of altitude and air pressure changes. These changes in pressure dilate your vessels and allow increased fluid volume to travel through these larger vessels. When the pressure returns to normal upon landing, your body may not be able to transport the excessive fluid out of the involved or at-risk extremity. The compression sleeve will keep the interstitial tissue compact so that the lymphatics can pick up larger molecules and clear out the area faster. Without the sleeve, changes in pressure allow more fluid to accumulate and tissue space to increase. And issues develop if the affected areas are unable to keep up with the transfer of fluids to the lymph collectors throughout your system.

Fortunately, all of these non-invasive treatments open up the valves that are in your lymphatic channel so that the fluids can be redirected.

As with all people who have had lymph nodes removed, meticulous skin care especially with my right hand and arm is more important now than ever before. If you develop signs of lymphedema, the risk of infection in that arm is increased. The lymph fluid that is collected is protein rich and such an environment can encourage bacterial growth. The lymph system is not in its usual defensive mode and is not properly filtering out the offending bacteria and viruses; therefore, any breakdown in the integrity of the skin results in susceptibility to bacteria, infection and cellulitis, the most serious of complications, but one I am sure I can avoid. With all of the traveling I have done, I am a nut case about washing my hands frequently and keeping as clear of germy things as I possibly can. Ask anyone in my family or anyone who has traveled with me. It's almost manic. What I really needed to worry about was the fact that I am such a klutz (remember my nickname "Bruizanne"?) and by moving faster than sometimes is necessary, I can easily envision myself creating a cut, scratch or scrape somewhere along the way. Now it was imperative that I immediately treat all cuts, burns, bruises, hangnails, ingrown nails, ingrown hairs, razor rashes, blisters, scrapes, mosquito bites, et cetera—as they are potential sites for infection.

I need to avoid heavy lifting: carrying purses, hauling luggage and bags or using over-the-shoulder straps on the side where I've had surgery. Strained muscles cause inflammation, so vigorous and repetitive movements against resistance can cause a rapid and sudden blood flow through the muscle and tissue, further impacting an already compromised system.

Therefore, I shall give up any thoughts of becoming a weight lifter or boxer.

Use of an electric razor versus a standard razor with a blade is recommended to decrease the possibility of cuts in my armpit. In my case, where numbness is present, this becomes pretty critical. Tight jewelry and elastic bands should be moved over to my left arm. Using hypoallergenic soap, deodorant and lotions without alcohol, dyes or fragrance that tend to dry the skin—are also a good idea. Extreme changes in temperature should be avoided (hot tubs), sunscreen is imperative and staying away from injections and needle sticks as well as chemicals in cleaning supplies is also important, as they dry out the skin and can create cracks that can become infectious entry points.

Safety can be accomplished by always wearing gloves (the same caution is needed for gardening, washing dishes and using knives or sharp instruments; I could really get out of doing *a lot* of stuff!). My blood pressure and blood draws need to be taken on the left arm, and should any signs or symptoms of infection or cellulitis be noticed, I need to contact the doctor immediately. Any delay in treatment will enable the infection to spread to other areas throughout my body.

In order to get rid of this Cord, I now need to call the Occupational Therapist. As if I really want *cancer* or a *cord* to become my new occupation. (I have yet another reason to abhor "C" words. The list is growing.) My first appointment with the Occupational Therapist would be on Monday, September 15th, when I would ask more questions.

The week before I was to meet with the Occupational Therapist, Dr. McCall and I talked again about this syndrome during our regular meeting. While she was examining my arm, she smiled and advised me that I could forget about OT, at least for now. Somehow, probably because I consistently worked out, the fluids had broken down and moved out all evidence of the Cord. It had been there a week ago. She had seen it before she had felt it, and now *poof!* Gone! Having quite enough on my medical plate, I was only too happy to agree to cancel those appointments.

Oncology breast cancer specialists work very hard to bring the patient and their lives back to a pre-cancer position and to provide them with the necessary tools, as well as the toolbox for the prevention of future issues. My short course on the lymphatic system included charts, plastic examples and diagrams on the wall.

I continue to be amazed at how complex our bodies and the world of medicine are. I now understand the fascination my sister has always had for the field of medicine even before she had become a doctor. I wonder if people had more knowledge about the inner workings of their bodies if they would make better choices for their lives. Once you receive an education like I had in the past nine months, you gain a newfound respect for the most incredible machine ever made.

On the fourteenth day of radiation, I had a mammogram appointment at the University of Chicago early in the morning. After getting lefty smashed to a tortilla in three different angles, I went back to the waiting room with other anxious women and awaited my verdict. My name was called again by Nurse Yolanda, a very compassionate lady who had been gentle with me during the procedure, explaining everything along the way. Although I'd been through this drill so many times before in previous years, it all suddenly seemed new to me and I appreciated the extra time and care. My previous experience was that if everything was OK, the nurse came back to the waiting room and said something like, "Suzanne, you are good to go." At which point I would already be half-dressed, peeling out the door and thinking to myself: *Clear for another year!* The only time I had been asked to see a doctor was on the day I was diagnosed.

This time, when I was asked to come back to see the doctor, I actually stopped breathing. I immediately imagined the worst, dabbed at the slowly falling tears with my ever-present Kleenex, followed Yolanda down a long hallway and readied myself for the news. Yolanda, just ahead of me, was talking away but I didn't hear a word she said. Had I heard, I would have learned that I should be doing a double back flip, as *everything was fine!* Entering the doctor's office, Yolanda and the doctor immediately recognized the confusion and assured me that I was OK and that their protocol was to always meet with the patient to talk with them and be available for any questions or concerns, and to show the film images. As if I'd even know what I was seeing or looking for! We had a great conversation. The doctor gave me her opinions on reconstruction surgeons that she has seen the "before" and "after" results of, and then away I went. Practically doing those double back flips back to the changing room.

My new post-mammogram mantra is: "Lefty is alrighty!"

Later that day, while in the radiation department at Edward Hospital, I was given more good news. My blood pressure is that of a nineteen-year-old and Dr. McCall would like to bottle and sell it and retire.

Rose graduated radiation today. She looked happy and very relieved. We traded phone numbers and e-mail addresses, promising to stay in touch. I gave her a plant that for me symbolized life. She introduced me to her husband; we hugged, we laughed and we cried, agreeing that life is good.

Chapter 68

When the Dark Days Come, Let Them Come

When my girlfriend Carol was diagnosed with breast cancer, I made sure to stay very close to what was happening to her both mentally and physically. I made sure that I was supportive without being smothering. I was convinced that I'd really gotten it; that I was intimately involved enough to truly understand what she was experiencing. I was wrong. You see, I could go home to my life. Become absorbed in other things once I'd left her or hung up the phone. *She* lived with it for twenty-four hours a day, seven days a week—and would for the rest of her life. It consumed you and in a sense, haunted you as well. It is just recently that I can honestly say that I truly get it.

Many of the people on my e-mail list have battled cancer of one kind or another and have openly shared their experiences and suggestions with me. Others, while not having had cancer, are still able to open my mind and allow whatever is in there to work its way out. It is amazing how similar some of their advice has been. Like allowing the dark days or moments to come, and exploring and not denying those thoughts and feelings, while at the same time reminding me of the importance of finding a way to keep them in perspective, never allowing myself to stay in that place for very long. I've listened and worked hard to stay honest with my feelings, thoughts and fears and everything they have said has helped. The support they've demonstrated provides a safe place to confront this stuff and not simply shove it all under the rug, leaving it alone in the darkness to be repeatedly walked on until the next dark day returns and it slithers back out. I am often in awe of how others handle it. Those who have little support or who choose to deal with their demons in silence because they feel they must or they know it is the only way for them. I've witnessed dozens of ways to continue life with this disease; some are quite noble while others are quite ugly.

For groceries, I prefer to shop at small specialty establishments where you get to know the owners and their employees and inevitably, run into the same customers every so often. I frequent a butcher shop, fruit store, bakery and a small family-owned grocery store that are all scattered within a few miles of our house. For me, it is akin to pretending that we live in Europe, shopping at each establishment for that perfect item—only minus the huge wicker basket in my arms, the mountains in the background and the music playing softly.

At the grocery store, there are four people who have worked there for many years that Larry and I went to high school with. Several months ago, one of the cashiers I do not know, noticed my hairless head and said, "You, too?" I looked up at her and immediately recognized that she was wearing a wig. So we talked and traded stories. She had had breast cancer five years ago, had gone through all of the treatments, several grueling reconstruction surgeries and now it was back. And it was back with a vengeance. One little microscopic fucker had slipped past chemo and radiation and it had returned and was in her bones, lung and brain. She kept losing her footing and breaking bones in her arms and wrist, which were sure signs of a metastasis to her bones. But she was fighting hard once again, as evidenced by the fact that we were talking while she was working.

It is difficult to adequately explain to you how emotional that moment was for both of us. As if propelled forward by a clock she heard pounding—not ticking—she quickly listed the things that she thought she might have done wrong, overlooked, accepted without question or didn't fully research or understand. Her words cut directly to the points she wanted to share, her voice imploring me not to make the same mistakes and her eyes, like mine, welling up with tears. In the middle of the day, in a grocery store, two strangers cried together while holding hands across the conveyor belt that continued to run with nothing on it.

What she had told me had taken on terrifying significance. How do you possibly learn all that you need to learn in order to make the best choices when cancer has accelerated the rate at which your own clock ticks? When decisions are measured and must be made in days and weeks, not years?

I asked my high school friends Sue Heinke and Tony Bellisario about her whenever I was in the store. When I asked today, they quickly looked at each other, wondering if they should tell me. That simple reflective gesture told me all that I needed to know.

It's a dark day.

I would like to share with you an insight I've had. You may consider these words as simple and trivial musings of a person looking too hard for answers to questions that have no answers. Or you may consider it as I do: just a personal insight. A thought, an idea, a semblance of words that some might look at more closely while others will brush quickly aside. No more and no less, as only you can decide if these words have meaning for you. But first, an explanation is in order.

People have asked me at one time or another, "How are you feeling?" I would generally answer, "Great," "Not bad" or "Doing pretty well." Once in a while, I might bring you into the gory details. But think about it . . . As you travel through your day, how many people ask you, "How are you?" or "How ya doing?" I would guess there are probably dozens. Do you honestly think that most of them really care, or want to hear the details about your kid throwing up this morning on the suit that you were planning to wear to that key presentation? Or that Mom or Dad is sick? That your aunt has cancer and your son flunked the second grade? That the dog bit the neighbor's kid over the weekend and they are now not speaking to you as they watch this child closely for signs of foaming at the mouth?

No. They simply want to hear that you are "Doing pretty well." That you, like them, are coping.

First, you must understand that timing is important here. I would not suggest you ask this question when the person is obviously having a really good day. My insight is this: when someone you feel comfortable with who is faced with a life threatening situation, presents themselves to you and you notice that they are not behaving as they normally would, if they seem to be lost inside themselves or overly quiet and reflective, and if you feel like you are ready to hear what may be a difficult answer, you might consider asking this question instead: "*What are you feeling?*"

Dr. McCall asked me this after she had caught wind of one of the more emotional days in the radiation changing room. Totally threw me off balance. This question places even the savviest individual in a place where "Great," "Not bad" and "Doing pretty well" just don't cut it. It forces them to confront and share their real feelings, if they can, about the situation. Those things that move far beyond what the doctors tell you that you may, should, could or might experience. If they are unable to answer the question at that time, for whatever reason, they at least know that you are a soft place to land on when they just might need one. They will know this because only a person who truly wants to get an answer, will ask this question.

The answers are sometimes raw, potentially unsettling and quite often when discussed in detail are not for the faint of heart. But in all cases, if the person gets started, they will be honest. And there will be opportunities for real human connections.

You might hear—

"I am exhausted and feel that I am placing too much on my husband's plate." "How can I afford this and still pay for food?" "I'm freaking out, it hurts so badly—one day mentally, one day physically then they both come together with a crushing blow." "My body keeps changing and I don't like it—how will anyone else?" "My kids are upset and are acting out and I am too weak to keep any of it in control." "I look in the mirror at the new me and it takes my breath away each time." "I am tired of crying and not being able to pinpoint why." "I have thoughts so terrifying that they stop me dead in my tracks while slowly yet steadily nibbling away at my mind." "I am weary of pretending to be stronger than I feel, and I am wondering if I might die earlier than I should."

The chick gang from radiation therapy was constantly consoling someone every day. There is so much anxiety wrapped around cancer that never seems to completely leave you. And because some of it won't easily fold up and fit nicely in a heavy box with a big bow that you can store away on the top shelf of a rarely used closet—we find ourselves becoming easily upset, frightened, medically suspicious and it often happens for no apparent reason.

I met Larry at a favorite restaurant the other night. We drove there and home in separate cars. I cried the entire seven minutes driving home. I have no flipping idea why. It just comes. Nothing was said, heard or imagined to upset me. It was a lovely dinner. It just comes.

It has been exhausting to put a happy face on this one all the time, so instead of being the Suzanne who motored around the world actively seeking the next new adventure and feeling comfortable engaging strangers in conversation, I kind of sequestered myself. Lately, I ventured out a great deal more than I did in the early days when spontaneous crying would erupt without warning, but I was still staying closer to home than I ever have before. For the first time in over twenty years, I traveled on just four airplanes in nine months and that was all on the same trip! It's kind of nice, but at the same time a little sad.

I smiled and pulled my bathrobe around me just a bit tighter, remembering that the dark days pass quickly, too. Then I gazed out the large picture windows at the crisp fall weather, knowing that winter was coming fast—and not long from now, one of us would be left behind; an expectation that, whether we like it or not, would inevitably be met. I savored the moment. Another season had passed and I was still writing.

Chapter 69

The Case of the Disappearing Tattoos

The last two weeks of radiation were the hardest, as you might expect. The treatment symptoms are cumulative and the effects add up faster and faster as the days move on. Towards the end, I had to just about force myself to get in the car and drive to the hospital. The good news was that I rarely had a runny nose or drippy eyes, my hair was starting to grow back and my eyebrows and eyelashes were closer to where they had been before all of this had happened. Neuropathy in my fingers and toes returned once in a while but never lasted too long. By the time I felt the tingles and knew that it had come back, I could sense that the symptom was easing up and everything would soon return to my "new normal." The lingering chemo symptoms were that my lower legs felt dead while lying down in bed. Kind of like the circulation in the lower section had changed somehow. I found myself doing leg exercises while lying down to keep any clots that might have been forming, fully aware of the fact that I was on to them and wouldn't let that happen; I would fight that, too.

For those experiencing this breast cancer phenomenon, the timeline to normalcy started in these areas about two months after chemo ended and continued to get better with each passing day. I was told that within six to nine months, they should all be a thing of the past. All of this happens in just enough time to deal with the challenges of radiation.

Imagine a large, fresh, fluffy, lemon meringue pie. (The flavor of pie doesn't make a bit of difference, so pick your favorite.) Now cut that pie into quarters. That was the shape of the radiated area for me. The pointy end of the pie was angled up to just about two inches below my right collarbone and then the pie shape traveled down under my breast for about two inches, around to the area in the middle of my chest and under my arm, spanning all of the skin inside. Other than my breast and underarm skin, it looked like I had the tan of my life, a color I was familiar with; whereas those other two areas, not having seen sun during my lifetime, were red, swollen and oh-so-very tender.

I diligently packed on moisturizing creams several times a day for weeks. The doctor had been pleased with my skin's response. It hurt like hell but she was happy and told me that she had seen so much worse—keep up whatever it was that I was doing. I remembered what Michelle had warned me about, and I went home to pack the moisturizer on twice as thick. I would soon learn that there was no escaping some of what Michelle had experienced, no matter how much or how often you put cream and moisturizers on. Daily radiation would wreak havoc on your skin; you could count on that.

Dry skin can also be aggravated by long and hot showers. Short showers with lukewarm water are recommended. This is one thing that Michelle and I had a hard time complying with, as we both love and look forward to long, hot showers. I must admit that we both continued to take them and just lathered on more cream than normal. It seemed to do the trick.

I was constantly cold, which had been the norm since chemo started. But during radiation, things became complicated, as the right side of my chest was a flame of heat and quite able to fry an egg, sunny side up. This to me was, and still is, an amusing thought.

The Mag 7 had had our monthly dinner at Marianne's house last week and I'd shown them the results of radiation ending at the fourth week. At first, they were afraid to touch me, thinking that their hands were too cold. But to me, those cold hands were amazingly soothing. When at home, I walked around the house in a get-up similar to what the Romans would have worn. I would fashion a toga-style ensemble made from an ultra soft and cuddly blanket from Vince and Amy, drape it around my left shoulder and pull it around my body, leaving my right side free to the cooling affects of the air around me. Thank God our house sits higher than those around us; you can't see into most of our windows.

Soon enough, the calendar marked the fifth week of radiation therapy. I was getting stabbing pains every once in a while that—believe it or not—continued to surprise me. They would pop up in a different spot each time. Then those aggravating, flutter pains that would run a circuit would begin, just like after surgery. This was normal, as was the tightness that I felt and the sudden restricted change in my range of motion. Although much to everyone's surprise, including my own, I continued to work out, which the doctor said had helped immensely.

Sleeping was a challenge, as anything that my skin came in contact with placed me in agony. I couldn't soak in a tub, as that would have made it worse, so I showered with my back to the water to avoid direct contact with the impact. That was something I really missed: letting the water pound my skin and muscles. Cold icepacks were not allowed, as they could create issues with skin being taken up along with the icepack or wet cloth too soon before the skin was ready to be released. My skin was thin and damaged and applying heat for relief—well, you know the trouble with heat from a few chapters ago. Therefore, moisturizer, old T-shirts, toga-like wraps and constantly searching for that cool spot on the bed sheets turned out to be my new favorite things.

You become quite creative in arranging pillows cooled by an open window into a tent-like design, which I found was the only safe way to get relief when trying to sleep. Placing several chilly pillows under and around my right side to allow a position change was also essential. Each night was a continuous process of cooling off and repositioning pillows until I couldn't take it anymore—many nights I would I give up and pop an Ambien.

At one point, I tried drinking vodka on the rocks with dinner (many, many glasses of vodka on the rocks) so I could avoid taking a sleeping pill. This worked marvelously until about 2:30 AM when I would wake up with the TV on to the show *Poker After Dark* and the *click, click, click* of players fondling their dwindling stacks of chips. It sounded much like my hospital roommate with her false teeth cracking or the sound the biopsy instrument made so many months ago.

I had the most strength in the mornings, and therefore I scheduled them fully, so sleeping at night became important. My concern was taking a sleeping pill at 2:30 in the morning, which might cause me to oversleep and miss a meeting—or, be so groggy that I might as well have missed the meeting. Right around this point, Ambien stopped working for me. So I often skipped it and continued to toss and turn while checking the green glow of the alarm clock announcing that yet another minute had slowly passed while I grew more frustrated by the second.

After four nights of this battle with sleep, the radiation therapists, Becky, Jessica and Hilary all recognized that I was not my usual cheerful self and decided to advise Dr. McCall. Their well-tuned communication protocol once again at work. A few questions later, the good doctor reprimanded me about not taking something to sleep, stating that maintaining a normal sleep pattern during this period was essential, as was giving in to rest during the day when feeling tired or worn out. After several days of hoping that a sleeping pill would work and when it didn't, attempting to do it my way (lots of vodka) to no avail—I had to agree. Since Ambien was no longer working, she prescribed Ativan. On those days that I felt that I wouldn't be able to sleep—either because I had slept too much during the day or because I just knew it—I was to take an Ativan. I listened to the doctor and it made a huge difference.

On Monday of the fifth week, they were unable to locate my tattoos, which were important to the proper alignment of the equipment. All three radiation techs were brought in. Several lights sources were used and yet, the little buggers were lost to everyone. They were totally hidden within my tanned skin. The thought of having four new tattoos placed on this ultra sensitive skin scared the hell out of me. My skin was beginning to peel in places here and there. I kept thinking, if only more skin had released in just the right places, we might have had a better chance; or if I could have stomached the pain of exfoliating in the shower to uncover the tattoos. The thought of that was worse than the thought of getting tattoos all over again. The "fright and flight" response began to work up within me as I planned the best and the fastest escape route.

They finally found the tattoos. They marked all four with a black marker and away we went.

The next day, the same problem surfaced as the marker had washed off in the shower and through my constant moisturizing. We went at it again and this time a template was made so we could quickly move to treatment and skip this search and recovery activity for the balance of treatments.

Dr. McCall gave me a cream used for burn patients called Thermazene (Silver Sulfadiazine), as well as several long and narrow bandages that were non-stick, and a post-surgical bra that closed with Velcro in the center and in front to keep it all in place. After she applied this cream and covered it with the bandages and bra, instructing me along the way with what to do at home, I had instant relief. This was to be my new undergarment outfit for the next several weeks as I began to heal. I now had areas that had peeled and were super sensitive, swollen and raw, others areas that were in the process of healing, spots here and there that were peeling off in sheets and then there were places where it would remain red, sore, raw and swollen until well after treatment ended. I would see Dr. McCall one month after the last radiation treatment so she could check the healing process.

There are a few things that I failed to mention earlier in the book that occur during treatments and would be interesting for new breast cancer patients. What I had previously thought was a poultice that the technologists place on the area to be radiated, is actually called a "BOLUS." It is a gel-like, malleable material encased in flexible plastic. It acts as an intensifier of sorts, bringing the radiation rays as close to the skin surface as possible. They always warm it up for me before putting it on—as the first time it was applied right out of the drawer, it created quite a chilling shock. Remember to ask for that, or get ready for a major reaction.

You are also given X-rays once a week to be sure that the prescribed treatment area is actually the area being treated and that there has been no movement on my part or setup errors on the technicians part that could be problematic. It took just a few more minutes and was done while I was on the table during a regular treatment.

Generally, most women get tired (really, the word should be *exhausted*) around the third week of treatment. It hit me on the fifth week like a ton of bricks. It was hard to concentrate; I had difficulty remembering things that I was told and communicating on subjects that I should know well. I couldn't sleep at night but that is all I wanted to do once I arrived back home from radiation every afternoon, and it was very hard to fight off.

During the last week of treatment, things changed a bit. Instead of radiating the entire quarter pie area, I was now getting what is called a "Boost." The Boost is directed at the incision site, as that is what they have found to be the area where latent cancer cells tend to mingle, and is the highest rated area for recurrence. It is attached to the radiation equipment and they would snap and slide a cone onto it. The end that was closest to me was like a round-ended rectangle that precisely matched the area of the incision. They marked me yet again with the black marker and lined the gizmo up, ran out of the room to escape the harmful rays, gave me several long and loud blasts and we were done. This latest setup was a huge respite, giving the other areas a much needed break and some time to heal.

The risk for skin cancer is six times greater in areas that have previously been radiated. If you notice any changes in skin spots or moles, contact your physician immediately. And always use sunscreen.

Yesterday was my thirtieth treatment. I had three more to go. After finishing a teleconference call at 9:00 AM that lasted until around 10:30, I took a shower and lay down for just a second to warm myself up. I went out like a light and woke up with just enough time to drive to radiation. Once I arrived back at home, I fell asleep for a few more hours. This was precisely why sleeping at night was not such an easy task.

The reason you get so tired is that radiation, like chemo, is killing off both good and bad cells. Your body, in reaction to the assault, comes to the rescue by sending what it can to the area to aid in the healing process. This takes a great deal of energy and the body seems to exhaust its normal resources in coping with radiation's effects. It is a body function that you cannot feel happening, although it results in a reaction that you can feel happening as it throws you directly into la-la land. Radiation, at this point, pretty much knocked me right out. Resting or sleeping provided the necessary quiet time that was needed for my healing army to work even harder, as I wasn't wasting energy doing anything else but cooperating through rest.

Due to the fact that I had had chemo first and then radiation, I would probably feel quite tired for several weeks after treatment ended.

I asked Dr. McCall a question that I knew the answer to but was hoping she could offer me something—anything—some glimmer of hope that what I had just willingly subjected my body to was the right decision.

I asked, "How do we know if radiation was successful?"

"We don't," she answered.

Just like chemo, this is all just a crapshoot, a game of numbers, a flip of the coin at your gene pool and how it will react to the drugs and the treatments that have been tried. The hope is that all of those little microscopic cancer cells have been caught and eradicated. There is no surefire way to know if breast cancer will return. All we can do as patients is to wait, watch, monitor our bodies carefully, alter our lifestyles and continue to live.

I had an appointment scheduled with Dr. Nanda, my chemo oncologist at the University of Chicago in early November, when we would talk about the next step: Tamoxofin, which is a drug that I will need to take daily for five years to ward off estrogen production. Suddenly, what used to be my friend is now my enemy.

I sure hope I don't grow a beard!

I left for a five-day business meeting four days after radiation ended. One of the events required black tie attire. There would be a special dinner this year, as it marks the seventy-fifth anniversary of the association. I had so wanted to wear this extraordinary dress that I'd bought fifteen years ago for some other event. As they say, everything comes back in style and this one would have been a winner. I was hoping that my generally strong healing powers would allow me to wear it, but my heart told me: *Probably not a chance.* When I tried on the dress, it was impossible to hide the redness from the radiation burns, as the scars were so high up my chest. Accessories with this dress would have been overkill so a high-necked, little black dress with my little boy haircut, paired with absolutely fabulous shoes would be the best that would be presented this year.

Then I remembered: at least I would be there. That was all that mattered

We celebrated the end of my radiation treatment with another lunch brought in for the whole department. I will never forget these ladies.

Note: for those going through radiation, here are other creams that may be helpful (lotions usually contain alcohol, so steer clear of those for now):

- *Aquaphor* can be purchased over the counter at your local pharmacy. It's inexpensive but I did not like the way it felt. It was too greasy.
- *Eucerin,* which was recommended by the doctor and can be purchased over the counter at your local pharmacy. It's inexpensive but I've never tried it.
- *Crème De La Mer* can be purchased at the beauty counter of your local department store. It's expensive but a little goes a long way. The founder of this beauty line had been burned very badly and had worked a good part of his

life to find a cream that would soothe and regenerate his skin. I've used the entire line on my face and the lotion on my body for years. I have a very strong sense that this is what worked best for me during the burn stages of radiation. My healing after Treatment No. 30 was pretty remarkable from just a week prior. I used Crème De La Mer religiously over those six and a half weeks in conjunction with the Thermazene and a lotion that Larry had found called Kiss My Face (found at health food stores and grocers) that is organic and free of all chemicals.

- *Thermazene* (Silver Sulfadiazine) for radiation burns.

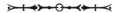

Dr. Song's Corner

Moisturizing cream is extremely important and a mainstay during radiation therapy. Some may have ingredients that can potentially interfere with the effects of radiation, so it is very important to run them by your radiation oncologist and her/his team before using them. The ones listed above are safe and already vetted.

Chapter 70

Lately, I've Walked More Than a Few Miles in My Italian Leather Slingbacks

It had been several months since I'd sent off a chapter from my book. I'd been writing a little here and there, snips and snaps and several starts and stops but nothing that had been worthy of my friends' time. While I won't claim that this chapter is necessarily worthy of their time or yours, it will catch you up on the medical aspects of the last two months as I walked miles and miles in various slingbacks, stilettos and pumps for each appointment, being grateful for every step I could take.

Now that my primary cancer treatment had ended, follow-up medical care would become crucial to maintaining my health and managing any treatment complications, drug complications or side effects. It is also a critical step in detecting early on when it is most treatable, whether cancer has returned or if it has spread to another part of my body. This is what is called a metastasis.

The cancer that I have requires lifelong management.

It had been eight weeks since radiation therapy had ended and in that time frame, I had had four follow-up appointments: one with each of the ologists and one with my surgeon. It was hard to believe that nine months had gone by since surgery. In November, I met with Dr. Connolly for that milestone visit. He agreed to meet me for lunch to be interviewed for the book and then we went back to the office and he did the exam. I'd wondered if the transition from lunch, where we had time to get to know each other better as people, to the doctor-patient scenario would be awkward for either of us, but it wasn't at all and it was nice to see Donna and Diane again.

In addition to seeing my surgeon, chemo oncologist and radiation oncologist, I also paid a visit to a dentist and my gynecologist and received a recommendation for a doctor in order to schedule the old roto-rooter colonoscopy, since my get-out-of-jail-free card would soon expire. Somehow this all seemed pretty normal; although when I consider my previous excellent health, I am amazed that in all the years of living, never have I seen so many doctors. Take any month in these last nine months and I would need to count a minimum of five years of normal time before I would have seen the same number of doctors.

My definition of normal continues to evolve.

Fortunately, as I continue to live, I am able to drop off a doctor here and there along the way. At this point I still need to see each and every cancer-related doctor for quite a while.

I suppose the most important appointment this month was with Dr. Nanda, my chemo oncologist. Our discussion on that day was all about Tamoxofin. This is the drug that I must take for the next five years as a continued method of treating breast cancer. It blocks the effects of estrogen; or reduces them, at least. It is the anti-estrogen drug for pre-menopausal women and those unnaturally thrown into menopause due to chemotherapy. It may also reduce the risk of getting cancer in my other breast.

I had what I thought was a great idea and asked her if simply removing my ovaries which is where estrogen is produced, would be enough to allow me to skip taking the drug. Her answer was no. Since chemo had thrown me into early menopause, my ovaries were already beginning to shut down, so why go through the risks of a surgical procedure to remove them? Dr. Nanda also told me that men and women produce estrogen in the body through the adrenal glands, which are just above the kidneys. A hormone called androgen is produced here. Another enzyme in our bodies called aromatase is found in our muscles, fat, liver and also in breast tumors. Aromatase turns androgens into estrogen, which is my enemy. While estrogen remains present in my body even after my ovaries shut down, at least we can block its activity.

Once eighteen consecutive months had passed without my getting a period, Dr. Nanda may switch me over to another drug for post-menopausal women. These drugs act as both antagonists and modulators. Sounds like a very confused drug to me!

Like all drugs, Tamoxofin carries all kinds of risks and potential issues. While these next few symptoms are scary, they are also rare, but Tamoxofin may increase the risk of a stroke, blood clots and endometrial or uterine cancer. Circulation is something to be critically aware of; I need to avoid grapefruit and grapefruit juice, and cannot use St. John's Wort, as these products may lessen the effect of Tamoxofin. Dr. Nanda also suggested limiting the use of alcohol and to use birth control to prevent pregnancy. Wouldn't that be special—getting pregnant!

Other symptoms are flushing, hot flashes, nausea or vomiting, change in sexual ability or desire, yeast infections, lower cholesterol, ovarian and uterine cancer. And the signs of a life-threatening reaction include wheezing, chest tightness, fever, itching, a bad cough, blue skin color (which would make me a shoo-in for the first female in the Blue Man Group review on Broadway), rashes, and fits (hmmm—what kind of fits?), swelling of the face, lips, tongue or throat, chest pain, difficulty breathing, swelling or pain in the leg or arm, diarrhea, changes in strength on one side greater than on the other, difficulty speaking or thinking, change in balance or blurred vision.

Damn!

Incredible, isn't it?

My sister told me years ago that when drugs go through clinical trials, all symptoms must be reported even if they affect only a small percentage of the trial's population. While the list appears daunting, I may never experience any or most of what they legally needed to warn me against.

There are two kinds of hormonal treatments used to fight breast cancer: anti-estrogens like Tamoxofin, which interfere with breast cancer growth by attaching to estrogen receptors in breast cancer cells, so that estrogen cannot attach itself. And the second hormonal treatment, known as an aromatase inhibitor, works by blocking aromatase, the enzyme needed to make estrogen. In post-menopausal women, aromatase inhibitors are generally used to reduce available estrogen that is necessary to stimulate tumor growth.

I did learn that Tamoxofin is used to treat a variety of cancers and has been used for many years. I also learned that probably both of these drugs would be in my future, one after the other.

The side effects from chemo that continue to this day are: silver halos that appear in both eyes and last from three to fifteen minutes, occasional dizziness, difficulty staying asleep every night, shortness of breath, hot flashes and this weird flushing that appears for ten seconds and then stops, occasionally a runny nose or weepy eyes, a spaced-out feeling (also known as "chemo brain"), and having a hard time concentrating. All of these are expected, and they all will hopefully subside within the next two months when I will have reached the six-month-after-chemo mark. Every day it seems to gets easier so I would agree that in two to four months, I should only experience the side effects associated with Tamoxofin.

It is much like being a gerbil and being placed on a gerbil wheel that you can't get off of.

To those who are interested in the timeline to "normal"—it had been nine months since surgery, five months since chemo had ended and eight weeks since radiation had ended. The burn scars from radiation were gone and the only visible mark was a weirdly shaped tan and that thin puckered horizontal line left from surgery that was now the color of my newly tanned skin. While the radiation area originally showed itself as the shape of a quarter of a pie, it ended up being a large rectangle spanning a much larger field.

There is one lasting silver lining to having had radiation: I might never have to shave my right armpit again. All of the hair follicles were damaged, having been totally fried every day for six weeks.

Dr. McCall told me that I was about a month ahead of schedule, as far as mobility and skin repair went. She mentioned that the skin massaging techniques that Dr. Connolly had told me to use, which I had been diligent about, had kept the scar tissue issues at bay, as well as reduced the hardening of other tissue due to radiation. I was in good shape physically.

I had my second haircut to even things out one month ago. I asked the local stylist to trim it just around the ears and the edges at the back, much like a teenage boy would do. In other words: don't cut off too much! These days, my hairstyle was going through a negative growth spurt, so it was quite unmanageable. It was long enough to be troublesome but too short to really style into anything. The color that had once been an amazing cornucopia of colors that tended to go towards platinum overall, had changed; it was now salt-and-pepper. The texture had changed as well, and it was a bit wavy, which reminds me of hair on a poodle. I did not like this in-between look at all, although others told me it looked chic. But honestly, what *could* they have said? "You're right, Suzanne—we shall now call you Fifi"? All I can say is—while I was not particularly crazy about this intermediate stage, it was far better than the Yul Brenner or "Chia pet" look. It was almost time for an intervention from Toni, my hairstylist downtown.

My appetite was back, although occasionally something would not taste the way it used to. This, too, shall pass. And for the first time in my life, my ears were freezing in this cold winter weather without having hair to cover them. I hadn't had to shave my legs or left underarm in thirty days and I had lost a crop of eyelashes a week ago, which really pissed me off. Of course, even in sickness, I had to have symmetry and some aesthetic balance, so the left eye was sparse on the inside corner while the right eye was an issue on the outside corner. Lovely! I must have had a bit of that chemo poison whirling away inside of me for my hair to have stopped growing—all over my body—and all of a sudden. I hoped that was all that it was.

I say this as a very good customer of Larry's had died over the holidays. She had been a single mom, sixty-nine years old and had been a total delight to be around. Whenever she called needing help, even just to hang a picture, Larry would drop everything to come to her assistance. She had been easy to love and you just wanted to help her and to be around her.

Anne had developed ovarian cancer at a time that was very close to my diagnosis. She had gone through chemotherapy sometime after I had; and five months after chemo had ended, she had been diagnosed with leukemia. I had been warned of this potential, as well. It is a rare reaction to chemotherapy but if you are unfortunate enough to get it because of chemo, it is harder to fight than acquiring leukemia in the usual ways.

Anne had been diagnosed and given *four days* to live. Can you imagine hearing those words?

She'd fought valiantly; eventually needing a tube in her throat and then tubes and lines seemed to appear everywhere, all over her body. She finally decided to leave us. The pain and the constraints must have been pretty bad for Anne to have made that decision. She had lived just three days after being diagnosed.

I know my cancer is different. I know this will not be my fate—but all the possibilities and unfairness of life came crashing in during that period of time that we mourned Anne.

It would be hard to describe or overstate how important it is to continue to dare to dream when you have been diagnosed with cancer. Do I have a future? Will I look in the mirror and be amazed at a sagging and wrinkled face that proves the life behind it and shows the vast geology of time unto itself? Short of a face lift—which, if needed, I am not opposed to—will I even have the chance to make that choice? Will I be able to look down while reading a book and notice knobby hands speckled with age spots and unfortunate curves, five full inches lost in height, hair greyer and now wiry, unsteady on my Louboutin shoes, no longer wanting to get all dressed up? Or, will I stand straight even if I am five inches shorter, looking slim and confident and feeling like I am sixteen and wondering who that person is that stares back at me as I pass a mirror? Considering the countless people who have passed through my life, most of whom, thankfully, have stayed—I have lived a full life.

For the first time, I think about a legacy without children of my own. I so badly want to pass something of lasting value on to the kids in my life, to those who call me Auntie Suze. Will I have the time to complete that journey? Will I be able to gather the energy? Will I come up with something so scathingly brilliant that it will be remembered for generations after I am gone? Is that too vain of a question to even ask?

There you are, diligently walking a straight line, or maybe a straighter line than you would have traveled in the past, when you briefly look up to check your course and you notice—always a great shock—that currents you can't feel or see have pushed you way off course. The challenge is to always recognize this change in enough time to correct it or refine it. Will I make that timeline?

Yes, I believe that I will.

Precisely three hundred sixty-five days ago on January 8th, my life had been changed forever. It had been a cold January afternoon, much like the one we were having today, when I had been diagnosed with breast cancer. A different set of surgeries and challenges were what I faced this year. My appointment with the reconstruction surgeon was for late January, so I push on for that, a new experience—and for so many other reasons, most of which start with my family and my friends.

This year had gone by fast.

I finally understood what Grandma had told me so many years ago: "Don't rush your life; it all happens way too fast, anyway. In an instant, it can all change. Stay awake and aware and savor each moment."

Chapter 71

Nutrition, Drugs and Their Amazing Interactions

If I wasn't the one experiencing this phenomenon, I may have had a hard time believing it myself. But once a week over the past four months, I had talked to at least one woman who had been diagnosed with breast cancer. Most of these contacts had been made through this manuscript, which was constantly being revised. Someone had a sister or a friend or learned that their kid's teacher had been diagnosed, and that someone had put the two of us together either on the phone, through e-mail, or both.

Today, two people contacted me asking how to best get through the various stages of chemo and place something of nutritional value into their body at the same time—without throwing it up, burning their mouth or having a hard time getting it down their throat.

Eating when going through chemo becomes a job in and of itself, and navigating some of the changes when experiencing certain combinations of therapy can be exhausting. I've never had a problem eating, although some call me a picky eater. I was never one of those girls who were afraid to eat in front of a new date or suffered any teenage eating disorders. I've never had a weight problem, although as the years moved on and I became less and less physically active due to laziness, I did gain more weight than I was happy with. What woman hasn't? But it was never enough weight to concern me. After my diagnosis, all of that had changed and it had changed in different ways and for very different reasons every few months.

The first change in diet arrived due to my fears and overactive imagination. I was, as you may remember, quite terrified of not only the prospect of having cancer or the terror of surgery and all things medical, but the surgical location simply took my breath away. In the days and weeks before surgery, I was totally uninterested in everything. I never seemed hungry and nothing tasted all that great, so I rarely bothered unless I was pretty much forced. My pants became loose and another notch in my belt was used.

Chemotherapy placed a whole new spin on things, and continual changes to the nutritional aspect of care for me were becoming a tad more challenging. With side effects such as fatigue and nausea, the swift change in the taste of foods, the fact that things that I once loved to eat were becoming unsettling to my stomach or taste buds or burned my mouth, and having to deal with a constricted throat—it was simply a constant struggle to figure out what would work. I had a strong intolerance for almost everything food-related. It drove Larry crazy. When talking to others, they have had similar issues but everyone has their own solution.

My nutritional solution became Bob's smoothies and the smoothies made by John Yurchak at the Hinsdale Fruit Store. John would also deliver fruit and vegetables to the house so I could make my own smoothies and have vegetables available when I was unable to drive. These healthy drinks would easily pass through my constricted throat—as would popsicles, sorbet, yogurt, fruit that was juicy and not dry and cut up into tiny pieces, and homemade chicken dumpling soup. I pretty much lived on those things for several weeks and then gradually moved up to Italian food that came from Capri, a favorite local restaurant. All the other restaurants or foods that we would make at home just didn't do it for me. For the most part, I existed on smoothies, fruit, soup and Capri's Italian food.

Timing became another issue; especially on the day of chemo and a few days after. You were not allowed to eat anything until after you had had your blood taken, tested and proven to be within the necessary ranges before chemo could begin. Once we were given the all-clear and told that my blood had passed the tests, Larry would bring me fruit, yogurt, soup, and sometimes I could get down half a sandwich. I drank gallons of liquids in all formats while the chemo poison was being dripped into my veins.

I was told to avoid high-fat, fried, spicy or greasy foods for the first twenty-four hours following treatment.

As treatment progressed, my taste buds and cravings changed again and again. I tried to power-pack my meals when I could by eating foods with a higher calorie count without sacrificing nutrition, whenever I could drag myself to the table and force myself to try. This wasn't very hard for me to do, as I love the "no-carb-left-behind" kind of mentality, which is not the best food to eat when you are healthy, let alone while going through cancer treatments. But eating higher calorie foods helped to maintain some weight.

They asked me to find a way to include protein in my diet. This was my largest challenge as I do not like red meat or milk. I tolerate chicken but only the breast part, of course. I enjoy fish immensely, along with veggies, fruit and cheese and just about anything spicy (Italian, Mexican, Spanish and Thai). For most of my chemo experience, my throat was so restricted, so small in circumference that only liquids could make it through. And I was never able to get into those nutritional drinks that everyone raves about. Their consistency was too close to that of milk.

The following is a list of some foods that have worked for others whom I have spoken to in the early stages of chemo: peanut butter on crackers (this would never have worked for me; it would have meant certain death as I would have choked), cheese, chopped hardboiled or scrambled eggs, nuts, avocado, oatmeal, grits, cereal, cottage cheese and pudding would probably have been perfect at one point or another.

It is essential to be aware of, sensitive to, and definitely ready to adjust the timing when taking your meds. It is critical to figure out early on, when to take each drug and in what combination, as the combinations of drugs often collide in their fight to cure you. And you must learn what you need to eat before taking those meds. The doctors never warn you about this; it would be impossible, simply because it is so individual. But beware: you will need to do a little experimenting. I needed to eat something like bread or waffles when taking any drug, at any time of the day or night and I had to carefully space it all out or they collided like atom bombs.

At this point during treatment, I was in a new weight class and I needed to buy smaller sized pants and belts and take those that I really loved to the tailor for resizing and the cobbler to get a notch or two added on the belts.

Hydration was critical during chemo. Being on a mostly liquid diet and consuming all the smoothies, sorbet and popsicles I could, made it a simple item to comply with. But sometimes that wasn't enough. I also found that I was insatiably thirsty and Pepsi (limited to one a day, which I coveted and made sure Larry stayed clear of, as he always wanted " . . . just a sip, babe!" Yeah, right.) and lots of ice water was the only thing that seemed to satisfy me. Fortunately, my love of ice water continues to this day.

During the first four days after chemo, a low white blood count (called neutropenia) occurred. This usually becomes more prevalent after several chemo treatments, and lasts from four to seven days. Larry gave me the dreaded Neulasta shot after each treatment to help in offsetting this problem and I was told to stay away from lettuce, honey, fresh fruits and vegetables and raw or undercooked meats and absolutely, positively *no sushi*. During this time, you are highly susceptible to infections. During this time, you also feel like shit. I found it impossible to eat for forty-eight hours after the shot anyway, so compliance was easy.

If you acquire mouth sores due to chemo, which I thankfully avoided, you need to stay away from acidic foods like tomatoes, citrus, saltine crackers, soft drinks that are carbonated and alcohol, while avoiding extremely hot or cold foods. Try using a straw for liquids to better direct the flow towards the back of your mouth or towards the other side of your mouth. That worked wonderfully for me. I found that alcohol and spicy foods were irritating and burned like fire and I never even had mouth sores—just a sore and sensitive mouth. There are several levels and you may experience one, none or all of them.

Other foods that were soothing and easier to get down during the middle stages of chemo were cottage cheese (which can be mixed with fresh pineapple, strawberries, raspberries, mandarin oranges or peaches and nectarines), Jell-O (although this was not for me, as I had learned years ago that gelatin is made from horse toenails or something equally gross and that was enough to end any future desire), applesauce, mashed-up bananas, scrambled eggs, mashed-up veggies and lukewarm soup. Should you get that metal taste in your mouth, try using plastic utensils.

I eventually moved to eating several small meals every day; a little snack every few hours. By this time, my weight had settled to a much smaller number. I had taken more of my favorite things to a tailor but had decided to keep several pieces of clothing in their original size, just in case.

There is one thing that I can say that would be true for all cancer patients going through treatment: anything that you can get into your system is good; ANYTHING. If you find something that works, then eat just that until you can progress to other things. It won't kill you to *not* dabble in each of the food groups or follow the perfect nutritional triangle like we were taught in school. In fact, it is impossible. Listen to the nutritionist, who should be a member of your medical team. Do your best in this area and don't let it freak you out, trying to eat so many ounces of this or grams of that.

The nutritionists I've spoken to, while extremely informative and intelligent, have never gone through cancer treatment and all they can tell you is what they learned in school; they will encourage you to eat as much as you possibly can of the good stuff. The reality is that your energy is best used in rest and healing and while nutrition is huge, these crappy side effects don't last forever. Most dogs eat the same thing all their lives; you can do it for a few months and I promise that every month or so, it all gets easier. It gets easier—unless of course, you feel the need to challenge yourself yet again, as I would this New Year.

On January 1, 2009, I began my latest and hopefully my last attempt at becoming a non-smoker. Eight days from now, I would celebrate my first "cancerversary." I hoped to celebrate my second "cancerversary" next year and my first year as a non-smoker.

This time, I fully prepared everything that I could think of during the month of December. All of the carpets, drapes, pillows, cushions and bedspreads were cleaned and I readied my previous prescription from last year's attempt for Chantix, the stop-smoking drug. I'd cheated four times using a non-menthol cigarette so it would taste crappy enough for me to not crave another. In the beginning few weeks, you are allowed to smoke while taking this drug; I'd decided to mix it up and do it my way and had only had those four. It has been very hard.

I was always hungry, so I kept a lot of fruit around me and I found that chewing gum seemed to help a great deal. The trickiest part had been figuring out precisely which drug to take and when to take it and with what combination of food was necessary, and which other drugs could be taken together; all of this without erupting Mount Vesuvius. This brought me to my newfound interest: amateur pharmacology. Until I figured out the secret combination to managing all of the drugs that I was taking, I had several episodes of throwing up quite explosively.

Two mornings in a row, I woke up, started my morning routine and took the Chantix. I went happily through the next forty-five minutes doing whatever it was that I had been doing that day when *wham!* Nausea hit me fast and furiously. The second day, I was working out in the basement with Tammy and just made it over to the sink next to the washer and dryer before it all came gushing out. I did continue working out once I was done throwing up; I am not a total wimp.

The thin, incredibly small type-styled instruction leaflet inside the Chantix package warns that you need to eat something before taking this drug. I am not a big breakfast person. Unless, of course, I am out of town, on vacation, waking up at 10:00 AM or later and then eating a cooked breakfast that someone else has cooked. The first day, the best I could do was to eat a few strawberries; it wasn't enough. On Day 2, I tried strawberries and a banana. This was clearly still not enough to protect my stomach from the hurlie-whirlies, so on the third day, I added a waffle to the banana and strawberries and that made all the difference. I suppose it was necessary to have something more solid in my stomach; something that would not as quickly be absorbed by my body.

Then one night, I forgot to take the Chantix pill and the next morning when I realized it, I wondered if maybe I could forgo the second pill of the day as I never really did learn to smoke while I was sleeping. I decided that this would not be a smart move, as I clearly recognized the need to have this stuff running around my system on a consistent basis, especially in the beginning.

Last night, I was taught yet another lesson. Larry and I had fallen asleep on the couch watching TV and when I woke up it was late enough to just go to bed. I went upstairs and took a Chantix and the required daily Tamoxifen pill. I was told to take Tamoxifen at night just before bed as it allowed me to sleep through some of the crap associated with its side effects. Because I was asleep on the couch when I normally would have taken the Chantix (at around 8:00 or 9:00 PM), I took them together. Ten minutes later, it felt like a tsunami was whipping through my body. I ran to the bathroom. Dinner and both pills spun wildly around and around in the porcelain goddess.

I took another Tamoxifen, as missing that is a major no-no. I skipped the Chantix, deducing that this had been once again the culprit. I went to bed prepared for my usual nighttime antics. Up every few hours, clothes on, clothes off, covers on, covers off, windows open, windows shut and then moving through various combinations of all of the above. I have had other incidents at night with nausea, so I am not yet sure if my pharmacological research has ended; but I am getting awfully close.

As far as the urge to light up a cigarette and the issues with a changing metabolism that makes it impossible not to gain weight, I was doing better than I had expected. I was being careful about what I ate and continued to work out three times a week. Now that I no longer traveled all over the place every other week (when I often ate three meals a day because I could squeeze another customer contact in or lengthen an important meeting by attaching a meal to it), my new schedule has helped immensely with losing weight.

Cancer is a force that leaves a person helpless and impotent with no say in the matter at all. Therefore, when you have a chance to have a say or make a choice, you need to seize that opportunity, no matter how fleeting or small that issue may be. I am working hard at my latest goal: to not eat things that are packaged. Think about the kinds of preservatives that are needed to allow a can of veggies to sit on your shelf for over a *year* and still be safe enough to eat! All of a sudden, consuming preservatives doesn't ring true for us any longer.

Don't worry, I despise people who become Evangelic in their newly changed lives. Those who preach and never stop talking about the sins of their past and how awful, unenlightened or literally crazy *you* are to be continuing down that path; that path that they have somehow magically or otherwise successfully traversed. I will not ever become that way, although I do invite you to consider a few things.

When I was a kid, everything we ate was made by my mom or some other family member, neighbor or friend. Back then, we did not have the money to buy potato chips and soda or Oreo cookies or eat at Burger King or McDonald's, all of which were considered a real treat. Plus, my mom was, and still is a fabulous cook and preferred to handle things in her kitchen, making sure that all food groups were properly represented at the table. We ate fresh foods with zero preservatives. Trans Fats? Hell, who even knew what those were until a few years ago? We were very healthy kids who had turned into very healthy adults.

I do remember a can or two being in the pantry, and we certainly loved Campbell's soup, tuna fish and Spaghetti-O's. But those were all consumed in a much more limited way. I can't help but wonder if my desire to cut a corner here and there and save a bit of time by using packaged foods or slamming down a quick-fix dinner, eating fast food on the fly while running to or from some meeting or catching another plane or cab for so many years—may have a part, not in my cancer necessarily, but in my overall health.

We aren't going overboard or anywhere near Evangelic in this house, but we are becoming more conscious of what we bring into it and we are largely limiting our intake of packaged food or food with preservatives. Even eating soup in cans is a thing of the past. If I don't make soup at home, Kramer's, the local family-owned grocery store makes two kinds every day.

I used to hope that smoking a filtered, "low tar and nicotine," "light" cigarette was something you did because you thought you were reducing your risk. I know—it sounds pretty stupid. In the first few days of not smoking, I was completely prepared, ready and able to smoke the stuffing inside the couch and roll it up into any paper I could find—the newspaper, if necessary. Mixing herbs from the kitchen became a thought I entertained more than once. And then I remembered my ashtray in the car. Not the car's actual factory-installed ashtray, mind you, as I would never put an ash in the ashtray itself and devalue the car. How silly that sounds: don't devalue the car by using the ashtray, but go ahead and mess up your lungs! This ashtray is shaped like those tall coffee cups with a lid; it fits snugly into the coffee holder molded into the car and collects all the ash and butts in the bottom. The first cheating I did was to smoke any prematurely extinguished butts in that thing. Gross, huh? I didn't get very far—as those of you who are, or were smokers, know that relighting a previously extinguished cigarette is, like, disgusting. And it wasn't satisfying at all when I was able to suck up a decent drag. Maybe I have a chance at beating this addiction, after all.

It was suggested that I meditate. It seems that every healthy person I know either meditates, does Pilates, works out, plays tennis, runs or practices yoga to assist them with life's big challenges. The really motivated people do more than one of those things. I've tried all of them at one time or another and I continue to wonder where in the name of all that is healthy does anyone find the time for all of this? When you factor in seven to eight hours of healthy and restful sleep, and making sure that you keep up with the suggested goal of having sex more than once or twice a week, then you add in eight hours for your job, planning meals and buying groceries, paying bills, dealing with the house, the laundry, the kids; I could go on and on. The hard part was that I needed to quit smoking far in advance of reconstruction surgery, while taking care of most of the above, working out, writing and editing the book, contributing to the business, working on the family Foundation—and all on one glass of vodka, less than one thousand five hundred calories a day and no menthol cigarettes?

God, help me.

I would definitely need more than one glass of vodka a day.

Karl's thoughts

The pharmaceutical companies would like us to believe that for most, smoking cessation is a monumental feat due to nicotine's highly addictive nature, and that the best way to quit smoking is to take their drug. What I have gathered in the years I have been interested in this issue is that even though nicotine (in combination with all the other chemicals in cigarettes, most of which are considered poison and ought to be banned) may be addictive, the withdrawal from those chemicals is quite mild, particularly in relation to withdrawal from other abused substances (heroine and alcohol, for instance—which can be quite severe and dangerous—must be done under close observation lasting up to a week or more).

The chemicals from cigarettes are out of the body within seventy-two hours, and what really needs to be dealt with for successful cessation is the habit of smoking and the associations (part of the habit). Also, the actual nicotine is out of the brain within forty minutes of the last puff, so the real addiction is the dopamine (the release of which nicotine triggers). We can train the brain to release dopamine all by itself—how is that for a natural "high." That is based on dealing with beliefs and emotions and the associations. People need to come to terms with what smoking represented for them; for some it was an emotion suppressant, for others it was to look cool or look older (when they first started), etc. Others have to break the associations: smoking after a meal, with a glass of wine or beer or a drink, at a bar, with the cup of coffee in the morning, when they drive or write a letter or talk on the phone, etc. And for some, it is important to get to the unconscious belief about how smoking is actually "serving" them. There is more to it than this, but you get the gist. The habit of smoking is the real issue, not the chemical dependency as Pfizer and others would have us believe.

Chantix blocks the brain receptors so that the brain doesn't "receive" the effect of the nicotine. That is why it's okay to smoke for a few weeks, while you continue to pay them for their drug! But what the hell good is that when in actuality the person trying to quit is almost encouraged to continue smoking! That is so contraindicated for someone trying to stop smoking. Also, Chantix is a drug that affects the brain in a similar way to nicotine and other chemicals, so people who take Chantix (or other like drugs) to quit smoking are merely replacing one chemical for another. Some people suffer withdrawal symptoms when they stop taking the drug abruptly. It sounds to me like Pfizer just wants to sell more drugs. What gets me is that there is no consideration for the habit, the emotional component, the associative element, and helping the person deal with the likely replacement issue (most people will replace a broken habit with another habit). That is why people gain weight—the decline of metabolic rate is actually minimal and can easily be eliminated with the right kind of cessation program and counseling/coaching (read: hypnosis).

Pfizer isn't the only one. The makers of Wellbutrin, Zyban, (anti-depressants—also used for smoking cessation, though Wellbutrin isn't prescribed often anymore even though its active ingredient is the same as that in Zyban) and others do the same, and they have spent so much money on misinformation and lobbying the AMA and FDA, it makes Enron look like a lemonade stand selling water with artificial flavoring.

Chapter 72

I've Decided That Much of What You Want in Life, Lies Right Outside Your Comfort Zone

I've been asked, "Did you have any epiphanies? Did you gain insight into how best to live life?" I am sure this will disappoint a few, but the answer is honestly "no." I have always lived life as large as my salary and very strict self-imposed savings plan would allow. I was constantly driving and pushing myself, defining my own terms, conditions and boundaries and being comfortable with displaying passionate intention. I was never one to back down from the next challenge, and I never minded walking into a dark room, confronting the unknown.

Since childhood, I've been most comfortable when putting myself "out there." Occasionally, I would find myself balancing on the edge. But more often than not, I was simply testing the waters by challenging and questioning it all, always helping or encouraging others in the process to grow along with me. I did not discover any magical wisdom or profound knowledge beyond these things because of cancer; but I learned so much. What I can promise you is that cancer has provided me with an in-your-face dose of perspective, real fast. I learned that anger, properly directed, is a far more productive emotion than sadness. Wallowing takes way too much energy and would make me feel as if I were giving in to the disease—and I'd much rather kick its ass! If I was going to feel real grief and sadness, then I couldn't allow it to be over losing a *boob*.

I've learned to stop focusing on the outcome—the result—as living with cancer holds far too many outcomes and its results and futures are much harder to predict. Once cancer comes into your life, while it can be cut out, chemically bombarded and burned to death, the day-to-day fact is that it never really leaves you and you are always held in anticipation of that next doctor's appointment.

I am a planner, an organizer. I continue to plan and organize and have simply stopped worrying about what is going to happen next week or next month or next year, as I have finally accepted the fact that I can't control everything. Lately, it is more than my body that has become flexible.

I've learned that opportunities are never really lost; someone will take the ones you miss and act on them, and that when you harbor bitterness, happiness will dock elsewhere. Early on in the experience, I was also very often reminded that to ignore the facts does *not* change the facts.

This has been said so many times before, and I try so hard to avoid obvious clichés, but the truth is that there are no better words to describe it—you learn to peel off all the things you *thought* would make you happy and find out what it is that *really* makes you happy. This can be as simple as a nice day without pain, or a nice day without a plan or being with people who care about you despite their flaws and yours.

You cultivate a taste for life's simple pleasures. Like the sounds the spoon makes when cracking into the hard, sugary crust of a perfectly made crème brulé. Or fresh garlic hitting a pan of hot olive oil and filling the air with that fabulous fragrance that screams "I'm home!" Or the smile that erupts on my face every time I see one of my nieces, nephews or godchildren. Or, when reading a particularly brilliant passage in a novel over and over and over in order to allow the words to become a part of me and then, devouring that book in one day, all the while mourning the loss of having it all end too soon; not being ready to let go.

Remember when the world was populated with telephone booths, before everyone carried a phone with them? Have you ever passed a phone booth with a ringing phone? Did you stop? Did you answer it?

I've had the chance. But I was always rushing to or from somewhere, and I never stopped. Frankly, that image has always reminded me of the stuff of old black-and-white movies. That chance encounter. That moment when going left or right would determine or alter the rest of the history of your life.

Nope, never went there.

But I am rethinking that position now. I've decided that much of what you want in life lies just outside your comfort zone. And sometimes you discover that it has always been there, closer to home than you thought. Even the familiar can offer the possibility of discovery.

Chapter 73

Tissue and Needles and More—Oh, My!

I was back at the University of Chicago today, one year and several days after my diagnosis. This year, the goal was to put a boob back in place; last year's goal had been all about taking it off and doing all that there was to stem the continuation of cancer reaching its tentacles elsewhere inside of me. I guess everything *does* always come full circle.

Halle*frickin*lujah!

Today's plan was to meet Dr. David Song—the Associate Professor of Surgery, and the Chief and Program Director for Plastic and Reconstructive Surgery at the University of Chicago Hospitals—and his team of plastic surgeons and nurses. My overall plan was to interview three plastic surgeons, all at different hospitals, but after the usual exhaustive research I generally amass, I had a sense that I would end up coming here for righty's rehab.

Today was also the day for Dr. Song to meet me. To take a look at the baseline body he had to work with and offer his opinion on my next best course of action. I walked into this meeting prepared with not just my research; I'd seen several videos, a few pictures, actually seen and felt live breasts of women who have gone through different reconstruction options and I'd viewed a partial surgery online and on TV. I was excited and scared to talk to Dr. Song and I was praying that I wouldn't pass out while he went through it all in his words.

I had been swinging wildly back and forth between the quick and easy solution as far as time in surgery, and pain and recovery after surgery, which would be implants, and a surgery that involves using my own tissue—this would take longer to get on the schedule, would be six to eight hours longer in surgery, would be four times the recovery time but would last a lifetime and answer a few other issues.

Let's go from the easiest to the most difficult choices in breast reconstruction, which, I promise, is nowhere close to your typical boob job. I'll start out with sharing my research and then I will tell you what the doctor had to say about my options.

First off, by now you are probably comfortable with the fact that while I have a particularly odd sense of humor and a fun-filled, self-depreciating way of looking at myself, I am also a bit vain and terribly particular about how I present myself and how I am perceived. With the help of Tsiona, the breast priestess of all boobie accoutrements at the University of Chicago, I was able to wear just about everything and no one would have known that underneath the fabric, I was not what they might have expected. I had also become quite comfortable with my battle scars and fully aware of the fact that if I didn't use Tsiona's magical accoutrements, you could still see the sinking area of my chest that surrounded the skin left by Dr. Connolly. Sometimes I was OK with that and sometimes I was not. This made the next step in the process all the more important, as after a year of living with both options—a boob and a boobette—I knew for certain that I wanted my landscape back.

I remember being in meetings at the office or other places where my situation was known and noticing people trying to find a moment in time when they could sneak a peek to figure out—*which one was it again?* It made me giggle because I knew that if it had been me on their side of this situation, I'd be sneaking a peek and asking that question, too. The specialized bras and the boneless, skinless chicken cutlets are simply amazing. But unclothed, there is before reconstruction and will be afterwards, a noticeable difference between the reconstructed breast and my natural one. For instance, my new breast will definitely not have the same shape as lefty, and much like it is now, it will have very little (if any) feeling and it may not "feel" the same as my natural breast when touched. And a nipple and areola—my God, wait until you hear about those alternatives.

While there are several options for reconstructive breast surgery, there is nothing currently available that will make a new breast look exactly the same as the original one. And, unfortunately not every breast reconstruction option is available to everyone. There are two instances when breast reconstruction can happen: immediately, when you are already undergoing surgery for a mastectomy; and delayed, which can mean a time period from any time after cancer treatments end, until years and years later. If you are not completely sure what to do about reconstruction, don't worry or feel pressured. You are not missing your chance if you decide to wait or not to do it at all.

Just to be clear though: immediate reconstruction does not mean—clap on, clap off—we are done. It simply means that reconstruction begins during your mastectomy. It takes several operations after the first to reach the end result.

Let's say you've decided to use implants. At the time of surgery for a mastectomy, some women will have the option to be fitted with a device called an expander, which is placed just under the muscle. It is much like a balloon that is not yet inflated. At the time of surgery, the surgeon will inject just a little saline into the expander so the woman wakes up with a start of the future of her new breast (think pubescent buds). The saline is injected through a port that is left inside your breast for this purpose only. My friends Carol and Michelle have told me that there is absolutely no pain when receiving these in-office injections over the following months. For most women, everything in that area is dead to feeling anyway, although some feeling has returned in a few places for me.

Over time, the surgeon injects saline into the expander to slowly increase the size and to stretch the skin in that area to prepare the space needed for the implant. It sounds terribly painful, and while it is uncomfortable according to those I have spoken to, it can be described very much like when a woman's tummy stretches and expands during pregnancy. It is expected that you will feel sore and weak and your doctor will likely prescribe medications to help you deal with this.

Once the skin has stretched to the size that will accommodate the breast implant that you have selected, the expander is removed and the implants are placed under the skin, fat and muscle through yet another surgery and the saline port is removed. This process of stretching the skin through an expander and then having the final implant surgery can take three to four months. But you aren't done yet. You still need an areola and a nipple.

To make things look balanced, similar, and pointing in the same direction—many women opt to have an implant placed in the other breast as well. My fear was lying down and having righty pointing north to the heavens while lefty was looking bored or uninterested, staring off to the west. You really need to have them both looking like a matched set and in most states it is a requirement of insurance companies to pay for the adjustment of the unaffected breast so that a woman ends up looking as close to normal as possible.

Implants have tough rubbery shells that are made of a material called silicone and are filled with a silicone gel. Some shells are filled with saline (sterile saltwater) but I have been told that if you've seen and felt a saline implant, you would most definitely prefer the silicone. Saline does not look or feel as natural. That is something I have yet to confirm personally but I intend to at some point before my surgery.

Some women are unable to have their implants placed during their mastectomy. For example, those women who know right away that radiation is in their treatment plan. Radiation, as noted in previous chapters, may wreak havoc on implants through shrinking, shifting and hardening. This does not always happen but it happens enough for me to remind you yet again—don't push for immediate reconstruction if radiation is in your future or might be in your future.

The cautions and risks are that breast implants are not meant to last a lifetime. Some women need a tune-up at the ten-year mark, while others can go on for fifteen or twenty years and not have any issues at all. Sometimes an implant can rupture and the materials (gel or saline) can leak out. In the case of saline implants, if it ruptures—the saltwater leaks out and the body absorbs it and your issue then becomes "The Case of the Mysteriously Shrinking Boob." If a silicone implant is used, the gel inside is very thick so the material doesn't really leak. Instead, the gel kind of bulges through a small ruptured hole that looks like a tiny cyst from the outside, if it can be detected at all. Many times you, your partner or your doctor won't even notice it; therefore, special MRI's may be needed to check everything out every few years. If these possibilities occur, most women opt for a replacement boob.

You may have heard that silicone implants were banned for cosmetic use for some years due to suspected links to health problems. A great number of studies have looked into this and no connection has been found between silicone gel implants and health problems. That being said, you and your surgeon need to talk about this to clear up any questions you may have and to learn of the up-to-the-minute data on this subject. As of this writing, it appears to be a very safe option, but you are required to sign off on certain hold harmless documents and you are automatically placed in a study. Each implant has its very own serial number that will be documented in your files in case of future issues. The reason for all of these cautions is that the FDA (Food & Drug Administration) won't completely sign off on its safety due to insufficient data. Don't let that put you off, as chemotherapy and radiation are also practices that have insufficient data. Currently, breast implant surgeries take one to two hours and seem to be the way that the majority of people I have met have gone.

The next set of options revolves around using your own tissue and fat to create a new breast. When using your own tissue you will have a more natural look than if you use a breast implant. Unlike implants, a tissue breast will last a lifetime.

A ten or fifteen year tune-up is off the calendar. And because it is living, breathing, metabolically active tissue, a breast made from your own tissue acts more like a real breast. What I mean by that is, if you gain or lose weight later in life, your reconstructed breast will get bigger or smaller right along with the rest of you. It sounds like the way to go, but read on. The decision becomes really complicated because there are options within the overall option and you need to find a surgeon who is skilled and experienced in micro vascular surgery.

Tissue operations are way more complicated for a surgeon to perform and they take longer, quite a bit longer. They are much harder on your body due to the length of time under anesthesia, the multiple surgical sites and the extended recovery times. Most tissue operations use the word "flap" somewhere in the description. I have come to learn that this is simply a word to describe tissue that is being moved from one part of the body to another.

A tissue flap can be taken from several places to rebuild a breast: the abdomen, belly, upper back or butt. When I was working through viewing the multiple research sites I had found for these operations, it was as hard as researching the various breast cancer surgeries I'd faced last year. Several times, I had to hit the pause button on a video and walk out of the room. I'd glide into the kitchen and fix myself a long and strong pour of vodka on the rocks, sit down and look out the windows and then put my head between my legs and take deep, lung-filling breaths before I could return to my office and continue. I could actually sense the hot and constricting fear that was bubbling up just below the surface of my skin—and that was happening just through writing about the procedure. Or was it just another hot flash?

One option is called a latissimus or "lat flap." In this case the latissimus (lat) muscle along with skin and other tissue is removed from your upper back. There is a great risk of muscle weakness in your back after this procedure because a piece of your muscle has been removed. This is not a problem if you play golf on weekends; but if you are active, have little children that need to be picked up and moved around throughout your day, or if you enjoy vigorous tennis or working out, then this may not be such a great option. Additionally, a lot of women don't have enough tissue in their upper back to make the sized breast they want, so often an implant is thrown in for a fuller, more balanced look. After thinking about it, I quickly decided that this was not a good option for me unless the doctor had a really convincing reason. Why go through a surgery to remove tissue from your back if you need an implant anyway? Plus, Larry loves my back and I looked forward to wearing backless dresses and gowns again, without having to conceal a scar and a back with weakened muscle tone. I later learned that Dr. Song is able to perform what is called a "TAP flap," which is a new surgical option that removes the same skin and fat but attempts to spare the muscle, although you may still need an implant.

Let's move it down south and consider tissue from my butt. This is called a "GAP flap" (Gluteal Artery Perforator), there is a SGAP (superior or upper part of the butt) and an IGAP (inferior or lower part of the butt) and it all depends on your anatomy as to where the tissue will come from. A butt lift is the result of this process for one side (the side to be used for breast tissue) and of course, the surgeon has to balance things out so the other side is thrown in as well. This operation is not one that is usually selected and therefore not done as often. It is more complicated, not all surgeons are trained to do it and it can take up to twelve hours. I can't imagine having a sore butt and a sore boob and only finding comfort for six to eight weeks on one side or the other. But who knows what the doctor may say.

Okay, flip me around to lie on my back again and let me tell you about a TRAM and a DIEP flap. A "TRAM flap" (Transverse Rectus Abdominus Myocutaneous), takes a section of skin, fat and muscle from the lower belly. Now hang onto your dinner for this one . . . Once the doctor has a firm hold on that precious chunk of flesh that has been expertly separated from its original location, he or she tunnels that tissue under the skin and up to the chest area to form a new breast. It reminds me of the crafts I used to do: stuffing things into little crevices with a knitting needle. Pushing and stuffing and cramming away, trying to develop a shape that I was satisfied with. I shuddered, just thinking about this being done on my body. The tissue stays connected to blood vessels in the belly area that it was taken from and continues to get blood from its original source. Due to the large cut that is required, a TRAM flap leaves a long scar that goes from hip to hip; and because muscle is taken from the belly, you are extremely sore after surgery. I've heard it likened to being hit by a Mack truck. The fact that there has been muscle taken also means that there is a risk of muscle weakness in the belly that could be with you forever. You are also at a much greater risk for an incisional hernia anytime after the operation. An incisional hernia is a hole that can form at the incision site where part of the intestine can bulge through. This can happen several months to several years after the operation.

Even though I am not planning for a spot on the Olympic team or even running a local marathon, I rather enjoy the feeling I get from working out and I want to keep in shape and have the freedom to be as active as I wish to be in the future. This sounds pretty nasty, cutting into muscle, and it was extremely hard to imagine the entire process without getting weak in my knees. But I digress, let's keep going; there is just one more option to tell you about.

The last option is called the "DIEP flap" (Deep Inferior Epigastric Perforator). It is similar to a TRAM because it makes a large cut and takes skin and fat from your belly or abdomen. But unlike a TRAM, a DIEP does not take muscle along with the other tissue. Because of that, there is much less risk of getting muscle weakness or incisional hernias after surgery. Also, the blood vessels are disconnected from the belly with this option—no tunneling! The surgeon then reattaches all of the tiny blood vessels, primary veins and arteries and occasionally a sensory nerve is located, found to be viable and that too will be reattached in an effort to restore erogenous senses. This means that if the doctor is able to locate my sensory nerve, I might regain more feeling than I already have. Remarkable! It is remarkable and very rare, as Dr. Song must painstakingly coapt the arteries and veins under a microscope, which is extremely delicate and laborious work. Having had radiation further complicates finding my sensory nerve.

Hopefully, my tissue would make a clean attachment and continue to live and act as tissue that has always been there. This surgery takes six to eight hours and the lion's share of it is done looking through a microscope; therefore, the patient and meticulous skills of an experienced micro vascular surgeon are critical.

I've been back and forth in the decision over implants versus a DIEP flap. I was hoping that I was a candidate for use of my own tissue but I knew that I wouldn't allow them to cut into muscle either in my belly, abdomen or my back. Additionally, I didn't wish to emerge from surgery looking like someone else. I simply wanted my boobs to look as close as possible to what I'd been given—if I was able to freeze-frame them at the age of about twenty-seven.

I had been warned against tissue surgery in the abdominal area by several women who've had it. The recovery is brutal, long and uncomfortable, but I am looking for a long-term solution accompanied with the fewest potential future alterations as possible—this is probably the way to go. The idea of being out for six, eight or ten hours freaks me out. But we'd see what the surgeon had to say once he had perused the old body. Dr. Connolly felt that I was a perfect candidate for this surgery. Plus, doing it this way sent a clear and positive message from my mind to my body that I am in this for the long haul; in other words, I don't want to be back in surgery at the age of sixty for a replacement boob job. I would prefer the trauma of surgery while I am young enough to better recover and then have the same boobs for the rest of my life with no future tune-ups required—and to know that they will shrink and grow right along with me, for however long that will be.

Janice Anderson, the Nurse Manager of the Reconstructive and Plastic Surgery Department at the University of Chicago Hospital, walked in. We went through the usual litany of questions and had a few laughs. She was easy to be with and to talk to in a medical setting and that helped immensely with the anxiety I always encounter in a hospital. I could have been just acting paranoid, but I had a sense that she comes in first to not only handle the required before-you-see-the-doctor protocol but to also evaluate what the poor doctor—and their team, for that matter—would soon have to be dealing with. I could only wonder whatever it was on my chart that had precipitated her arrival or what she would be sharing with her team about her short visit with me. In any case, I put my best boob forward and could only hope that we would all click well together.

Exit stage right for Janice and soon after, a resident named Dr. Aaron Pelletier walked in and talked with me as well. This was definitely practice for him, of zero value for me and probably an opportunity for Dr. Song and Janice to talk before Dr. Song entered the room to finally get this show on the road. Dr. Pelletier seemed very capable and asked the right questions and even told me a thing or two that I wasn't aware of. If he already has or can acquire the necessary skills in surgery, he will be a very good surgeon because he had certainly aced the bedside manner part.

Dr. Song entered the room and I immediately liked him, which had been the same response I felt with the rest of his team, including his head nurse Bernadette—who, at this point, I'd only talked with on the phone. It was the three of us in the room: Dr. Song, the resident and me. Dr. Song wanted to know what I knew about my options. I told him briefly about the research I had done through their website, my Internet and book research, my conversations with other patients and reading everything I could find on the topic. We talked briefly about those options and then we quickly move to my typed list of twenty-seven questions.

He was visibly relieved that I was prepared to wait for the effects of radiation to subside, that I had a realistic expectation and that I had listened carefully to and executed all of the suggestions by the doctors that had come before him. He said that they would just briefly leave the room so I could change into the gown so he could make a complete examination. At that point, I did not want this guy to get caught up in any hallway dramas or delays, and I simply never understood why they leave the room only to shortly return and see everything anyway.

I asked him, "What's up with that?"

He answered that this protocol was designed to provide the patient with some level of privacy. I asked him to mark my chart that for me that *that* is a total waste of time, and I started peeling off my sweater. He laughed, the resident appeared totally shocked and away we went.

Dr. Song said that I do not have enough skin or tissue on my back to make a latissimus flap possible and I do not have enough skin or tissue on my butt to make a GAP flap possible. Considering the fact that I refuse to do a TRAM flap—taking muscle along with everything else—this left implants and the DIEP flap. Marvelous; we had arrived at the same place that I'd arrived at weeks ago on my own.

He said that I was a good candidate for the DIEP flap because of my healing abilities and because I have firm skin tissue. He was very surprised at the level of healing that had been achieved with the surgical scar from my mastectomy and that I had kept the scar tissue down in a major way through Dr. Connolly's massaging techniques. I would imagine that my constant moisturizing throughout radiation was a part of the improved result, as well.

There is another option called an SIEA (Superficial Inferior Epigastric Artery flap) that Dr. Song performs. There are only a few people in the entire world who are capable of doing this surgery, and Dr. Song has a lion's share of the world's experience. An SIEA is taken from the same exact area as the DIEP but the blood vessels are in a superficial plane; unfortunately, only about thirty percent of patients have this blood vessel positioned in this area. He wouldn't know if I did until he had gotten inside of me. Superficial blood vessels are much more advantageous if they are utilized properly and precisely, because unlike the blood vessels for a DIEP flap, these vessels are located above or superficial to the rectus muscle (abdominal muscles) so that the dissection or harvest of this flap is less painful and recovery is much swifter than with a DIEP flap. Typically, they attach one or two arteries and one or two veins.

He then began to review my chart and noticed that about eight years ago I had had a surgery to remove fibroid tumors: a bikini cut location. He asked if I would show him that scar. I still had my jeans on, thinking that this exam had no reason to head in that area and I said that I hadn't been able to find the scar for years and not for lack of trying or the ability to bend myself in that position. It had healed so well that it had pretty much disappeared.

He muttered something like, "Yeah, yeah, yeah. I just want to see."

No harm in that, especially if he would ultimately be doing my surgery, so I yanked down my jeans and together we tried to locate this scar. We were both searching and feeling and laughing. He asked me to move a little bit this way and relax my muscles and then he saw it and was once again very pleased. I heal extremely well, so I should have little problem expecting the same results again.

He expected that the surgery would take six to eight hours. I would be in the hospital for three days and on an automatic pump of some wonder drug. I should expect to feel like roadkill for several weeks. I would leave the hospital with two drains. Dickie the drain shall make a return appearance for the new boob, and his brother Dwayne would be introduced to tap off the liquids in my abdomen. After being released from the hospital, I would have two weeks of required bed rest. Working out would be on hold for six to eight weeks. Approximately two to three months after surgery, the tissue should be well-anchored and adjusted.

I asked how many of these surgeries he had performed and how many had been successful. Out of over five hundred surgeries he had performed, three had failed. By "failed," I mean that the blood vessels, veins and whatever else that must be attached had not formed lasting connections, or had never formed a connection at all. Or, there had been an infection.

In any case, the tissue flap must make a seamless marriage with the tissue already there, reestablishing blood sources—or it simply dies away. Once everything has settled down, several months down the road, you go back in and get a tattoo of an areola. It is done in the hospital and I am told that the woman who does them is very, very good. She must be; Dr. Song had taught her the techniques. I couldn't wait to meet her and see her pictures.

After that had healed, I would go back into surgery for Dr. Song to construct a nipple and give lefty a little lift so that it would be at the same level as righty. And yes, I asked that, too . . . It would be an actual three-dimensional nipple. He told me that fashioning the perfect nipple is like Origami; and since he is Asian, he has that skill in his blood. Strike up the band!

Dr. Song would be fashioning my nipple using the skin already there. There are other ways of making nipples from your own tissue. Taking it from the upper inner thigh or the other breast or from—yikes!—I don't even want to go there, but use your imagination on tissue found elsewhere on a woman's body that would match a nipple's color . . . and you'll probably make the correct guess.

I am totally happy with his idea of Origami. I'd heard that he is an artist, extremely precise, very careful and totally into what he is doing. I do not want another scar in another spot on my body.

The reason you must wait several months before having the tattoo and the nipple reconstructed is that your breast tissue needs an opportunity to settle into its final form and place. It is equally important to provide the blood vessels with ample time to fully anchor in, figure out their new pathways and to make sure that the center of your breast continues to remain the center of the breast that you will live with for the rest of your life. In this instance—precision, artistry and accurate placement are very important; but first, adequate time must pass so that everything settles into its natural position.

Which led me to another question; one that Dr. Song told me he has never before been asked in his career. I imagined that the surgery would be carried out while I was lying on my back with all the needles and tubes and lines attached to the many places where they attach all that stuff. When a woman who has natural boobs lies down—no matter how young and firm her boobs are, they have a tendency to, well, spread out to the sides. But once that same woman sits up, things settle back to where they should be: front and center. So, how do you compensate for that when doing a breast surgery when the patient is lying down?

What they do is place you on a table that is designed like a cross. You are positioned on that table with your head strapped back and your arms spread wide so that when they move you and the table into a sitting position everything falls into its natural place. Isn't that simply ingenious? This is the position that I would be in while Dr. Song performs his work. I'm impressed that they had actually considered this and that a workable solution had been found. I would be able to work on my core strength muscles while under anesthesia, and while Dr. Song is working on everything else.

Tammy, my trainer, would love that.

I asked Dr. Song about smoking, and told him that I was a recent convert who occasionally fell off the ashtray/wagon. His response was swift and spoken with amazing clarity and strength—in other words, this was no bullshit he was serious—"I insist that the patient is free of nicotine-related products (cigars, cigarettes, nicotine gum, etc.) for thirty days, as nicotine can cause issues with healing at the donor site and the mastectomy flaps. It typically has not been found to affect the microvascular anastomises (vessel connections). Additionally, they must remain smoke-free for the healing process." Having heard from Dr. Connolly that this is a huge requirement for a successful outcome, I had found myself not cheating as much these days.

As with most women experiencing breast cancer, it was important for me to know of any new developments. Dr. Song told me he was developing many new options and that for women who select a lumpectomy, he performs oncoplastic immediate lumpectomy reconstruction. This is huge. Many women opt to have a total mastectomy if their lump(s) is large or encompasses a larger area, as they may as well take it all off and start over. But for those women who have a small tumor and decide on a lumpectomy, this is a major opportunity. Dr. Song's latest breakthrough procedure means that even after a lumpectomy, plastic surgeons can immediately intervene prior to radiation to help reshape the breast into a more aesthetically appealing shape. Additionally, the after-effects of radiation that I have spoken of in many chapters are lessened, as the doctor can immediately make the shrinking and shifting adjustments ahead of time. The limitation is that the area to be reconstructed in this way, in most women, can be no larger than one-third of the breast volume.

I asked him: If he could tell the women who will read this book one, two or three important issues that they should know about relating to breast reconstruction, what would that be?

He carefully considered this question then said, "That any and all women are candidates for breast reconstruction; age is not a criteria. Clearly, one's underlying health condition and body habitus (the shape of one's body) is. Additionally, a prospective patient must really like and be able to tolerate her plastic surgeon, as she will see him or her for a long time. I often say that one must like and must tolerate my style, as we will have a lifelong relationship. Trust your gut; if your plastic surgeon gives you the heebie-jeebies, then you have the choice to seek another opinion. I feel that most informed women, who are looking for the best result, should seek multiple opinions before deciding on this partnership. You also need to have realistic expectations—as these breasts, once the reconstruction is complete, will be sisters and not identical twins. Finally, breast reconstruction is a passion of mine and I feel privileged to be doing what I do. A patient should seek out a plastic surgeon with this mindset, but more importantly, one who is aware and sensitive and puts a singular priority on curing and treating breast cancer first, because it does no good to create a wonderful breast if the cancer is not treated properly in the first place. Thus, a team approach is extremely important."

Can you see why I like this guy?

He also has a very good sense of humor and was willing to play along with mine, which I have found to be an important part of the process for me.

By this time, Janice had walked back in the room—probably wondering what was taking so long, as she should have been in there as well. I asked if I could see photographs of women who have had implants and the DIEP flap right after surgery, three months later, six months later and a year later; and also if there was a list of women that I could talk to who have had both surgeries. Dr. Song was more than happy to get this together for me through his nurse and assistant Bernadette. He then asked if I would be willing to do the same for other women when I was on the other side of this surgery. Of course, I said yes. And then I just couldn't resist telling him more about the plans for the book. He agreed to help me with the medical aspects of my writing, regarding reconstruction surgeries.

This is one very busy guy. He told me that I would probably not be able to get on his schedule until September. If I didn't want to wait that long, he suggested that I consider seeing his colleague, Dr. Parks—a brilliant surgeon he had hired about nine months ago. I thanked Dr. Song but said that I really wanted him to do this surgery; I would wait.

Unfortunately, this would delay my plans by five months and I was so looking forward to retiring the boneless, skinless chicken cutlets before summer. If another patient did cancel their surgical time slot, as sometimes happens, Dr. Song would place me on the list to report for surgery on a moment's notice. I sure hope I wouldn't be traveling if this chance ever opened up. I highly doubt that American Airlines has a special fare for emergency boob job travel.

Before ending this chapter, I would like to caution you about something else. I was originally told by my breast surgeon, Dr. Connolly that I was an excellent candidate for the DIEP surgery.

One of the plastic surgeons I had interviewed months later, prior to meeting with Dr. Song, had told me that I was not a good candidate. This really bothered me so I questioned him further asking him to explain why he felt that way. After some discussion, I came to the conclusion that it was not that I was not a good candidate for this surgery—*he* was not qualified to perform it. This is another example of why seeing more than one surgeon for an opinion is a good idea. On the day of surgery, you will enter the operating room with confidence that you have left no stone unturned or question unanswered.

Chapter 74

Dreaming with Your Eyes Wide Open
& the Transition from Patient to Advocate

It's ironic that cancer begins with "can" when there is absolutely *nothing* about cancer that allows you to feel comfort in that generally positive word. Cancer can be seen lapping at the edges of the entire world's toniest and most privileged zip codes, as well as the darkest and dreariest of slums and tenement homes; and slurping up all of that lying in the middle. It is a bipartisan type of disease; one that is able to infect any person walking the earth in just about any part of their body. Lately for me, it has become insidious. It seems to be happening all around me and I, like so many others, am helpless to stop it. All that I can do is wait on the sidelines and watch as it creeps and crawls into the lives of so many women and their families every day, and then I carefully mark the appropriate time to step in and hopefully be of some assistance. The thought that overwhelms me the most is that those that I learn of and can somehow reach, are only a miniscule percentage of the numbers that I—or anyone, for that matter—could ever hope to reach.

I retired at the end of February. That sounds as odd to say this year, as it was last year when I'd said I had cancer. My days of entrepreneurship are over and I now maintain the position of Investor; although those who know me can already say without question that I am not the silent investor type. Therefore, while

I still have some skin in the game (Bob and I continue to own a bit of stock), I will continue to check in and attend meetings here and there. While this was a planned event covering a five-year period after we had sold a majority position in our company, where each year I dropped a day from my work week and moved further and further onto the sidelines, it is nonetheless bittersweet for so many reasons. But that is a subject for another book.

I am fairly confident that most people would agree that this is definitely not the best time to retire—with the stock market tanking and at historical lows, everyone's 401K's shrinking into 101K's, credit markets almost frozen solid, home prices collapsing and unemployment rising. But these issues aside, I am really excited as I face the unknown once again. For the immediate future, my work week will smoothly morph into working on the family Foundation, this book, and the requests to talk to others who have been diagnosed with not just breast cancer but *any* cancer.

In recent months, as I've spoken to countless people experiencing cancer, I have come to notice a universal similarity. When a crisis strikes, people go from living their lives for the future, to living in the *now*, right at this very moment; and that many things change or alter in their importance. When life moves at its natural and expected pace, we are no longer philosophical; we are anxious and hungry for what's next, swiftly moving from one experience or event to the next, never satisfied and always eager for more. Why must it take a catastrophic event to slow us down enough to recognize that the frenzied pace at which we had been running, was taking such a large toll? Consuming so much of our lives that we might not have been fully living them? All of a sudden, you open your eyes to the fact that you may have missed huge chunks of time, and important experiences and connections. When a crisis strikes, everything seems to move to a heightened level of awareness and immediacy, and things seem to shift to the moment at hand. I would call this Phase One: your attitude begins to shift dramatically.

Today, I had lunch with my long-time friend John Kuhlman and the woman he had put us in contact with fourteen months ago: Mary Ellen Connellan, who is the Executive Director of the University of Chicago Cancer Research Foundation. Mary Ellen assisted me and Larry in getting to the right team at their hospital for an opinion and that first meeting with Dr. Connolly.

Mary Ellen passionately described her involvement in the Cancer Foundation. She said, "I have the honor of overseeing the fundraising activities of the boards and auxiliaries of the foundation. I work with board members, their friends and families, other donors and grateful patients in a variety of ways. Sometimes I am engaged in fundraising; sometimes I am helping to find the right physician for someone to see. We are as much advocates for the cancer program at the University of Chicago as we are fundraisers. It is very rewarding work because I interact with basic scientists as well as clinicians, all of whom offer a rich perspective in the field of cancer treatment, care and research. Since 1946, the UCCRF has been a part of funding some of the most innovative research conducted at the University of Chicago, and for that we are very proud."

I believe that I have met my match; Mary Ellen is a Type-A personality on steroids, just like me. I told her about the book, my story and spoke of my desire to work more closely with the hospital. As I recounted the past fourteen months in a Readers' Digest version (short and sweet), I was clearly remembering in blaring Technicolor how blown away I had been at the start of my cancer drama; and since then, having gone through everything that is medically available, I'm certain that I can help others get through their experience a bit more easily, and help them remember not to give cancer permission to take over their lives. I think I may have just found the next great experience in my life!

What a difference a year makes. I was actually telling this person that I, Chicken Little as far as medical stuff is concerned, would be willing—and even happy—to come back to the *hospital,* on a *regular* basis and work on the surgical, chemo and the radiation wards, providing support to anyone who wanted it. She seemed very happy to accept my offer, and promised to get back to me with some ideas on where I might like to start.

Without having to leave the house, I continue to speak to at least one person a week who has been given the same challenge to fight for his or her life. When talking to others at the beginning of their cancer journey, I always need to ask myself: *Are they ready for the next piece of information?* Is she/he ready for the next step and then the ultimate decision that must be faced and made based on knowing that next step? Is this the moment to press or try and break through the denial and the fear and expose the horror of what has just been learned?

I think about this while I fight with myself; a strong and brutal internal struggle that forces me to consider both sides of each question over and over and over again, balancing the options I know to offer and causing me to pause much longer than normal in my response, as I remember that the scars of hearing the words "You have cancer" are still very fresh for this person.

Or, is it time to pull back, review progress and consolidate everyone's thoughts and the real options at hand? It is such a sensitive time; and if you want to help, you have to help in the way that individual needs it, which is not necessarily what you may have needed. This has been the hardest part for me: knowing just what to filter out, as everyone handles their disease in such a different way. And in looking back at my own journey, I've noticed that the way I handled things continued to change for me as I continued to live. I would call this Phase Two: facing the truth and gathering information.

At one time, I mapped out a blueprint of my life, to which Fate had little choice but to conform. Fate, as fleeting as it is, forced me to consider experience. My life story has shown me that strength is generally earned through experience. I suppose *that* is the strongest bit of help that I am offering lately; getting through the daily nitty-gritty, moment-by-moment constant struggle for mindfulness, living in the "now" and allowing the advantage of your experience to lead you ahead of your ego and your fear. And most importantly, accepting that you have a responsibility to positively reframe the inevitable disappointments in life in a way that impacts others and freely passes on to someone—anyone—that attitude is *everything*. If only to get others thinking or considering another way; or better yet, challenging me so that I can further explain or apologize for my actions. It's true—no one lives an unchallenged life and no one has ever said that life would be easy; they just promised it would be worth it.

With the completion of surgery, chemotherapy and in some cases, radiation therapy for cancer—you need to be able to get to a place where you realize you've done everything you can from a medical standpoint to beat cancer head-on. And then you need to boldly move on with your life. Noting the experiences you've had with a huge punctuation mark on a piece of paper that is then safely tucked away in your trivia box; while you rebuild your strength, learn again how to sleep at night without assistance from drugs, watch your nutritional choices, and exercise. At that point, your focus must shift to living each day to the fullest and making the necessary lifestyle changes to promote a healthier lifestyle overall.

As this is happening, you are simultaneously aware of the constant day-to-day job of reducing the risk of a recurrent cancer. You need to remain mindful and not assume your journey has ended. Medicine, technology, techniques and skills are improving every day and being right in the middle of it, I am amazed at the new information that is now out there that hadn't been available just fourteen short months ago. You must continue to stay tuned in to these changes in medicine and all changes in your body. You must continue to learn and then to share what you've learned. This is Phase Three: continuing to fight the good fight by staying actively informed.

The final part is never really completed until you die, so it becomes more like a new reality and can't fairly be described as a phase. The reality involves the inevitable doctor's appointments that will continue for years and years and years to come. While for now, cancer may have left the building, there is not a lock and key strong enough to ensure that it will never again return. Recent graduates of cancer treatments worry about cancer's recurrence quite often; at the same time, they are both happy and reluctant to let go of the security net that weekly visits with various doctors provides, to be sure it is all on track. This simple fact requires that the phases I have just mentioned continue to repeat themselves. They move in a smoothly flowing circle; and while the circle gets larger each year as you continue to put another year of tests behind you, I have been told that it never completely leaves you. I believe that. It has not left my mind, either.

At this point, you must be very careful about lingering too long in what I call "perpetual limbo land" as you wait for the next test or scan or thumbs-up from one of the doctors on your team. You will find yourself moving smoothly from fight mode to man-I-hope-it-doesn't-come-back mode, more often than is comfortable. For most of us, it is much easier to fight than to hold your breath. And you begin to realize that sometimes the best presents come in the ugliest package.

If you figure out how to think in a completely different way, pay close attention to all of the new things that you are learning about, and ask all of your questions; then you will surely discover that there are always options and new methods that are being brought to the forefront. You will also discover that it will actually be within your power to experience something that before would have thrown you into high gear, high blood pressure and high anxiety and move you through it more easily than you ever thought possible—with confidence, peace, strength and sometimes elegance. Walking boldly through it; first learning and then absolutely knowing, literally feeling it in your bones that you are stronger than you ever thought you were, and allowing yourself to dream with your eyes wide open.

Chapter 75

All I Need to Do Is to Show Up

May 5, 2009

It was another smooth landing as the plane kissed the runway in Chicago. I was returning from a surprise birthday party that had been given for my sister, precisely thirty days before my next surgery. The original date in September had been moved up to June 5th. As soon as I walked from the plane into the terminal, it hit me hard like an unexpected wave in the ocean. The next thirty days would be a mix of excitement and horror. Could I be willingly walking into a nightmare? Or was I simply and finally landing at the beginning of the end to this drama?

The next thirty days were full of beautiful spring days, and I found my thoughts wandering aimlessly at least several hours on each one of them. I would jump abruptly from being completely scared to being absolutely terrified. At times, it was almost impossible to write; and although I sequestered myself at the lake house for a week to work on the book, the words did not always come easily. I even tried to place myself in the third person, once removed from the real experience. Unfortunately, that didn't work, either; most of my time was spent going back to the very beginning, polishing words, changing punctuation and making major edits to the copy I had originally sent via e-mail. I needed to work hard and really concentrate in order to maintain a presence of mind large enough to do justice to the subject. It was simply too soon for that walk down memory lane, even in the third person. Everything remained all too real and fresh. I only figured that out when the job of editing became so focused and intense and after I had been at it for several days in a row.

I had a hard time tearing myself away from my office when I would finally arrive there each morning directly from bed. And far too many times, I found myself looking up at the clock only to realize that the day had gotten away from me, as I was still quite comfortable in my pajamas. I spent that time diligently tapping away at the keyboard. Occasionally, I would allow myself to zone out with all thoughts focused on the beauty of the lake or some animal foraging around outside my office window. On several days, I would linger far too long in bed; much like it was last year before surgery.

The lake house was well-stocked with food, vodka and silence. All I needed to do was concentrate and focus on the big picture. I filled my days with at least eight hours of writing, which was considered Priority One. Once I was comfortable that I had given proper attention to the book, I caught up on reading that had been stacking up, took care of a laundry list of to-do items at the house, and ate well and never missed the cocktail hours at the end of each day. Even though I was alone, I felt that I had a great deal to celebrate; starting with the fact that I was alive.

Once in a while, I would wander into town for a visit with a favorite art gallery owner or walk through the kitchen gadget store—anything to keep my mind occupied with thoughts other than the book and the upcoming surgery. I did not exercise as I would have, had I been home, but I did give it a passing thought each and every day as I quickly walked by the free weights, exercise mat, stretching bands and weight balls. I was thinking that I needed to fatten up so that Dr. Song had enough fat and skin to make a reasonably sized boob.

I continued to feel confident in my doctor, the selection of the type of reconstruction I would have, and the hospital. I just had this underlying anxiety that I couldn't seem to shake off.

Fear had grabbed me firmly by the buttonhole of my shirt and was whirling me around like a tornado in Kansas. I knew that I had not yet mastered the medical stuff but I also knew that I had become so much better at it than last year.

Now, if you'll excuse me, I have a glass of vodka being chilled that won't be swallowing itself.

May 27, 2009

Today was all about pre-operative meetings with Dr. Song, his surgical team and the anesthesiologist. Once again, all of my questions were asked and answered, vital signs were taken, and Bernadette Schmitt—Dr. Song's nurse—took five pictures. The cameras were set up in their very own room, complete with those professional black umbrellas surrounding the area. If it hadn't been a photography session for breast surgery, I might have had some fun with it; but it wasn't fun at all. It was sad. These pictures would be used as documentation of my "before" status.

I was able to see "before" and "after" pictures of previous patients who had made the same surgical choice; I found them interesting and terrifying all at once. It was my turn to give back. These pictures of torsos only, are not only used for showing future patients the potential "before" and "after" results, but for Dr. Song to refer to when teaching and to have something to compare to as we move forward with each procedure; first, allowing Father Time to have his way.

Several weeks earlier, I'd had the pleasure of speaking with two women, Dolores and Judy, who had been Dr. Song's patients. They confirmed that my selection of surgeons was excellent. They answered all of my questions in frank and colorful detail and offered to be available should other questions pop up later. In my experience, I have found that women are usually generous souls when things are "normal" but when a sister meets another through breast cancer, the ties drive so much deeper, and so much faster. And all barriers are quickly removed.

June 4, 2009

Tomorrow would be the first of a minimum of two surgeries and one "procedure" dealing with righty's rehab.

I was grappling with multiple fears. Will my life end on the operating room table? Will the incision be exceedingly large? Will my general good healing abilities fail me now? Will I wake up in severe pain? Will I be one of those who become aware, actually wake up in the middle of surgery but are helpless to alert anyone due to the paralyzing drugs? Therefore, having to suffer the searing pain of a sharp knife or needle tearing through my flesh, and listening to machines that are whining, beeping and sucking in the background and having to handle it all in terrified silence?

Then I remembered. This would be a positive surgery, one that would most probably have a happy result and so unlike last year's surgery that had been riddled with fear and uncertainty.

Calm down, I told myself. *What's the real problem?*

If I wanted to regain my original landscape, I would either accept surgery or accept a life that would require me to wear those prosthetics—boneless, skinless chicken cutlets—for the rest of my life. What's the point of lamenting about fear and pain and squealing about it like a group of teenage girls at a sleepover? What makes this situation positive? Remember your assets. And remember that the liabilities have all been discussed and completely understood. Options? I'd done the research and it was a tad too late to change things now.

When I was a little girl, my dad used to tell me, "Remember to die only once, sweetheart. It is a complete waste of time to die multiple, slow and agonizing deaths when the experience you fear will probably be just that—an experience."

Dad also reminded me that someone had once said, "Cowards die a thousand deaths; brave men die but once."

I took another deep breath and tried to remember that I'd been there and done that; I'd bought the T-shirt and even considered joining the fan club. I really wanted to walk into this surgery with a smile and a positive energy field around me. And I looked forward to trading in my "cleave-edge" for a cleavage!

This next bit is extremely important for anyone taking Tamoxifen and having surgery. Dr. Nanda, my chemo oncologist told me that I MUST stop taking Tamoxifen ten days prior to and ten days post-surgery. Evidently, this drug is associated with blood clots and can produce these clots during reconstruction surgery and cause a failure of the flap.

Dr. Song agreed to allow Tsiona, the lady who works in the hospital with her own breast cancer accoutrement store, to view the surgery from the enclosed theater above the operating room: just like in the movies. And I agreed to allow a doctor from New York to join the party as well. He would be learning Dr. Song's techniques; we need to spread this talent everywhere we can to provide more women with this option. The surgery would take six to eight hours. It's a long surgery to stand around for. I wondered how long they would last.

I signed up for a research study whereby a sensor would be placed inside the breast flap after surgery. It's a virtually non-invasive, near-infrared spectroscopy to quantitatively measure blood flow. The monitor would be next to my bedside for me to see as well as for the nurses, who would be paying particular attention. It would beep if the level got too low. It measures the entire flap and not necessarily an individual blood vessel, but obviously it is a reflection of the total blood vessel repair. By taking part in this study, I was also allowed to go straight to a regular room and avoid Intensive Care (IC).

IC would normally be necessary without the sensor, as the flap would need to be continuously monitored and IC is the best place for that type of care. This study is a blessing for me, as I would be in the hospital for three long days and I would do just about anything to avoid IC. Not to mention the fact that there are really sick people in IC and germs run rampant. And it's a scary place to be if you don't have to be there. I planned on being home on Monday, as bright and early as possible.

Tomorrow, my life would begin again; complete with new challenges and changes.

And all I needed to do was to show up.

Chapter 76

Measure Twice, Cut Once:
Reconstruction Surgery

The entourage for today included Larry, Mom, Dad, Shere and Bob. We arrived in three cars, one after the other; much like in a caravan. Why did this remind me of a funeral procession?

It was 5:45 in the morning. Not the best time of day for me. I am a night person. At least I *used to be* a night person.

We checked in and I filled out a short form. Hmmm. This was the shortest form I have ever been handed at a hospital. They have just about everything on me stored away in the hospital computer. Today, at check-in, all they wanted to know was who to update during surgery. Shit! I was starting to get a little edgy.

I barely had time to take in the new surroundings when they called my name. I gave everyone a hug and kiss and carefully considered how I must look like to them. I attempted to look hopeful. I am certain that I'd failed miserably.

Larry and I walked into pre-op, dutifully following a nurse. We were ushered into a little space that separated us from other people by a thin drape that slid nosily around a trolley in the ceiling. You know, privacy and everything. It was an attempt at privacy, yet I could clearly hear conversations all around me.

"Please take everything off and put on the gown."

"What is your first and last name?"

"Date of birth?"

"What kind of surgery are you here for?"

"May I see your arm?"

I gave Beth, the pre-op nurse, my left arm. Since breast cancer surgery last year, my right arm had been forever rendered a "no-poke zone." Three needle sticks in my left arm with no good result forced her to move to the top of my hand. Three or four more needle sticks followed. I was unable to relax, which made the nurse's job all the more difficult. Larry was trying to distract me and held my hand more tightly. I could tell that this was as painful for him as it was for me. Our quick and shallow breaths mirrored each other.

This was a pre-op nurse. She was very good at her job; I just have crappy veins made possible from the last year of intravenous chemo drugs and blood tests.

Beth called over one of the anesthesiologists, a nice-looking resident who would be with me during surgery. He tried a few more times; I lost count. It was decided that in order to start a line, I would need to have my hand numbed so he could dig around more freely. With one hand, he gave me the numbing shot, while his other hand held onto my hand as it prepared to receive the needle. Our fingers were locked together. It felt comfortable. The needle slid in. That human connection and his gentle touch provided the calming moment that we both needed. My hand immediately became numb. The shot had worked fast. He then proceeded to dig around for a vein to get things moving along.

The head anesthesiologist, Dr. Stephen Cohn, arrived next. He introduced himself and asked if I had any questions.

"Please make sure I don't wake up," I pleaded.

I also wanted to know if he or the other anesthesiologist would be there with me throughout the entire surgery. He assured me that at least one of them would be there at all times. I trusted them.

Next, we met with Dr. Song's microsurgery fellow, Dr. Michael De Wolfe. They have worked together for nine years. He asked me to take off my gown as he whipped out the human version of a Sharpee pen and began to mark me up with black ink. Circles, arrows, zigzags, horizontal lines and little shapes like poufy clouds traced from my pubic bone, all the way up. I kept looking down, fascinated with my new body art.

"Suzanne," Dr. Wolfe said, "You need to stand straight so we are assured of symmetry."

He needed to tell me this only once, twice . . . maybe three times. When he was done and was satisfied, we talked a little, shared a few laughs then he announced, "Dr. Song will be in shortly with a red pen for his turn to paint you."

In walked Dr. Song. This guy is so cool. He wasn't in his scrubs but in a golf shirt and khaki pants. Did he do this to provide me with a sense of normality? Did he have an early round of golf or had he overslept? I decided that he had done it to normalize things for me. Out came the red pen and he made a few markings of his own and I knew by now to stand straight and tall. He made the fatal mistake of asking, "OK, Suzanne, before we start, what are your questions?"

Larry groaned. He knew that I had made a list of several requests.

Dr. Song smiled and answered each and every question, acknowledged my requests, admonished me not to worry and said he'd see me on the other side of surgery. I later learned that he had arrived in pre-op in a suit and tie and not golf attire—*that* had happened on Saturday. Good drugs!

The nurse readied a few other documents that I needed to sign and I overheard the resident anesthesiologist say to the head anesthesiologist, "That vein will never survive this surgery."

I froze.

What did *that* mean?

My right arm was taped off so there was no question; it couldn't be used. My thoughts jumped to the jugular vein. Or would it end up being the carotid artery? Damn, I wished Shere were in here with us. *Edgy* had turned quickly into abject fear.

Someone else approached and asked us to follow them out of pre-op and into the operating room. I expected a short jaunt.

I expected to enter a room with huge lights like you would find on a dark road at night, lit up to allow workers to fix the road. I expected to see several people smiling at me through masks. What happened was that we were taken on what appeared to be a tour of the hospital.

"This is probably better than a short jaunt," I said, "as I would never find my way out of here now."

Bailing was not an option.

We eventually arrived in the operating room, but I couldn't remember much after walking down the hall with Larry and the nurse. Later, Larry would tell me that we had made "the walk" before pre-op. He is probably right, but this is *my* story and besides, it matters little to the results. I do remember being asked to move from the gurney to the operating table. Thankfully, they not only provide drugs that land you directly in la-la land but paralyze you and erase your memory. *Ahhhh*, thank God for current drug technology. Better living through pharmaceuticals is the only way to go when you are sick.

It was an eight-hour marathon surgery for the surgeons, nurses and anesthesiologists. I couldn't remember a thing. I was told that I woke up easily in the recovery room, but I remembered nothing until I was settled into my very own room (Thank you, David Hefner and Suzanne Kopp). What surprised me the most was that I felt better than I had expected. I immediately checked out righty and my tummy to be sure that surgery had really happened. I was expecting a raw, black-and-blue and savagely disgusting disaster that would follow the crooked road map left by the magic marker. Instead, I saw several lines of very narrow surgical tape along my abdomen, running from hip to hip, and more tape that was in the shape of a shield on my right breast, a breast drain, an abdominal drain, and no bruising. I had never seen anything more beautiful when it came to my body. It was warm and swollen but for the first time in sixteen months, I had symmetry. I had *cleavage*. I also had a sensor sticking out of my breast, attached to the monitor that followed the blood flow of the breast flap skin. But I was so happy that I had to be careful not to pop a stitch.

I was being taken care of by Lucy Ferraro, Registered Nurse, during the first twelve hours; and Susan Forest, Registered Nurse, the second twelve hours of each day. They were in the room every two hours, taking a Doppler reading on three points of the skin transfer, delivering pain meds, checking vitals and providing encouragement. The Doppler sounds like the heartbeat you would hear when monitoring a pregnant woman's tummy. A smooth *squish, squish, squish* sound that says, "I am alive and well and pumping blood where blood is supposed to be active and moving." It was a glorious sound.

On a separate schedule, I had to have a blood draw from the phlebotomist. Xylia, the nurse's assistant, measured and emptied my urine bag and occasionally, housekeeping arrived to keep things nice and clean. Xylia was encouraging and helpful and full of good information and housekeeping was very diligent about keeping everything spotless. Being a clean freak, I completely appreciated their attention to this important detail. I didn't get to know the phlebotomist. That person would quietly arrive in the night or early morning. Maybe it was a resident vampire. If it was, they probably enjoyed the morphine, too.

Shere had decided to become a fixture in my room, and she monitored the comings and goings of anyone entering it and talked housekeeping into limiting their visits to just once a day. She stood guard, asked the questions I wish I could think of, made sure I had water, rolled me over, helped me in and out of bed to go to the bathroom, placed pillows around me for comfort, adjusted the leg cuffs they placed on each leg that loudly puffed air into them to keep my circulation going, and conferred with the nurses—all while keeping me company. I was so happy that she was there as I could completely concentrate on nothing but healing and leave the rest to her.

I loved the morphine delivered through my IV, and I had another pain device attached by two very thin wires that poked into the skin of my abdomen; it constantly delivered a soothing smack of something. I happily pushed away at the button even when I didn't need that smack. I really didn't need it, but I pushed the button every once in a while anyway. Why not? I was paying for it!

Early Saturday morning, Dr. Song stopped by for a visit. This time he was really dressed for the golf course. He wanted to see me and talk before he played that well-deserved eighteen holes. We discussed the criteria for getting released from the hospital, talked about the success of the surgery and shared a few "gentle" laughs. I was still a bit groggy but I had a huge smile on my face that matched the joy that I saw on his. It was another of those patient/doctor moments when everything had gone well and had been smoothly handed over to the hands of God and the angels of healing. I asked him to raise one for me on the nineteenth hole.

I was told that I must pass several tests before I would be allowed to leave the hospital. The day after surgery, the urine catheter was removed. The first goal was to pee on my own. Check. Turning on the water did help to get things started.

I was sweating profusely and was unable to regulate my body temperature. My neck began to itch and it was very tender on the right side. I gently scratched at it and ended up with a thin line of liquid that I felt trickle onto my hand. It looked clear and smelled odorless. I felt a loosening of sorts or a release, and my hand uncovered a needle that was attached to a plastic catheter that was attached to a thin tube. I was touching a *needle* and some sort of vessel in which it sat, staring right at me.

What the hell—?

Shere walked back into the room after a much needed break and told me that they had had to access my external jugular vein, as the needle originally placed in my hand was not able to handle the assault of eight hours of surgery and the delivery of pain relieving drugs afterwards. It was also used to provide fluids throughout the operation in a safe manner and would be available when and if the hand vein collapsed. I remembered what I had overheard the anesthesiologists discussing the day before, and it all made sense.

This was a common vein that is used for people who have frail arm or leg veins because it is of a larger caliber and less likely to infiltrate. The anesthesiologists preferred to have a reliable IV for a long surgery like mine. I couldn't have agreed more. Especially when it was accessed after I was asleep. The unique thing about this IV is that nurses are not allowed to place them, so the doctors must do it.

Dr. Aaron Pelletier who is Dr. Song's senior resident and the guy I met at that first meeting with the great bed side manner said, "It is not uncommon for patients to accidently remove the IV because it feels awkward to have something taped into your neck and it is easy to reach up and scratch at it, especially after waking up in the hospital after surgery. I have placed many in my days of junior residency and been frustrated when they were pulled out! Also realize that there was no real "needle" in your neck, just a plastic catheter."

Okay, a catheter—a needle. It was *still* something stuck in my jugular vein.

I could never be a doctor.

I could actually feel a hole: the catheter's entry point. I was afraid to look at it. Shere helped me to completely disengage myself from the IV and told the nurse that it was out. The second test to pass was to get off all IV drugs. The needle in my neck was out and I had to pee . . . again.

Shere, the nurse and I waddled into the bathroom. I was trying to aim directly into a gizmo that they called the "hat" that measured urine output, while hovering above the toilet as I would not actually sit down. The cleanliness freak emerged even when drugged. Shere was hanging on to the drains; and the nurse was keeping the portable IV stand, which was attached to my left arm, from getting all tangled up. Suddenly, I felt this rush of heat in my hand and looked down to see it puffing up like a popcorn kernel in a microwave oven. The vein had collapsed; liquid was rushing into my hand; no longer being restricted to a vein. The nurse told me not to worry. We could access a new vein once I returned to bed. (*Not* happening.)

As long as I could keep needles for intravenous drug access completely away and rely solely on oral drugs, I had passed Test No. 2. Check!

The third test to pass was to eat without throwing up. Not a problem. I was starving and thoroughly enjoyed the hospital food before Larry arrived a bit later with yet another dinner, my favorite: Italian food. Triple check!

The hospital floor I was on was for transplant patients: people who are really sick and recovering from a kidney, liver or pancreas transplant; serious stuff. The reason for my being on this floor was the level of aftercare required for the skin flap.

The man in the room next to mine was having a particularly difficult time finding relief from his pain. He would cry out in sheer agony every few minutes. The nurses, Lucy and Susan, who worked twelve-hour shifts for three days in a row, were kept busy all day and night trying everything in their toolbox to help him. They were running around throughout the entire shift. He would find relief for a few moments and then it would start back up. It was very hard to listen to and several times Shere and I would almost cry out along with him in sympathy and solidarity.

This always seemed to happen to me: whenever I thought that whatever was happening was going wrong or badly for me, God would send a message to remind me that it could always be worse.

During the day and night, Lucy and Susan were kept very busy by this man and others who were in a similar situation, and they felt secure in the knowledge that I was doing really well. Shere and Larry were in the room, standing guard and making sure that everything was moving along. There was not much that the nurses could do for me but monitor and maintain and they did that extremely well; along with being encouraging, helpful, kind and loving. I felt completely safe. They voiced their concerns and we assured them that we were completely happy with the ways things were and encouraged them to take care of those who truly needed it.

Shere actually stayed at the hospital for sixteen straight hours on Saturday. Don't get me wrong; the nurses totally did their job and I did not feel in the least bit ignored. It was a simple understanding between all of us as to where their expertise was really needed. Shere would have been there in any case. Since being freed from the IV drugs, I had to take everything orally and at one point needed to wait over two hours for a pain pill. The level of anguish from the man next-door had elevated, and Lucy and Susan really had their hands full, yet they continued with their stellar attitude. This was the perfect time to pass Test No. 4.

Off we went, Shere and I, drains in hand and me bent slightly at the midsection as we waddled down the hall looking for someone to hand over the relief. I aced that last test by walking unassisted without passing out.

I received a visit from Dr. Aaron Pelletier right after surgery and again mid-morning on Saturday. He shared with Shere and me the details of the surgery. I was there for a DIEP surgery which was a transfer of skin and fat and minimized the damage to your abdominal musculature. In the majority of cases, this surgery can involve some dissection of abdominal muscle. There are several major arteries that must be located and harvested from the abdomen, and moved up to the breast in order to establish proper blood flow. In a previous chapter, I mentioned that thirty percent of women have one of these major arteries lying directly above the muscle plane of the abdomen. It is an SIEA artery (Superficial Inferior Epigastric Artery). Patients who have this artery in this position have a much faster recovery and the surgeon has an easier time, as he/ she does not have to dig around in a search and recovery effort. I was warned that this was very, very rare and that I shouldn't get my hopes up. Most women have that artery buried deep within their abdominal wall.

"We opened you up and like a gift from God," Dr. Pelletier explained, as he gestured with both hands opening up like a priest. "There was that beautiful artery staring us right in the face. It was an adequate SIEA (Superior Inferior Epigastric Artery), the artery that is superficial to the muscle in thirty percent of women. We also located a beautiful DIEP (Deep Inferior Epigastric Perforator) artery that miraculously wrapped around the abdominal muscle. As such, we were able to capture both arteries with their corresponding veins, without touching the muscle at all, and move them to your chest to reconstruct "righty." This special DIEP vessel anatomy is extremely rare. We said a silent thank you and cheerily moved on."

I loved the fact that he was using my lingo: "righty." Priceless. It made these doctors feel all the more accessible to me.

Dr. Pelletier also told us about an observation that was made by someone in surgery. "The surgical team was intrigued with the shape of the skin panel to which we ended up tailoring from your abdominal tissue," he said. "This was the shape that fit best after we had lifted and removed some of the scarred mastectomy skin (from radiation treatments). It just happened to look like a Superman logo; an upside-down triangle, if you will. This isn't necessarily common for us."

Later in the day, I spoke to Dr. Song and he said, "Due to the internal scarring you had from the mastectomy, to merely place the flap within your remaining breast skin would have left an indentation . . . like that of a clothesline. So I opened this up and replaced it with the Superman shield of skin from your tummy."

I now refer to the scars that will eventually go away as the Superman shield. The metaphor seems totally appropriate for the experience I've had and pays homage to the surgeons and nurses involved in my care. Shere teased that instead of a tattoo of a "normal" areola maybe I should reconsider the shape. I'm giving that a great deal of thought, since I am resisting any signatures and dates to mark the artistry now displayed on my body.

Sunday morning, I woke up to Larry walking into the room. His timing was, as always, perfect—especially when it involved food, as breakfast was just being delivered. We shared breakfast and eagerly awaited word from Dr. Song. He had promised to spring me from the hospital one day early if I promised to stay in bed as though I were still in the hospital. We received and signed post-op instructions, a stack of prescriptions and a list of people to call in an emergency.

Dr. Pelletier asked if I would like to take the Vioptix automatic pain monitor home with me. Considering that I already had two drains to deal with, I decided to forgo this, as it was an optional accessory. I remembered Coco Chanel's rule when accessorizing: you always need to take one accessory off before leaving the house. Plus, I couldn't imagine dealing with three things attached and protruding from my body. With a few quick snips, I was released from the breast monitor and a few more snips released me from the abdominal pain monitor. Absolutely no pain was involved in either case. This left me with a return performance from Dickie the breast drain, and his brother Dwayne the abdominal drain was introduced.

Larry had wrenched his back and was grateful for the wheelchair they provided us to take me to the car. It allowed me and all the detritus of the hospital stay to be carted away much easier through the labyrinth of hospital corridors.

Once back home, the family arrived for a visit. After a while, Shere threw everyone out so she could take care of "both" of her patients. Armed with a cache of drugs, I made my way up to the bedroom where everything was set up and waiting. Larry decided to lie on the floor next to the bed, hoping to keep his back straight. I looked up at my beautiful sister and together we laughed. She had never signed up for this but she happily made us all dinner. She delivered it to me in bed and on the floor for Larry, and she hung around talking and laughing before she tucked us in and hopefully, finally, got some rest herself.

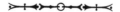

Dr. Song's Corner

While Suzanne had an uneventful post-operative period in the hospital, with minimal pain and discomfort, this experience is not necessarily one that everyone shares. Each individual patient has different levels of pain tolerance, anatomy, potential sets of setbacks and experiences. A good rule of thumb is to ask your plastic surgeon questions as to what the typical hospital course is for his/her patients and to also ask to talk with patients of his/hers; a patient can tell you in more vivid detail what she has gone through. While we, as plastic surgeons, perform surgeries like Suzanne's on a regular basis, we must all remember that we haven't personally gone through it. It is one thing to treat patients and help them through this operation; it is completely another to have experienced it.

Chapter 77

The Waiting Begins Again

During the first night at home, I slept like a baby. I had several visits and phone calls from family and friends and was continually fascinated with what I could see in both surgical areas. I would check everything out at least a few times an hour. It changed and improved daily and I documented it all with photos.

If I moved too quickly or in the wrong way, I would get a sting so debilitating it would take my breath away and stop me dead in my tracks. When that happened, I would be moving against the drains that were sewn inside of me and were very creatively attached. I remembered as a kid, playing with a braided hollow object where a finger from each hand was inserted into each end. The trick was to find ways to get your fingers loose. Dr. Song had sewn in what has medically been called a Chinese Finger Trap. These drains would not easily come out of your body. They were sewn into my skin inside of me in a way that reminded me of the fine details embroidered on couture dresses.

When I moved the wrong way and too quickly, I was also penalized with a stinging, burning pain in my thigh. Not just at the drain sites, but several inches down my thigh. What's up with that? I wondered if this was Dr. Song's way to keep me down. He assured me that it was all related to the SIEA flap that was harvested from my lower abdomen and that the pain would stop in a few weeks. I could deal with that, especially since I'd been able to walk since the day after surgery and had become a tad more erect each day after. I'd started out looking like Cro-Magnon man all hunched over, and had slowly returned to the straight and tall stance we all enjoy today.

My arm was black and blue and yellow from the continuous needle sticks; it made me look like an amateur junkie or a seamstress who preferred to use her arm as a pin cushion.

Two to three months must pass before I could get the areola tattoo and the nipple reconstruction. At this point, lefty was totally jealous and looking forward to the time when the swelling had gone down in righty, making things a bit more balanced.

The waiting began again.

Chapter 78

OK, So How Fast Is the Speed of Dark?

With the speed of light, it appeared that I had easily slid past the most difficult pain and discomfort. Then on Wednesday afternoon, five days after surgery, I learned the speed of dark.

My girlfriend Donna had just left after dropping off a home-cooked lunch and visiting with me. I had a conversation with a nurse about an upcoming appointment, and the next big event of the day was to be present on a teleconference call with the office. It was an important call. Bob was already downtown in person, and I wanted to be sure that I showed up, if only by phone, to support him and our position. It was a long and complicated discussion.

Even though this call had absolutely nothing to do with what I am about to say, in retrospect it did mark the occasion. It became really helpful to mark time with an occasion, as I had been just hanging around the bedroom and in bed for five very long days. They tended to blend all together after a while.

Halfway through the call, I began to have an occasional sharp pain in my right breast. It also appeared more swollen than in previous days. I could feel the unnecessary liquids being sucked out of my abdominal cavity and around the breast area, boiling and rolling somewhere below my skin. It was freaky-weird. When I looked down at it, it appeared as though an alien was slowly setting up shop inside. I noticed my abdomen moving up and down like a percolating coffeepot, on a totally separate pattern from my breathing pattern. Then, *swoosh*—a mucous-like clot appeared in the tube and was sucked into the drain. Totally gross! It wasn't easy to be on a teleconference call while trying to stifle the sounds of pain and make a reasonable contribution at the same time. All I really wanted to do was to groan, loudly; completely simpatico with my floor-mates' groans at the hospital just a few days earlier. Somehow, groaning always seemed to move things along.

This was not agonizing, ready-to-kill-yourself pain. On a scale of one to ten, it was probably about a two or a three, but I was hyper-aware and it forced me to tune in to my body and temporarily leave the teleconference call in spirit. I believe that any pain medications that may have been slowly releasing in my body, left inside of me from surgery, were waning in my system. It started to hurt and become terribly uncomfortable at the drain sites. I took two Oxycodone pills and waited for them to find their place in my body.

A few hours later, Larry came home. He brought up a glass of ice water, a plate of cheese, crackers and grapes and we sat in bed like two little kids. Unfortunately, wine and vodka were off the menu while taking pain pills. For me to say no to a cocktail, demonstrated self-control. I was impressed with myself. I found it exciting to believe my own growth in another way; eating this stuff in bed would not have been acceptable a few years ago. In this case, it was a private picnic on blue sheets instead of green grass.

We went downstairs for dinner. At one point, something went down the wrong pipe and I began to cough. It hurt so bad; my entire chest and abdomen were straining against the self-dissolving stitches and the painful spasms. A tear fell from my left eye as Larry stood next to me in horror, not quite sure how to help. He wiped my tear away and we waited for me to regain some control.

That pretty much completed that evening's dinner experience for me. I went upstairs to the bedroom and took off my bathrobe, which had perfectly positioned pockets that allowed the drains to hang without pulling. I carefully stretched out.

Larry voiced a concern that my breast looked more swollen today than it had the previous three days. That, coupled with the fact that the previous night my abdomen drain had pushed out ever so slightly and had begun to bleed, and the stuff I'd experienced earlier in the day—I started to worry. Was the skin flap showing early signs of a rejection?

I sent an email to Dr. Song. This was all normal, completely expected, not to worry.

I was so relieved.

I asked if the surgeon from New York who had sat in on my surgery was as impressed as I was. Dr. Song told me that the week after my surgery, the techniques that this doctor from New York had learned were put to the test; he had done his first SIEA surgery. That was music to my ears. I wish Godspeed for my "sister" in New York on her recovery; and I pray that the New York doctor is watched over by the angels on Dr. Song's team.

I continue to be amazed at how quickly these doctors and nurses respond to my emails. I never abuse that privilege and I pray that other patients feel and act in the same way. Accessibility is important for a patient, but abuse is all too common. While all of my health care providers have agreed to review the medical aspects of the book for accuracy, Dr. Song consistently responds with lightening speed.

Two nights before surgery, I sent him a chapter to review at around 11:00 in the evening, and I received a response within half an hour. I emailed back and asked if he ever slept.

He replied, "Duty calls."

I was impressed and a little worried. I asked him not to pick up the phone or check e-mail when "duty called" on Thursday night, as I really would prefer that he have had a good night's sleep before he cut me open on Friday morning.

I took two pain pills and a sleeping pill, worked a bit on the book and eventually grabbed five hours of blissful, healing sleep.

Chapter 79

"Stress Is When You Wake Up Screaming and Then You Realize You Haven't Slept Yet"

Two of the women from the radiation chick gang, Michelle and Jane, stopped by yesterday bringing lunch, and we had a council meeting of the "Brave Babe's Boob Brigade." I just made that up—the boob brigade comment. Rose had to work. Michelle brought our leading man: her fifteen-month-old son Aiden, who was the only bright light during our long days of being radiated. We had become very close, forever connected and continual support for each other.

As we sat eating, I was faced with the usual challenge of adjusting Dickie and Dwayne for comfort. Michelle and Jane offered the perfect solution: instead of pinning the drains to the oversize T-strap shirt at various points, depending on the position I was in, they suggested pinning them onto a shoelace tied around my neck. Brilliant!

The following morning, while getting ready to see Dr. Song, I pulled out a shoelace from my sneaker and tied it around my neck, attaching the drains by their safety pins. It was instant relief from the weight and the painful sting I felt at every movement of my body. Additionally, it allowed me to feel more confident that the two-foot long tubing wouldn't get caught on a cabinet door knob or something similar, which had happened several times.

The problem? It was a shoelace from a sneaker that wasn't clean, and I didn't have any new laces in the house. While in the shower sitting on the marble ledge with the drains lying alongside me, a light bulb went on. Christa, my goddaughter had made me a chain of crystal stones a few years ago to attach to my eyeglasses so I could keep them handy. I slipped each safety pin through both loops and made a necklace out of it. Not only did this work, but it was a re-purposed gift and was well-positioned for the drains. And it was clean, fashionable and matched today's outfit. I wish I had heard of this solution twelve days earlier; but now anyone reading this will know, and the idea can be passed on. While Dickie and Dwayne were still with me, this necklace helped—a lot.

My girlfriend Jeanne Brommer stopped by with a handful of lanyards she had, which are used to attach a name card when attending a trade show. These will be provided to Dr. Song's team for future patients. They are the perfect length to attach drains to, and to allow them to hang freely from your neck.

Wearing underwear or my now-famous thong was not possible due to Dwayne's position. I put on a long skirt, hiked it up over the "girls" and the drains that were now hanging from my neck, picked out a cute sweater, and then we took off. I was going commando. The first thing I thought of while Larry helped me into the car was what mothers have told their kids for decades: "Be sure to have clean underwear on whenever you leave the house." I smiled, feeling gloriously wicked about my secret. My secret—up until now.

Every pebble we drove over caused excruciating pain against Dickie the drain. For the last twelve days, I'd been moving around like a spider. I would slowly lift myself from the bed or a chair, and lightly touch the floor with my left foot. While one limb made contact, the other three remained suspended, perched mid-air. I would cling to the mattress or the arm of the chair, preparing for each limb to slowly follow to its natural position.

Getting in and out of the car was not pretty. But the breeze was pretty nice, and my skirt was long enough to ensure that I wouldn't pull a stunt like those of some young actresses who are caught by paparazzi and whose pictures are put in grocery store magazines.

After being called into the examining room, we waited just a few minutes before the nurses—Janice and Bernadette—and Dr. Song arrived. I had been crying in the waiting room from an upsetting email, the pain and total exhaustion. Larry told me that as soon as I'd seen the trio, my spirits had visibly changed.

My first course of business was to get Dickie the hell out of me, and fast. Dr. Song took a look, asked me about its output, and agreed. Janice, who was obviously not used to my sense of humor, whispered to Bernadette, loud enough for me to hear: "Who are Dickie and Dwayne?"

Bernadette whispered back, "She's named the drains."

Last year's mastectomy drain had been positioned in the part of the skin-sparing mastectomy where all feeling had ceased, and removal was pain-free. This year's drain needed to be placed differently and was in the zone of feeling: to the right of my breast and approximately five inches below my armpit. Hence, the last seven days of on-and-off pain; it hurt to breathe. Dr. Song was very gentle but I could feel each inch as the tube slid out. Although it continued to throb, even after being removed, the relief and freedom I felt was overwhelming. I hoped that the throbbing would soon subside. Today, I would breathe freely and tonight, I might sleep more easily.

Dickie the Drain had passed away. He was such a bastard during his life that we decided that we wouldn't be having a memorial or a funeral and we definitely would not be sitting Shiva. He was immediately cremated.

Dwayne, who had been trouble-free and lately draining 85 cc of liquid daily, was holding steady at that number. Until the output reduced to 30cc over two consecutive days, I would need to maintain our relationship.

As everyone expected, I had a list of questions. But noticing that the waiting room was filling up fast, I suggested that we discuss only those questions that would be too difficult to email back and forth. I would email the rest of the questions later in the day so that they could move on to the next boob who was patiently waiting in the room next-door. I do believe the nurses were shocked once again by my insolence. Dr. Song, quite used to it by now, didn't bat an eye.

No big surprise, but the first several questions were of a business nature. I asked if he would be willing to collaborate with Dr. Connolly, Dr. Nanda, Dr. Chmura, Dr. McCall and me—to determine where the money earned from the book would be used. He agreed.

I then mentioned a friend of mine who is nine months behind me in her cancer journey. She lives in another state and wanted to meet him and discuss her situation. She had located a surgeon she liked in her area but was not yet skilled in this surgical procedure. If it was determined that she was a candidate for a DIEP, and they connected as patient and doctor, she would travel to Chicago, have the surgery by Dr. Song or Dr. Park and recover at my house until cleared for travel back home. The hometown doctor wondered if he might handle her follow-up care and collaborate with the team at the University of Chicago. A huge smile erupted on Dr. Song's face.

He said, "Just this Monday, I saw five new patients all of whom flew in from other areas of the country. There are just not enough of us to take care of everyone in a timely fashion and provide time for me to train others. Like Dr. De Wolfe and Dr. Pelletier. I hired Dr. Park to improve that imbalance. She is brilliant, talented and a skillful surgeon with extraordinary results. Many patients prefer a female doctor, as they bring an understanding into the mix that a man could never have. She has been very successful here. Lately for me, collaborating with and training other surgeons, being Vice-Chairman and Chief of the department, Associate Professor of Surgery, Department of Surgery Chief and Program Director leave me with little time, and if I am to follow my vision and patient needs, then more doctors must be trained in these skill sets. Our team would be honored to help her and collaborate with her doctor."

I then learned that righty was considered out of the woods seventy-two hours after the surgery and would die only if *I* died or was in a major accident. What a relief; I was terrified of a skin flap rejection.

I asked, "What would have been necessary if the monitor of the breast flap had beeped while I was in the hospital? Or if the flap dies next week?"

"I hate to think about that," Dr. Song replied. "We would have taken you back to the operating room emergent, removed the flap and then replaced it with another flap from your back or your butt. That situation is very rare, so take it off your mind."

His answer sent shivers up my spine.

Once I left the hospital and my morphine friend, I had a virtually pain-free experience except for maybe five days out of the last twelve. Larry, my family and friends weren't too comfortable when they observed me folding my legs, all crisscrossed; or if I dared to reach down, albeit carefully, to pick something up. I hoped that Dr. Song would sanction them to get off my back. I am naturally very flexible. Always have been, and I expect I always will be. I felt *great*. I went so far as to show him and the nurses what I could do after only twelve days. I was quite proud of myself.

Dr. Song was not at all impressed with my demonstration. Although he approved of my sitting in *some* unconventional positions, he made it very clear that flexing my abdomen would present future problems and impede present healing. He also reminded me that working out in any way, even the arms and yoga, was not to happen until he had released me. I could lift nothing heavier than a gallon of milk. I could take a five-mile walk if I wanted to, but nothing else. That was all it took—Larry saw his opening and went off and told Dr. Song all the things that he felt I was doing much too soon, and the two of them had a wonderful few minutes double-teaming me.

I was told to use Neosporin, an ointment and topical pain reliever, twice a day (day and night). This would assist the scar in healing and would keep those areas moist and flexible. The scars felt a bit tight; later in the day, when I tried Neosporin it was very soothing. I asked about using cocoa butter or scar cream to help fade it all away faster and Dr. Song replied, "That will be possible, but only after I've seen progress on the healing of the scar in future weeks."

Later that evening, I sent Dr. Song the balance of my questions. I am adding here those questions and answers that are not specific to me, so that others will know what to expect.

Today, Dr. Song removed all of the surgical tape that hadn't released on its own and he trimmed up the self-dissolving stitches that were sticking out in a few places. Once home, I stood in front of a full-length mirror, checking everything out, and I noticed a lumpy bump at the left end of the abdominal scar. It looked like a small pea. Hmmm. That would certainly show through some blouses and T-shirts and would bug me terribly.

Dr. Song assured me, "Lumpy should go away, but if not, I'll use the excess skin to stuff the nipple."

I thought that this was a pretty darn creative solution. I remembered and rejoiced in the fact that I would be asleep when this "stuffing" business occurred.

I wondered if I was imagining the ability to feel both drains pull liquid, clots and mucous out of my body, as I've mentioned a few chapters before. "Nice thought," Dr. Song told me, "but chalk it up to your active imagination. You wouldn't be able to feel that."

Q: When can I travel by car and by air?
A: Once Dwayne the abdominal drain has been removed.
Q: Is it a bad idea to go on a boat during the Fourth of July lake house party?
A: That would be fine, as long as the abdominal drain has been removed by then.

This one surprised me. While on a boat, you employ abdominal muscles to keep yourself upright from the waves and all of the bouncing around. It must be a time issue, as that would mark twenty-nine days from surgery.

Q: Do I need to wear a special bra once you give the OK to wear one?

A: No, a regular bra is fine.

Q: Is wearing an underwire bra bad for breasts, reconstructed or not? Or is that urban legend?

A: At this point, any bra is fine—underwire included. Just be sure to check your reconstructed breast after using an underwire, as your new breast does not have sensation quite yet.

Sensation. Did I hear you say "sensation"? I thought sensation was a thing of the past for righty!

Eventually, I can expect to get some feeling back. While it wouldn't be the same sensation as before, I was thrilled that I would have a return of feeling at all.

Q: Will I need to wear an abdominal truss?

A: No, never.

Q: How soon until I can sleep on my tummy without hurting righty?

A: When I take your last drain out.

Q: The drain site where Dickie used to be on my breast, leaks. Is that normal?

A: Yes, that is normal and may last up to a week. It all depends on your anatomy.

Q: Since Dickie has been removed, I continue to get stabbing, painful jolts. Certainly not as bad as the last three days, but they hurt. Is this normal and when should it subside?

A: For most patients, this subsides in about a week after the drain is out. But again, everyone is different.

By midnight on the day Dickie was removed, I was in brutal, agonizing pain. It lasted for twelve long hours. When Larry arrived home for lunch the next day and came upstairs, he was confronted with quite a shock. My color was wrong, my breathing was shallow, my body temperature was elevated, and I was sweating all over and shivering as well. My breast was more swollen than any of the days before. I was crying, streaming tears and moaning like I was in labor. I wanted to die. The pain was not being controlled by the Oxycodone. At one point in the morning, it hurt so badly that I found myself talking out loud to all of my grandparents and my aunt in heaven, pleading with them to petition God on my behalf.

Larry called the nurse. Evidently, Oxycodone has side effects that we were not aware of and two of those are that they impede healing and do absolutely nothing for swelling, which Nurse Kelly Retzlaff felt was causing most of my anguish and pain. It was suggested that I stop the Oxycodone and take one to two Vicadin for pain, which I had on hand from last year's mastectomy; and for the swelling, a 600mg Ibuprofen, which I had on hand from a dental procedure two years earlier. That appeared to be the answer.

In actuality, the physiological response was that the nerves were firing off as they sought after the new connections that they needed to make. Swelling was a direct result of that activity. After taking the pills, I slept most of that afternoon, that evening and the next day; waking up only to go to the bathroom, change the dressings from the leaking drain site and take reinforcement pills.

Thursday night when Larry came home, he changed the dressings; it was impossible for me to be sure that everything was properly covered and taped. During the night, I could tell that the bandages had soaked through, so I changed them. I must say I did an awful job as far as aesthetics were concerned but at 2:00 AM, all I cared about was sparing my sheets and the mattress.

I would like to share a few helpful hints that we learned through this experience. The suggestions sound so simple, so obvious—but for those in the same place, they may provide a valuable head-start. Because it is impossible to know just when the drain site will leak after the drain is removed, and how much will come out at any given time, it is a good idea to place a towel over the bottom sheet on the bed to catch any residual "liquid stuff" leaking out of the bandages. Use a white towel so you can clean it with both soap and bleach.

The second thing we learned was that using surgical tape to keep the gauze or fabric bandages in place, hurt like hell when you pulled it all off. Larry put a butterfly bandage near the drain site—which was a fairly large, puckered, red, tender-looking hole—and he placed gauze bandages on top. We did not close up the hole but rather reinforced the area around it; the liquid had to have a way to come out. Larry put a stretchy, tan-colored Ace bandage on top of the gauze bandages and wound it around my body until the length of fabric ended. He kept all of that in place with three metal clips. It worked perfectly and made it quite simple, pain-free and easy for me to change all by myself when he wasn't around. (Warning: do not wrap anything on the reconstructed breast. Compression of this tissue, at this point in time, is a bad idea. My drain site was low enough to wrap the elastic bandage loosely around me without compromising that area.)

The last bit of advice is to wear a large or extra large T-strap shirt. They are also known as Dego T's; being half Italian, I feel comfortable using that slang. They will keep the Neosporin from rubbing off onto your sheets, pillows and other parts of your body as you move around. The consistency of the ointment is thick and a tad greasy and it lasts on your body for a very long time. It is unlike a cream or lotion that soaks in quickly. Unless you want to stick to yourself or anything else that you come in contact with, this "uniform" works best—and because it is sleeveless, your drains are not in any way restricted.

It was now Friday evening. Two weeks ago, I had been in the hospital, having just completed surgery. I'd come a long way, baby. I no longer need to say, "The *breast* is yet to come."

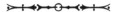

Dr. Song's Corner

It is not unusual to have clear or blood-tinged fluid leak from an incision or drain site. It is perhaps a bit more common after a delayed reconstruction, wherein the skin and chest wall have been previously radiated, as the lymphatic channels that drain the lymph fluid have been permanently damaged. However, once this passes, the new DIEP/SIEA flap like Suzanne had, will often help the entire site—as a new set of vessels and lymphatics have been transferred to the area.

Chapter 80

Love Means Never Having to Say You're Sorry

After a challenging weekend, I had a scare on Monday morning, the seventeenth day post-surgery. Dwayne the abdominal drain had more than doubled its output from the three days prior. This was a major setback, as it had been steadily going down and had hovered at around 40cc; 10cc away from freedom, before soaring back up to 90cc. I was moving in the wrong direction. Larry was convinced that there must have been a clot of some kind damming up the hole of the drain tubing that had finally let go or moved out of the way. Two hours later, I delivered a long stringy thing—a clot that probably *was* the cause of the backup.

I was sick and tired of being sick and tired. I was worn out from constantly cleaning up the oozing open breast drain wound and redressing it, draining Dwayne and occasionally having to push the bastard back inside of me (as it would sometimes slither out an inch or two), gasps of pain, issues with back spasms and constipation from all the drugs. I'd just about had it. I began to doubt my decision in placing my body in this state. To say that I was feeling completely sorry for myself would have been an understatement. I could see that seventeen days of who-knows-what-will-happen-next was wearing out Larry, too. Once again, my tears began to flow as steadily as Niagara Falls.

All cancer patients question a full life after diagnosis, and on that day I was convinced that I would probably be dead in five to ten years, anyway. Why should I be any different from so many others? Maybe having implants would have been the best, less traumatic choice. It sure seemed to be the more popular choice. I was exhausted by my own choices and the price that needed to be paid because of them.

What was happening to me?

I was depressed. What else could it possibly be? After calming myself down by taking an extra long shower and just hanging out, letting the water pound soothingly on my tightened muscles, I remembered that I'd felt like this before—last year after the mastectomy; simple cause and effect.

Depression seems to be as rampant as cancer these days. Turn on the television and in any given hour, there will be several commercials about depression and cancer. The symptoms of depression can start out to be subtle, but they add up quickly until you begin to assume that that is normal for you, and you just accept it. I am not claiming to have expert knowledge on this subject, but I know enough, and have worked through helping several friends—and these dark and negative feelings were not normal for me.

I apologized to Larry for dragging him along with me through this hell. He had responded as had been the case throughout our relationship. When I am weak, he becomes stronger; he pulled me through the process by reminding me that I had just experienced a major surgery in two places on my body. That it had only been seventeen days. That yes, I was probably depressed, but I wasn't in a full-blown depression. I decided to believe him and began to relax.

I mention this only because I hope to remind others going through the same experience that this is not something to be ashamed of. But it is critically important to confront it and to deal with it. I was able to snap out of it once I had recognized its root cause. But if those feelings had lingered, I would not have hesitated to talk to my doctor and seek help.

They were very difficult and exceptionally long days after Dickie the breast drain had been removed.

The breast drain site continued to drain several times a day for precisely seven days, and the pain continued on and off for the same length of time. Tomorrow would mark the third week post-surgery.

I remembered a movie I had watched when I was a teenager: *Love Story*. I loved this movie and had watched it several times. At one point, Ali McGraw says to Ryan O'Neal: "Love means never having to say you're sorry."

I started to cry all over again. But this time, they were happy tears.

Chapter 81

Wondering What Happens When You Get Scared Half to Death—Twice

Today marked three weeks since reconstruction surgery, and a year from the day that I had completed chemotherapy. Wouldn't you know it, but I had an emergency trip back to the University of Chicago hospital this afternoon. I spent most of that morning productively sitting around being nervous about what might come next. And then it came.

The breast drain site had stopped leaking and had closed up quite nicely on Wednesday late in the evening; right on time with Dr. Song's estimate. Thursday, Day 20, there was not a drop of liquid. By that evening, I had started to feel warm, then cold, then pain would begin rolling in and the skin flap on righty would go from warm to cool and then cold. The color seemed to have changed. I was perspiring and had the shakes. What the hell was happening now?

Friday arrived. At 1:00 in the afternoon, I began to feel a chill on my entire chest area. But being used to constant temperature changes, I did not immediately connect it to anything out of the ordinary. Then I looked down to check things out and saw that my entire T-strap shirt was literally drenched, and a yellow liquid that looked like what used to come out and flow into the drain was dripping onto my legs. I was covered with this stuff and it took three large towels and several washrags just to keep up with the continuous flow.

I pulled out a mirror and took a look. It was much like a small geyser, spewing out this garbage every few seconds. It wasn't coming from the drain site hole but was leaking from the breast flap in between the stitches, at the lowest point of the breast. I called the hospital and asked that the doctor on call, phone me as soon as he could; Dr. Song and Dr. Park were in surgery. Mega seconds later, the phone rang.

The doctor on call asked me several questions. Do you have a fever? Are you sick to your stomach? Has your appetite changed? Does the discharge smell? What color is the discharge? What is the consistency of the liquid—thin or thick?

The doctor agreed with my assessment. The liquid, unable to discharge from the drain site, was now seeking a point where it could be released. He said this was far better than if the liquid had stayed in the breast area and festered, as the only recourse at that point would have been a needle aspiration. It was OK to take a shower.

"Keep it clean," he said, "and call should anything change or begin to concern you."

Not five minutes later, I was calling the hospital again. The discharge now had an odor. The consistency of the liquid went from watery to thick. The color of this new liquid had changed a bit and was tinged with red. It had a glossy sheen to it that hadn't been evident before. The verdict: "Get in here so we can make a proper assessment."

Larry had left the house after lunch, and I knew that he had a very full afternoon with many critical appointments. I called Mom, the "Roadrunner" I've mentioned in previous chapters, also known as the original muse for the Energizer bunny. She broke every traffic law in the state of Illinois to get me to the hospital as quickly as she could. Traffic was heavy. We were terrified.

They took me in faster than ever before. Debbie Davy, a reconstructive surgery nurse, checked it all out and proceeded to squeeze (express) out as much of the garbage as she could that was still broiling inside of me. It hurt, badly. Debbie told me that after only three weeks post-op, she felt that all my surgical areas looked amazingly good—giving me at least a spot of good news. She took a culture of the liquid to have it tested to be sure that there was nothing else growing in there but a raging infection.

I met nurse practitioner and Registered Nurse, Kelly Retzlaff who would make the decision as to what to do next. Kelly is also the tattoo artist I would work with for Part 2 of righty's rehab. She tested the skin flap on the Doppler machine; it appeared to be within the necessary limits. She gave me a script for an antibiotic called Clindamycin. I asked her what I could have possibly done wrong to get an infection. I had been vigilant about keeping everything clean and sterile. Thankfully, her answer was, "Absolutely nothing. Sometimes this happens."

Kelly added, "The shiny discharge was a fat necrosis that had broken down to liquid and was no longer needed."

Whenever I coughed or breathed deeply, I felt a pain in the upper chest area above my breast. I asked what that was about. The answer surprised me. In order for the doctors to properly attach the arteries and veins to establish a new blood supply, they needed to take off a section of cartilage on my rib to make room for the work to be done. The discomfort would soon subside but the idea still grossed me out.

Nurse Debbie bandaged me up and we went home.

I was concerned that this infection would place the flap at great risk. Dr. Song eased my mind later in the day, the infection had occurred three weeks after surgery when the flap is known to be firmly anchored and LIVING! Having a breast flap issue at this late date, although possible, would have been absurdly rare.

Later that evening, Larry went to pick up a few groceries and I took the antibiotic as directed. Within an hour, my heart was racing so fast that I was sure I was having a heart attack, although the other classic symptoms weren't present. I chewed a baby micro-aspirin just in case and made sure that some of it went under my tongue for a faster delivery. My heart continued to pound, and could be felt racing by simply placing your hand *anywhere* on my chest.

I called Larry, grabbed all my scripts and went downstairs. In case I passed out before he arrived, he wouldn't need to carry me down the stairs. I had the cell phone with me and kept pressing 911 but not hitting the send button. In case things got worse, I wanted a fast way to get help. My heart seemed to slow down a bit so I called Larry back and told him not to rush and to be careful. The episode was probably at its end.

As soon as Larry arrived home he listened to my heart and wanted to immediately get me to Hinsdale Hospital's Emergency Room, which was a mile away. I wasn't too happy about going to yet another hospital that day and I bluntly refused. I was beginning to feel better. He firmly stated that I was going to the hospital or I needed to sign a waiver releasing him from any lawsuits my parents would present to him if anything happened to me. He was serious. I gave in.

Once at the hospital, I was rushed into triage. My blood pressure was low (odd for me) and my heart was at 225 beats per minute (BPM), which is more than three times the normal rate. I could only imagine what the BPM was at the start of this drama. As soon as the triage nurse had told us what my heartbeat was, I looked at Larry. He had turned white. He later told me that he isn't able get his heartbeat over 170 BPM even after a rigorous run or workout.

Oh, my God, I thought. *I am going to die.*

After several attempts at starting an IV line, one of my veins finally made itself available. I have a tendency to hold my breath against pain or fear and Jill Ibrahim, the nurse, implored me to breathe deeply. I summarily ignored her. I could barely hear her through the fog that my mind was creating. I was only able to calm down after Larry held my face with both of his hands and told me to look at him and concentrate as he coached me through breathing correctly. It is hard to believe that such a strong person, as I believe I am, can become so lame in the face of medical issues.

The phlebotomist came in to draw blood. She had no luck in finding another vein. Jill was called in and together they tried to find a vein that was viable. Several needle sticks later, they sucked out five tubes of blood.

I was monitored for several hours and hooked up to all sorts of lines. By that time, Larry had called Bob and told him what was going on. A few minutes later, Bob and Lisa walked into the hospital room. They both looked really worried and I immediately wondered if I was being given the full story.

I was given an EKG and an hour or so after that, I had a CAT scan with contrast, via a needle push of iodine. The three of them attempted to get me to accept that I just might need to stay overnight in the hospital. I strongly resisted that, knowing full well that the vampire phlebotomist would make a return visit if I stayed.

Doctor Guth spoke to the doctor on call at the University of Chicago. After their conference, they agreed to change my antibiotic to Sulfameth/Trimethoprim and Cephalexin. While the antibiotic I had taken was probably not the cause of this little episode, and the real reason was yet to be determined; the cardiologist, Jill and Dr. Guth all said that after a major surgery like I'd had, this reaction was not uncommon. I was released from the hospital at 2:30 in the morning.

From one of the tests, it was noticed that I had a 7mm, pea-sized, lower left lobe pulmonary nodule on my lung. It was suggested that I get another CAT scan in three months to be certain that it had not changed in size. This new issue with a lung nodule really freaked me out. Would I be chasing yet another cancer soon?

My chemo oncologist, Dr. Nanda said, "We do not have a baseline for comparison because we don't routinely do such scans on patients at low risk for metastatic breast cancer. One of the reasons we don't is because we are much more likely to find benign nodules than metastatic disease. And once we find a nodule, it creates a lot of anxiety and necessitates that we do additional tests, biopsies, surgeries, et cetera; trying to figure out what the nodule is.

"I think that this nodule is most likely NOT related to your breast cancer, for the following reasons:

1. If Estrogen Receptive (ER) positive breast cancer recurs in only one place, that place is highly unlikely to be a solitary lung nodule. It most likely presents itself in the bones first (your bones were fine on the CT). Usually, when we see spread of the breast cancer to the lungs, we see multiple nodules, not just one.
2. ER positive breast cancer, if it recurs, usually recurs five years out from the completion of treatment. It is usually the more aggressive types of breast cancer (HER2 positive and triple negative) that recur early—usually two or so years out from the completion of treatment. You are not even two years out from your treatment AND you have ER positive breast cancer.
3. You only had one lymph node positive, and you were treated very aggressively with chemotherapy, radiation therapy and now anti-estrogen therapy. While there is no guarantee that your breast cancer will not recur, the timing (this early with just one lung nodule) just does not fit your clinical situation.

"But now that we know about it, we are obligated to follow it to confirm that it remains stable in size. While I very much doubt this is breast cancer, the only other possibility if it increases in size is that it might be a small lung cancer. If it does increase in size, then I will refer you to a surgeon to take it out. If it is stable in size on the next scan, then we will follow it for a bit longer just to confirm that it continues to remain stable in size.

"I don't think a PET scan would be of any use in this instance because the nodule is too small to be picked up on PET; nodules usually have to be about 1cm or larger for a PET to be useful."

"Bottom line: I would like to repeat the scan in three months at the University of Chicago. I asked your husband to have the CT burned to a disc so that when we repeat the scan here, we can have it compared to the old images."

I felt much better after talking to Dr. Nanda; yet, I didn't sleep at all that night. I was afraid to, in case I never woke up. My heart continued to race, although not as much as it had earlier in the evening. I even felt it pounding through my back.

I now needed to begin a relationship with two more ologists: a pulmonologist and a cardiologist. On Monday, I would be fitted for what is called an event monitor that would be attached by leads and wires to several places on my chest. These leads and wires would then be attached to a cell-phone-size machine that I would wear around my neck for thirty days. The monitor would record all changes in my heart and provide an indication of any future problems.

The data from the EKG would be sent by holding the monitor up to a phone after dialing their number. It would be submitted electronically through the airwaves. If I began to feel faint, lightheaded or my heart started to change in rhythm, I was to push a button and it would record an EKG which would be sent to the doctor's office. Once the information was transmitted, a human would pick up the call to ask me a series of questions. I would need to tell them what I had been doing or feeling when the "episode" had occurred. This monitor would also record data during the day even if I don't activate it, and a doctor would review the information frequently. It had to be worn twenty-three hours a day.

I know that several women on this email list are also challenged with breast cancer and are eager to learn how this surgery had gone for me. If it hadn't been for the infection, the whole experience would have been a breeze, relatively speaking. Don't be discouraged. This heart issue could very well be a one-time event and might not ever happen again. The monitor is a way to play it safe.

The Mag 7 were convinced that God had just wanted another exciting chapter.

I wondered what the next several days would bring. But I was grateful that at least I had made it to the next day. On Saturday morning, the schedules had been organized with Marianne from the Mag 7 coming to "booby-sit" and make breakfast and lunch and look after me. Then Bob and Lisa would arrive. Next, Mom and Dad. The following days, each of the Mag 7 dropped by with dinner, conversation and support. By then, I was hoping to be back on the road again; just driving a lot slower. Now I know that you can be scared half to death—twice—and still live.

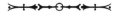

Dr. Song's Corner

While infection after breast surgery and reconstructive surgery is rare, it can happen. In my experience, patients who have had radiation therapy are slightly more prone to skin breakdown, fluid collections and infection. The theory is that radiation, while life saving, not only kills cancer cells but all cells in the area including lymphatics, blood vessels, skin and fat cells. Injured cells can't fight off bacteria as well as normal healthy cells, and despite meticulous efforts to antiseptically prepare a breast(s) for surgery; inevitably some bacteria can be introduced into the surgical site. Typically with antibiotics that are given at the time of surgery, this is not an issue. But even with antibiotics on board, those who have had radiation are more prone to having the minute amount of bacteria that may have been introduced, then go on to become an infection.

When the surgical site becomes warm, more uncomfortable, or the patient feels different with a fever, malaise or flu-like symptoms—this may be the first signs of an infection. Thus, after surgery if these things occur, your doctor should be notified ASAP.

Chapter 82

Life De-drained and Re-claimed

On the twenty-fifth day after surgery, and four days after the scare I'd had with the geyser leak in my breast, as well as an out-of-control heart rate, I had a follow-up appointment at the University of Chicago to check on everything relating to the reconstruction of righty.

I was very encouraged by what I heard. My healing was progressing faster than expected and I could finally begin to use body creams and lotions to keep everything moist and flexible on my abdomen. Due to the infection, I must wait to use them on my breast. What I needed to add to the mix was to apply just a pea-sized amount of Thermazene to the open breast wound. I'd used this cream during radiation. It should be applied to the open wound area twice a day. Then I was to position a soft cloth-like bandage over it and tape it all in place.

"Just know that it is normal for the cream to turn yellowish after coming in contact with the wound," Kelly cautioned me. "As long as the redness continues to be resolved and you are not having fevers or chills, this should heal quickly."

It did.

Ten days later, Dwayne the abdominal drain had completed his duties and we cremated him in the exact same manner as his brother before him. It was relatively uneventful. It had taken twelve days to get rid of Dickie and thirty-five days for Dwayne, as he'd had a much larger area to clear out. Dwayne had been forever getting caught on my foot while I'd been sitting with my legs crossed in bed, or he'd catch the bathroom or kitchen cabinet doorknob. It had been constantly getting in the way of one thing or another and it had seemed as though there were areas all over the house that I'd get caught on. After I'd calmed down from the pain that those occasions had caused, I would slowly push what slid out, back inside of me; the stitches holding it in had loosened a lot. It was never at risk to completely come out of my body, as a good eight to ten inches still remained coiled inside of me.

Last night, the drain bulb would not stay contracted and I learned that this was a surefire sign that it was ready to be removed. I was elated when he was removed and happy to have completed another colorful brush stroke on my personal portrait of torture; at least for the time being.

Kelly removed the drain. After I kissed Dwayne good-bye (in actuality, I gave him the finger), we talked about the next step. Kelly is also a very skilled tattoo artist for the cosmetic surgery department. She showed me pictures of women in the same situation: women with one real breast and one man-made breast, and it was nearly impossible to distinguish a tattooed areola from a God-given areola when looking at her work. She is very good at what she does. I asked about contour, the variations of color and shading, and the uneven hills and valleys found on unconstructed breasts. She knows just what needs to be done. Lefty would now become righty's muse. The procedure would take place in September.

I have to tell you that after meeting Kelly, I was enormously relieved that I did not need to face a big, hairy guy wearing a leather vest and dirty jeans splattered with ink, for my tattoo. Those guys scare me, and they have *needles* in their hands. Kelly is tall and slender, wears a clean, white doctor's get-up, and she is not hairy. She is super knowledgeable with a calming and comfortable way of dealing with people. Trust is important when you are allowing someone to draw that very intimate object on your breast.

I had reconsidered the earlier idea of tattooing a superman patch in place of a normal-shaped areola. Instead, I am leaning towards the conventional side of things. An image that I can still recall, an image that had been taken for granted so very long ago. I know and can see and will always remember my battle scars, and I've chosen not to allow my otherwise cheeky humor to get the best of me.

I was able to once again slather as much lotion on my entire body as I cared to. I asked Kelly about the name of the best scar fading creams to use. She said that there is no real evidence that these products help to remove scars any better or faster than keeping everything soft and pliable by applying the lotion that I would normally use.

There was a bit of scar tissue that was a tad hard in a few places on the rim of righty that concerned me. This was similar to the scar tissue that I'd felt after the mastectomy. I asked if I could begin to massage those areas to break it down. The answer was yes; massaging both scars with creams or lotions was the best way to break down that tissue and keep it soft, flexible and moisturized.

I was allowed to drive again, but I still needed to wait until eight weeks had passed before I could go back to my exercise routine. I was able to walk as much as I wanted to, and I planned a treadmill visit every morning in the basement. It was beginning to sound like the "can" in cancer was finally happening.

Both drains were history and now the only thing protruding from my body with wires that would catch on everything, was Milton the Monitor for my heart. Larry named it the Cardio-Pod. Milton would be packed up and sent away on the twenty-ninth day of July, thirty days after our first meeting. To this point, I had not had another "episode." While I've always been one to maintain relationships that last forever, I looked forward to saying sayonara to all this drain tube and monitor business. I looked forward to taking back control of my body and being able to wear anything I liked without worrying about how to attach things to my clothes or how to strategically place boneless, skinless chicken cutlets in my specially designed bras. Soon, I would be able to wear those hot Victoria's Secret items that had been carefully stored away, out of sight.

My collection of bandanas and scarves would once again be used as accessories that no longer needed to cover my head. I had stored the chicken cutlets, specialty bras, hats and wigs for the next person I would meet who had a need for them. I could now confidently step back into my former body, knowing that perfect symmetry in nature and in life does not exist.

Every fear, every struggle, every pain and concern had been worth it. My hair had returned to its natural-odd color, which I love. My body landscape had returned. Life was good.

Chapter 83

Nurses and Their Critically Important Role

Today's nurses have assumed an increasingly important role; and by doing so, have become the glue that holds the health care system together. In addition to having strong assessment skills and a solid theoretical base due to their college education, they now need to be experts in technology, informatics, and evidence-based practice (a fancy term for "patient reality," which I consider as knowing how to get to the core of each patient's unique bullshit factor; or to put it mildly, "their reality"). Nurses look at the patient holistically, are the managers of interdisciplinary care and they seem to be the people who are up close and personal with you, every step of the way. In a word, they are or can be—if you allow it—your "advocate."

Nurses work very closely with not only the patient but also with the patient's families. They instruct them on how best to manage their disease and better handle at-home care, and very often their lives become inexorably intertwined with their patient's during this very vulnerable time. It's a huge responsibility and often a difficult job; sometimes these nurses help to deliver difficult news at 10:00 in the morning, and then celebrate the end of treatment with someone else at 10:30.

At the same time, traditional nursing roles are expanding right along with technology, just as it affects all of us in our jobs. As a result, bedside (and "chair-side," in my case) nurses now use computers to document everything that is provided to a patient or happens to a patient. These portable computers are networked to the hospital's database.

Operating room nurses are now being assisted by the DaVinci robot, which enables surgeons and their teams to perform complex surgeries in a minimally invasive way.

They truly see, and must completely understand, the whole picture.

We are honored to have a nurse in our family: Leslie, my cousin Steve's wife. She, as well as others whom I've met, embody the spirit of nursing. They are quintessential caregivers who have demonstrated all the good that I have experienced in my quest to graduate from patient medical school. My experience with the nursing profession through breast cancer, my first foray into anything medical but the normal required check-ups, has shown me that quite often nurses are doctors without the certificate.

They are in there before the doctor is, asking questions, and evaluating your bullshit level while balancing it with the reality of your situation. They have seen and heard it all. I also feel that they are totally underappreciated by not just some of the doctors they work with, but by us: the patients.

In our business, we call them the "go-to guys." If you want something done, call a nurse. Please understand that I am not in any way discounting the value of a doctor. All of you know by now the admiration and respect that I have for Dr. Connolly, Dr. Nanda, Dr. Chmura, Dr. McCall and Dr. Song, and my sister and brother-in-law. But the reality of the medical profession is much like any profession: the doctor determines the protocol and the treatment plan, and performs the surgery; it is the nurses who coordinate, implement and monitor the entire process long before, during and after the doctor leaves the room. With my healthcare, I have found them to be the line of first defense.

During chemo, if I began to see a problem with my IV line or started to feel like I was leaving the planet, I wanted the nurse. She was the one who could alter the plan *now*; quite often, waiting for the doctor would just not have been possible or prudent. Before surgeries and procedures, they held my hand

and explained what was to happen and occasionally (actually quite often), wiped away my tears. After surgery, they checked important stats and monitored my pain levels, my healing and my comfort. They were encouraging and helpful and hopeful. They were critical to the success I can claim today.

Brigit Gallus, oncology nurse at the University of Chicago, said, "I guess the main point I want to get across to the readers of your book, is that I feel lucky to do the work that I do. We are curing cancer here and making enormous strides each and every day. I bear witness, watching my patients go from a terrible place in their lives, where they have just received the worse news ever, to hopefully getting the news that their cancer is gone. The tumor has shrunk; the CT scan is clear. And we all take a collective breath. I feel honored to be able to help patients get to that point. The losses we experience in our department are profound. We truly feel heartbroken when we lose a patient, but we can't let that outweigh the good we are doing. We're saving lives. I believe that I feel connected to my patients in a very special way because I am with them at such a vulnerable time. I am truly blessed to be healthy, and I'm thankful that I am able to continue to be touched by these truly special people. Our oncology patients are unlike any other patient I have ever met. They are strong. They have to be; they are fighting to live."

Elia Martinez, my oncology nurse for the last several treatments, considered things from another angle. She said, "Being a nurse is a rewarding profession, mostly because of the patients that make our work unique and special. While each person is unique, so is their experience, and everyone who enters our department both medically and emotionally needs something different. I treat everyone the way I would like to be treated and probably with a bit more compassion and understanding—knowing what they are facing. I am not sure if it is fair for me to say this to those who have cancer; because I am not sure if I could handle a diagnosis of cancer. I feel a strong connection to every patient I meet and I have met amazing people in my journey as a nurse and a fellow human being. Each patient has taught me to be better and to be grateful for what I have. I realize that I have a lot to be thankful for and I thank God for that. I love what I do and I know I am making a difference. Now, I live, I love and I laugh each and every day."

Leslie said, "One of the first lessons I was taught in nursing school was how to get to the "patient reality" or the bullshit level. We were told to realize that sick people are selfish. Not in a juvenile or spoiled way but as a means of survival. It is human nature to go into survival mode when we are hurt, sick or stressed. This knowledge allows nurses to get past the bullshit and to concentrate on each patient individually. We already know that each patient sees themselves as our most important. I had most of my schooling in a hospital setting and work experience in a doctor's office. In both cases, the nurses do develop a relationship with patients and their families. I spent many hours on the telephone listening to people's concerns and fears. One patient even called in to report the measurement of his daily bowel movement. We are told many things that even the doctors didn't know. It is our job to act as a liaison between the two. I was always a huge proponent of patient education and tried to make sure my patients understood how and why things were happening. Nurses today are dealing with technology that I never had. While this has many benefits, I sometimes wonder if it cuts into the one-on-one time with the patients. Nursing can sometimes be emotionally draining but it is one of the most rewarding things I have ever done."

Chapter 84

One Nipple Away from a Full Set & My Last Tattoo

August 5, 2009

Two months had flown by since reconstruction surgery. I was going to the hospital this afternoon to get a tattoo. I'd been told that the procedure wouldn't hurt. There was some feeling in righty except in the middle section; but I must be honest—I'd yet to *really* test it out. I simply couldn't work up the nerve to scratch, pinch or poke righty in any way.

My largest concerns about the procedure were twofold: the overall weirdness of getting a tattoo on that place and the fact that the placement of this particular tattoo must be accurate the first time out. They have yet to invent an instant eraser for tattoo errors. Although I am quite familiar with "White-Out," I doubt there is a product called "Areola-Out" available on the market. I had dutifully waited the required time to allow all of the tissue to settle into its final form, shape and position. Now I was required to once again hand over the reins to someone else and pray that they had slept well the night before.

There had been one positive change: Dr. Song would be doing the tattoo. That made me more at ease about the whole thing than I had been in previous weeks.

Aside from accuracy, I was also looking for a realistic color. A color that matched lefty's, visually displaying all of the subtle variations, contours and textures that would make it look . . . real.

I was Dr. Song's last patient for the day.

Larry and I walked into a huge, well-lit room that was way in back of the exam rooms that we were used to being seen in. There were all kinds of machines and odd-looking lines hanging from the ceiling and enormous picture windows on two sides. There were no drapes or blinds, from what I can remember. Debbie told me not to worry; we could see out but no one could see in. She also told me to ignore the hanging lines. We wouldn't be using them today.

Debbie and a resident I'd just met, began to select several small pots and little tubes that looked like they contained lip gloss but were actually filled with tattoo ink. By mixing one color with another, righty's color matches were made. Having been in the printing industry a good part of my life, I am familiar with color matching so this was an event that I was highly interested in. When a color was thought to be a close match, a cotton swab sweep was made alongside the nipple on lefty. We made several adjustments.

It is near impossible—unless you have a written formulation—to produce an exact color match the first time, so we experimented a little. Every woman's nipple and areola has a different combination of hues. There are no stock colors; these are very individual nuances.

Dr. Song walked in with a fellow micro-surgeon who was still working through his residency. Janice entered next with Dr. Parks and a few others. We now had the beginnings of a party. I was asked if I was comfortable with the number of people in the room who wanted to watch Dr. Song's artistry. Two years ago, I would have asked that they not be there. But as Art Bowers had told me at the beginning of this journey: you get used to being "exhibit A," and eventually it doesn't even faze you. I was at that place; it didn't even faze me. I was in a teaching hospital. I trusted Dr. Song. We made the best of it and pretended that this was the normal way to meet each other: with me naked from the waist up.

Dr. Song asked me to stand up from the examining table. He placed a tracing paper or cloth on lefty's areola and traced its size. This would be used as the template for righty's areola. The actual size that would be tattooed on righty would end up being slightly larger. The nipple would be added at a later date, during another surgery once the tattoo had healed. Because the nipple would be formed using the surrounding skin of the areola, there needed to be a little play in the size so that righty would end up being the same size as lefty. This reduction in size was predetermined to match lefty's dimensions.

This next step, the nipple surgery, which would not occur for several months, would be when the art of Origami became truly personal.

Dr. Song used the template and drew a slightly larger circle on righty, using a blue Sharpee pen. Larry and I both agreed that it appeared to be an accurate placement. The needle part was about to begin. I was, as expected, a tad anxious. The instrument that would be used is the same one that is being used in traditional tattoo parlors. When switched on, it pulses up and down. Dr. Song took a bit of ink from the final color-matched pot and began to draw the areola in. It didn't hurt a bit but it made my upper chest vibrate and caused me to cough. I could feel Dr. Song pushing down on righty to make the skin taut enough to better accept the needle's entry. Every once in a while, he dabbed at the blood with an alcohol pad.

We were talking throughout the entire process; all of us except Larry. He was standing next to me, totally enthralled with the whole thing. Dr. Song attempted to draw him into the conversation by asking if he agreed with the size and the color. Larry started to ask a few questions. They were questions involving technique; he could see that it looked like a pretty good color match. The actual color would start off a bit darker than what it would end up being because it would fade in the beginning.

After the preparatory color matching was done, the actual tattoo took about twenty minutes to complete. When Dr. Song felt that the job was finished, he placed a protective layer of A&D ointment mixed with tattoo ink right on top of the tattoo. The mixture ended up being the color of calamine lotion. Adding the A&D ointment to the ink color in this final step, allowed some of the color's pigment to further sink into the area, while being softened with the protective healing properties of the ointment. Dr. Song added a non-stick oval pad and covered the entire breast with a clear bandage. All of this needed to be kept in place for forty-eight hours. I could shower with it on.

After the requisite forty-eight hours, I was able to remove all of the protective layers. I applied A&D ointment on the tattoo and covered it with nursing pads—the kind that a woman who is breastfeeding, might use to soak up leaking milk. With adhesive strips, already attached, the breast pads stuck to the inside of your bra; they covered the area completely. You needed to change the pad and add the ointment three times a day for two weeks. While showering, the tattoo must remain covered. The best thing to use is a breast pad on your skin, covered by medical tape with an easy-release adhesive. The tape would ensure that the pad does not absorb too much water during your shower and would keep you from rubbing or washing the area accidentally. The ink is delivered only two layers down and therefore, in the beginning, should not be rubbed against anything.

At night, because I didn't want to wear a bra to bed, I used camisoles to keep the pad attached and the A&D ointment close to my body. This was much nicer to sleep in than tape. The A&D ointment smelled horrible but somehow I got used to it.

Many women will notice a scab that forms on their tattoo. That is completely normal. It is actually a sign of healing. Don't pull or tug on the scab; allow it to fall off naturally. Using the ointment and protective pads did an awful lot in keeping the scabs at bay.

Today marked the first week since I'd had my tattoo and all I could see and feel was a slight roughness and peeling, which would settle down in a few weeks.

Future mammograms for lefty would continue as all others before. Righty would never again have to experience that universally dreaded tissue flattening machine. Instead, Dr. Song would see me yearly to monitor for recurrence. He would give me a physical exam, and this would continue for the rest of our hopefully long lives.

The use of an MRI would only be ordered if the surgeon, doctor or ologist feels that something is awry in the reconstructed breast. Between my two surgeons and all of the ologists, someone would be checking me out and feeling me up every few months for quite a few years.

I had an appointment to see Dr. Song for a cursory checkup in two weeks. At that time, if everything looked good, I had to wait at least another two weeks before the nipple surgery could be scheduled. He is booked for months; it could take quite a bit longer for me to actually get in.

I was cleared to work out. And I was now one nipple away from a full set!

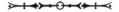

Dr. Song's Corner

The patient and I will spend a significant amount of time getting the color and position just right. This is a collaborative process in which the patient's wishes are at the forefront. Outside of unreasonable and aesthetically abnormal requests (e.g., skull-and-bones tattoo) the patient's input is just as valuable as the doctor's/nurse's tattoo and color skills. Be sure to speak up and voice your opinion.

Chapter 85

Origami's Fabulous Folds & Lefty Gets a Lift

Have you ever seen what a Japanese origami artist can do with a sheet of paper as they twist and fold and turn those flat slivers of pulp into a three-dimensional object? A three-dimensional object that is carefully sculpted into strong, yet sometimes fragile, but always amazing shapes that uncover intricate beauty? Those precise lines that evolve, quite often give way to unbelievable forms that are displayed in geometric designs, all kinds of sizes and shapes and incredible and real-looking textures.

For me, it's a lot different. I'm looking for a multitude of things. The weird part is that these things need to be fashioned on a human body—my body, not slivers of pulp. I am looking for the complex color of skin variations as they unfold into something that is not only stunning; but when texture is added with slanted slopes and smooth and uneven spots, transforms into a true work of art. In my case, quite a personal work of art and while I am a collector of art and unique blown glass pieces, I hesitate in asking Dr. Song to sign and date his work.

Even in retirement, I find myself on a deadline. In order for the book to be published in late October, which is the agreed upon end-date with the publisher, I have asked Dr. Song to schedule the final surgeries for September so that I can write about the experience and have everything "sewn up" and ready to go. Being the consummate professional, and not wanting to jeopardize the best possible outcome, Dr. Song wants to wait to do the final nipple surgery and the surgery for lefty's lift until more time has passed.

My challenge was to have the entire book chronicle every experience I've had: physical, emotional and medical, from diagnosis through to this point; and while the news of a delay in this final step was a setback, it reminded me of the art of compromise and the ability to be creative in problem solving.

This chapter will take on a different character than the others. It will be a discussion between me and Dr. Song, as to how the final stages should and probably will occur. I will be able to ask all of my questions and completely describe what will happen; when the time is right.

These last few steps will be taken care of in October or November; depending on Dr. Song's and my schedules. By the time of my next "cancerversary" in January, I expect to be well on my way to being healed. I also expect to be through with surgeries and caustic cancer treatments. At that point, the calendar will have moved forward by two years.

Some women decide to end their experience here—not moving ahead with a nipple surgery. One reason being: the muscles that contract to allow a nipple to become erect and then relax are no longer there. This means that you will have an erect nipple on the reconstructed breast 24/7, for the rest of your life. That could be troublesome but as in many things, there are simple solutions. There are ways to cover the problem by using nipple covers (also called "petals") that fit inside your bra and can be purchased at most department stores in the lingerie department.

Understandably, at this point, many women are quite done with surgeries, the adjustments and challenges because of them, and the scars that inevitably reveal themselves—at least for a while—and nipple surgery becomes an add-on feature, a luxury attachment, an option.

The Interview

In a few months, I will have the final surgeries. They will be done on the same day and will include the "origami" nipple surgery for righty and a lift for lefty, who has been patiently awaiting her turn for a little update.

Based on my research, the actual surgery sounds like a breeze compared to the last nineteen months of medical drama. I began my questions for Dr. Song with my largest fear: being awake for any of it. He assured me that I would be able to go on a brief visit to la-la land throughout this next step, although many women can do it under local anesthesia. The time in surgery for the nipple is less than an hour, and the surgery for the lift is around two hours. I'd rather be totally unaware during those three hours. Once you understand the drill, you might agree. I am hoping for an anesthesia found in many dental offices or when you get a colonoscopy—they call it "twilight sleep." I even like the name.

From a previous chapter, you may remember that at the left end of my abdominal scar, I have a small piece of skin. I have heard it referred to as a "dog ear." It is a result of closing up the area at the end of surgery, and coming to the end of the line. You can't turn a person inside out, like you would when making a pillow case, in order to make a clean closure. My issue is to have a flat profile at that end.

Dr. Song would excise the "dog-eared" skin by direct incision and then place a few sutures to close it up. Once that skin is available, he would take off the outer layer and use the dermis and fat to stuff into the reconstructed nipple. Next, Dr. Song would make a series of seven cuts along the tattoo. He would then place the "dog-eared" skin at the center, lift the now smaller sections that had been made by the cuts on the tattoo—and he would deftly roll, fold, snip and suture it into its final form: an Origami masterpiece. If necessary, color would be added to the tattoo several weeks later.

I imagined the process as being similar to making Crab Rangoon, where you place a bit of crab mixture, spices and cheese upon a noodle or thick pastry and then origami it closed. Minus the deep frying to complete the recipe, this morsel—the nipple—would then be considered done.

As for the breast lift, Dr. Song would make an incision around the areola on lefty, and an incision beginning at the center of the nipple going down vertically to the bottom of the breast. He would then raise the skin off of the breast tissue, moving the nipple up and cutting out any excess skin. He would complete the process with one of his expert surgical closing techniques. Any skin that had been removed from the breast would be used, if necessary, to augment it. This is a safe option; so far, my left breast is cancer-free. Any excess skin not required for an augmentation would be sent to pathology as a safeguard.

Would you want to be awake and aware during all of *that?*

The after-care for both surgical sites is to keep everything bandaged for forty-eight hours and then apply ointment twice a day for two weeks. I can see the purchase of more nursing pads in my future.

Complete healing for the nipple would be six weeks on a cellular level, but two weeks visually. The restrictions after surgery would include two weeks of activities such as running or cardio-type exercises.

The best news is that I would not see a repeat performance from Dickie the Drain.

As far as issues that could be expected post-surgery, there really wasn't much; they are quite simple procedures. And as far as scars go, it is inevitable whenever you cut into skin through several layers that a scar will result. The scars from the nipple surgery would be quite expertly hidden within the tattooed skin. For the breast lift, the scars would be evident in the beginning around the areola and down from the areola to the inframmary fold. But they always fade away; I've seen it.

I asked Dr. Song what types of stitches would be used. For the nipple, the deep stitches that couldn't be seen would dissolve, but the outer stitches would need to be removed in two weeks. This is a pain-free event. For the breast lift, the stitches are dissolvable.

There should be no major changes in the nipple after surgery except that at first, it would appear very large but would shrink in a few months. The changes in the breast lift are changes that I am looking forward to after the incision heals: a perky boob that matches righty. Dr. Song did mention that some women complain of hypersensitivity in their nipples for a week or so after a breast lift. There should be no change in sensation for the nipple reconstruction on righty.

My last question was about righty and the reconstruction. Would I need a revision?

Dr. Song feels that at this point, it won't be an issue for me until I reach the age of about ninety. At that time, I may need a breast lift. At that time, I fear I will need more than just a breast lift, although I would love to make that appointment.

Next Monday, I would see Dr. Song for a quick check on the tattoo. At that time, I would be able to see pictures of his work on nipple reconstruction and breast lifts. Considering that these are the easier surgeries but still require skill and technique, I am looking forward to another rewarding day as I dream of the future, just a few months away. I imagine myself back together again—unlike Humpty Dumpty—and I have a playful and sculptural formation that continues to fascinate me.

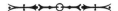

Dr. Song's Corner

The tattoo and the nipple are the final stages of reconstructive breast surgery. Even those who did not desire the final stages often feel whole again after having a new areola and nipple. Most plastic surgeons will create the nipple first and then tattoo it after the incisions (yes, *more* incisions) are healed, but I prefer to tattoo first and create the nipple after the color is right, for several reasons: 1) Any tattoo artist will tell you that it is more difficult to tattoo onto a three-dimensional surface like a nipple, but easier on a flat surface—I agree; 2) A tattoo is a dermal injury by the nature of how it's done. Tiny, sharp needles embed the correct pigment into your skin and thus, will cause some bleeding. Dermal (skin) injury can inevitably cause minute scarring, and scarring in a newly created nipple accelerates its collapse; and 3) Sometimes just the tattoo of the areola can restore the image of a breast. Several patients have told me to just stop after the tattoo. Here's why: a reconstructed nipple will always stay erect and show through clothing, et cetera. For those women who have battled a larger or erect nipple all their lives and have covered it up with Band-Aids or other cloth, to go back to an erect nipple can get in the way. For these select few, we can merely tattoo the nipple to give the visual appearance of a nipple that is relaxed (not erect/stimulated). "What a relief," they will often say.

As for the nipple construction itself, there are multiple methods for reconstruction—from using skin flaps (skin Origami) to borrowing part of the other side (nipple sharing technique) to using other body parts such as earlobes, toe pulp and skin from the groin region. Discuss with your plastic surgeon what you and he/she prefer. I personally prefer the sequence of tattoo first; and once the tattoo has healed, to then make the nipple using skin and fat already located on the reconstructed breast in an Origami-like folding. For a woman who has undergone surgery and incisions, I have found that taking from other body parts is less attractive, as many women don't like the idea of adding yet another scar.

Final note on nipples and tattoos: regardless of the technique, all nipples and tattoos fade over time and thus will most likely require a "touch-up" tattoo session or a small minor revision to the nipple. This is almost always performed in the office, not the operating room.

Chapter 86

When Support Moves Beyond a Bra

If you've made it to this page in the book, I believe you would agree that having supportive people around you is essential to experiencing a more bearable life during cancer treatment.

Some women are comfortable with being open about their disease, as I have been; completely losing it in the beginning and then slowly getting it together. Others cry often or are distressed, from beginning to end. And some can't even say the word "cancer"; they chose to refer to it as the big "C." There are those who handle diagnosis well. Sailing through surgery, chemo and radiation—and then they fall completely apart. The stories that I have been honored to be a sounding board for have run the gamut. I have learned that support is available in many ways.

The universal thread is that all of us need some kind of support. For me, it was my e-mail group. They would read my chapters; sometimes reading while traveling with only a Blackberry available, which blows my mind, as many chapters ran for seven to eleven pages. It would have driven *me* absolutely mad. Many would respond to these e-mails, sending words of encouragement, love and understanding. Then of course, there was Larry, Mom and Dad, Shere, Bob and the Mag 7, who were always doing something to help me.

Others I have met have found solace in attending activities held at local Wellness Centers, the Cancer Support Center at their hospitals or their church.

Our family had come to know the many offerings provided by the Wellness Community after my aunt was diagnosed with cancer. My dad, her brother, took the news of her breast cancer really hard and sought out the Wellness Community to learn more about the disease, and what could and should be done.

My parents live in Florida for eight months of the year. They went to the local Wellness Community in Sarasota, as suggested by their friend Sue Klauber. There, they learned of the resources available to cancer patients and their families.

D.R. Zaccone, my dad, had this to say: "The Wellness Community is a place of peace, learning and acceptance. They offer council, advice and complete support with a professional staff, as well as a staff of local people who provide the hands for touching and an ear to hear. It's a place to meditate and a place to heal as a patient. You will find a safe and comfortable environment for any family member or loved one who is or has been touched by cancer. Their web site is help@thewellnesscommunity.org or www.thewellnesscommunity.org. I encourage you to go there and learn what the Wellness Community can do for you. There are Wellness Communities in several areas throughout the continental United States. They can help you make a connection in your area."

I had the pleasure of meeting David Hefner during his tenure as President of the University of Chicago Medical Center. Mr. Hefner is now engaged in Washington DC with health reform, and has been involved with The Wellness Community on their national board for several years.

When speaking to him about support, he said: "How do you take this care-giving profession—now operating inside a high technology, wiz-bang twenty-first century platform of highly interdependent devices, pharmaceuticals and computers, that often neglects the patient's psycho-social needs and concerns—and close the loop in such a way that the patient experiences our humanism?

"While the neglect isn't intentional, it is just missing. Having enough time to treat the patient's disease as well as their psyche is nearly impossible in today's hospital environment, although improvements are constantly being addressed every day. That this important part of healing is even missing, and doesn't show up in the day-to-day environment as being missing, continues to be the challenge for most facilities. But if we acknowledge that it is indeed missing, we assume that the needs are somehow being met elsewhere and that healing the human psyche is not our role. Hence, the critical role of The Wellness Community & Gilda's Club Worldwide emerges as a bridge between these two worlds.

"Here we have the wherewithal to bring the nurturing side of humanity into the high tech milieu and have the two worlds actually complement and empower each other by bridging the fear and the unknown for both the caregiver and the patient.

"In an environment of health reform, we will inevitably have to confront head-on that our ability to treat cancer(s) will have to be balanced against the economic reality that we cannot provide everything to everybody, particularly when quality of life is factored in. Greater engagement by the patient and their family is a necessary imperative going forward."

Jay Lockaby, Executive Director of The Wellness Community in Sarasota, Florida, pulled it all together by telling me, "No one should, or has to, face cancer alone. At The Wellness Community, people affected by cancer find a place to connect with others facing the same raw challenges they are, *while* getting help with nutrition, exercise, support, and other individual information. Cancer can be especially saddening because one feels so alone and so frightened after a diagnosis—and burdening family and loved ones with these thoughts is often not an option. The Wellness Community is where patients and their loved ones can go and release stress, get information and just be themselves and talk with others who "get" the craziness of the cancer that they're dealing with. Nothing beats that for enhancing quality of life while fighting the disease and in many cases, enhancing recovery."

Resources
The Wellness Community International Office
919 18th Street, NW, Suite 54
Washington, DC 20006
Phone: 202-659-9709
Toll-free: 1.888.793.WELL
Fax: 202-659-9301
help@thewellnesscommunity.org
www.thewellnesscommunity.org

A friend I've made along my cancer journey gave me a business card for Imerman Angels. I never used it but when coming to the end of the book, I knew I had to investigate what they do—and if it passed muster, include it in the book. I called, spoke to the founder, who has quite an inspirational story himself, and I have decided that this is a place that can be of true assistance to those in need.

They provide one-on-one cancer support and will connect you to other cancer fighters, survivors and caregivers who have the same type of cancer that you do. Imerman Angels has an international reach, as well.

Please contact them at:
www.ImermanAngels.org
info@ImermanAngels.org
Imerman Angels
400 West Erie Street
Suite 405
Chicago, Illinois 60610
Phone: 877-274-5529

The pair-up process begins when Imerman Angels meets a cancer fighter in need. Once the initial contact is made, an Imerman Angels representative speaks to each cancer fighter, either by phone or in person. The representative, who is a survivor himself/herself, then searches the database for a survivor most like the fighter based on factors such as cancer type, treatments, age, gender and geographic location. The cancer fighter and survivor are then introduced. The relationship is in the hands of the fighter-survivor pair; but Imerman Angels is always available to offer further advice, information and guidance.

They serve *anyone* touched by *any type* of cancer, at *any* cancer stage level, at *any* age, living *anywhere* in the world.

Connect
Facebook: *http://luc.facebook.com/group.php?gid=18582449000*
Twitter: *http://twitter.com/jonnyimerman*
http://twitter.com/ImermanAngels
MySpace: *http://www.myspace.com/imermanangels*
LinkedIn: *http://www.linkedin.com/in/imermanangels*
YouTube: *http://www.youtube.com/ImermanAngels*

3. Love/Avon Partnership

The Love/Avon Army of Women is driven by two key partnerships that will accelerate the research necessary to discover ways to prevent breast cancer: a partnership between the Dr. Susan Love Research Foundation and the Avon Foundation for Women; and a partnership between scientists and women.

Heading the Love/Avon Army of Women is Dr. Susan Love, a distinguished breast surgeon, a trusted breast cancer authority, a best-selling author on breast cancer and women's health, and the President of the Dr. Susan Love Research Foundation. The mission of the Foundation, a 501 C3 non-profit breast cancer organization, is to eradicate breast cancer and improve the quality of women's health through innovative research, education, and advocacy. The Foundation works to identify the barriers to research and to then create new solutions.

The Avon Foundation for Women, a 501 C3 public charity, has raised and awarded more than $525 million worldwide for access to care and finding a cure for breast cancer. Support is also being provided by Avon Products, Inc., the largest corporate supporter of the breast cancer cause, which will work through its US Avon Sales Representatives to recruit women coast-to-coast.

Any female qualifies to join in this fight, whether they have breast cancer or not. I am a member myself. We need all of you.

Please contact them at:
Love/Avon Army of Women
c/o Dr. Susan Love Research Foundation
2811 Wilshire Blvd., Suite 500
Santa Monica, California 90403

In the United States and Canada, call toll-free: (866) 569-0388 or email at info@armyofwomen.org/ *www.dslrf.org*.

Chapter 87

Accepting the Challenge and My Future

I recognize and fully acknowledge my habit of and complete addiction to being alive. Over the last twenty months, I've encountered many boundaries. I've paused for a moment to consider their merit, and have occasionally had to step on them, squashing them good and hard, walking ahead with as much strength as I could gather. My fear of dying way too soon, and my faith in something larger than all of us, are what fueled this forward movement.

Along the way, I've developed a burning desire to change many of those boundaries for tomorrow, for the next woman, for the next family needing to travel a similar road.

I am working hard to figure out precisely what I am supposed to do with the rest of my life.

I continue to speak to at least five to seven women a month. Most of these women are newly diagnosed. Others have found me at a later point in their treatment. They learn of my journey from someone on this email list, and they ask that a connection be made. Speaking with others, helping them to navigate this puzzle called cancer and providing resources and hope—these will certainly be part of my future work.

But I'm still on the road.

I know it is on those side streets where the real magic often occurs. I know I had been missing some good stuff along the way. It's not just the scenery that you miss when you go too fast. There is so much more out there if you occasionally stop and experience the magic of the place, and stay long enough to visit with the people in the towns; the people who live off of the major roads that you generally speed right past.

I plan on shaking out, sweeping up and collecting all of those wasted hours that I've accumulated over my lifetime; and then carefully rethink how my future hours should be spent.

Throughout my journey, I often listened to people tell me that they would never be able to go through all that I have written about. Admittedly, I felt the same way before I was diagnosed. When the Mag 7 learned that Carol had breast cancer, and when we began to realize all that this would encompass, we had one of our monthly dinners. I took Donna aside and made her promise to just shoot me if this ever happened to me. She understood and agreed that it would be devastating, and we were both terrified, but I don't remember her ever promising me. I want to take this opportunity to thank Donna for not killing me.

That's the other beauty of this book. As I have said several times before, I am a medical Chicken Little. It was very hard for me to even walk into a hospital two years ago. Once when visiting a dear friend, Judy Greiman in the hospital, the nurses had ended up taking care of *me*—as I had gotten so weak in the knees that I'd almost passed out.

While all of this has become easier, I still cringe at the sight of a stethoscope or porcelain paired with needles and white hospital coats.

In the beginning, I didn't think I would live—let alone be able to do what I've eventually done. It was only by taking baby steps to get through each process; and because of the strength and support I received from my family, my friends and the staff at the University of Chicago, Edward Hospital and Hinsdale Hospital—that I am able to freely talk about this today.

I understand that I must act on all of the future requirements. I need to learn to deal with blood tests, attend the follow-up appointments with a myriad of ologists and surgeons, and continue having those mammograms and sundry other tests; so that I stay alive. Believe me—God forbid this would happen to you—while it might feel like your world is imploding in the beginning, if you are reading this book and if anything has resonated with your thoughts and feelings, then you are a fighter, and a lover of life and you will find your way.

I've been cut up, chemically bombarded and burned to death, provided air in an otherwise airless time from my support system, then put back together again. Somehow escaping the most deadly slings and arrows, I have come out on the other end of this journey feeling more whole and full of love and life than I ever have before.

Life is divine chaos.

Life is good.

As my friend John Kuhlman always says, "Don't give up. Don't *ever* give up."

Chapter 88

And This: My Final Chapter

DESIDERATA

Go placidly amid the noise and haste,
and remember what peace there may be in silence.
As far as possible without surrender
be on good terms with all persons.
Speak your truth quietly and clearly;
and listen to others,
even the dull and the ignorant;
they too have their story.

Avoid loud and aggressive persons;
they are vexations to the spirit.
If you compare yourself with others,
you may become vain and bitter;
for always there will be greater and lesser persons than
yourself.
Enjoy your achievements as well as your plans.

Keep interested in your own career, however humble;
it is a real possession in the changing fortunes of time.
Exercise caution in your business affairs,
for the world is full of trickery.
But let this not blind you to what virtue there is;

many persons strive for high ideals;
and everywhere life is full of heroism.

Be yourself.
Especially, do not feign affection.
Neither be cynical about love;
for in the face of all aridity and disenchantment
it is as perennial as the grass.

Take kindly the counsel of the years,
gracefully surrendering the things of youth.
Nurture strength of spirit to shield you in sudden
misfortune.
But do not distress yourself with dark imaginings.
Many fears are born of fatigue and loneliness.
Beyond a wholesome discipline,
be gentle with yourself.

You are a child of the universe,
no less than the trees and the stars;
you have a right to be here.
And whether or not it is clear to you,
no doubt the universe is unfolding as it should.

Therefore be at peace with God,
whatever you conceive God to be,
and whatever your labors and aspirations,
in the noisy confusion of life keep peace with your soul.

With all its sham, drudgery, and broken dreams,
it is still a beautiful world.
Be cheerful.
Strive to be happy.

~ Max Ehrmann—1952

Prescriptions & Over-the Counter Drugs that Were Taken

Prescription Drugs Taken

Xanax for anxiety (addictive; be careful)

Ambien CR for sleep (controlled release)

Ativan for sleep

Oxycodone (Percocet) for pain

Hydrocodone (Vicadin) for pain

Ibuprofen anti-inflammatory, 600mg

Neulasta shot to boost white blood cell count

Zofran anti-nausea drug taken for three days after each AC chemo treatment

Compezene for nausea and vomiting; the "emergency rescue" nausea drug

Colase for constipation

Dexamethasone steroid (one tablet daily for five days after chemo)

Doc-Q-Lace stool softener

Senna Lax laxative

Decadron (after Taxol) for bone, muscle and joint pain

Tamoxifen anti-estrogen pill (every day for five years)

Clindamycin antibiotic

Sulfameth/Trimethoprim antibiotic

Cephalexin antibiotic

Over-the-Counter Drugs Taken

Bayer Micro aspirin
Tylenol or Advil check with the doctor; sometimes these are
    contraindicated with cancer drugs)
Biotene toothpaste and mouthwash
cocoa butter for sore feet
eye drops for dry eyes
Sennokot stool softener
Thermazene silver sulfadiazine cream for radiation burns
Aquaphor cream for radiation burns
Eucerin cream for radiation burns
La Mer moisturizing cream for radiation burns; this was my
    favorite, purchased at a department store like Neiman
    Marcus
Neosporin ointment
A&D ointment

Vitamins Taken

Calcium with magnesium and zinc
Vitamin D
Co-Q-10
One-a-Day Vitamin

Some of the things I happily missed as symptoms, while going
through chemo, were thrush in my mouth and a metal taste,
mouth sores, a prolonged shortness of breath, a sustainable
high fever, low white blood counts, diarrhea, continued nausea,
heart pain and a lasting neuropathy (nerve issues of the hands
and feet; I only had occasional numbness and tingling). Watch
carefully for these symptoms and alert your doctor immediately
when and if they occur and join me in praying for those still
suffering these sometimes lingering and debilitating after
affects.

What Questions Should I Ask My Doctors?

Try to pay particular attention to the statistics. For example, thirty percent of patients respond to this procedure or drug. Follow up many of these questions by asking about statistics that *this* doctor has had with patients who have the same cancer as you. Ask about long-term and short-term side effects. They may help you to make a decision.

Some of these questions may not apply to you or your cancer but I have included them as they may spark a thought for your situation simply by reading them. Additionally, some of the questions in this first grouping may not be answered by a breast surgeon, and will need to be asked and answered by the chemo, radiation or reconstruction doctors. I tend to ask some of the same questions from each team member in my treatment field for a fuller scope of opinions.

I have a suggestion to make this entire process a great deal easier for you and for the doctor: arrive at the meeting armed, having done some basic research. Then look at the questions and highlight those that are most important to you at this point. Hopefully, you will be seeing (interviewing) more than one doctor; therefore, you want to know the answers to the questions that are most important for you, so you are better able to compare the answers. Leave the rest for later, when you are moving forward with the doctor that you have selected.

Questions for the Breast Cancer Surgeon (Pre-Surgery)

1. Is the closeness of the tumors to the chest wall of particular concern?
2. How do we know if it has metastasized? Could it be in my lung, brain, liver or bones?
3. Is the size of the mass, of concern?
4. Do you suggest a lumpectomy or mastectomy? Why one over the other? What are the stats of recurrence for each?
5. Explain the surgical procedure for each (lumpectomy and mastectomy).
6. Will I become disfigured? Where will the surgical scars be located?
7. Due to the calcifications found in my breasts, is it a prudent idea to have a bi-lateral mastectomy (both breasts removed)? Why or why not?
8. What percentages of patients have calcifications that turn into cancer?
9. Does my body produce or retain more calcium than necessary and is that why I have had calcifications? Where do they come from? Can they be avoided in the future?
10. How soon after you take the lymph nodes will they be tested and the results are known?
11. I am concerned about lymphedema. What are my chances of getting it? What are the symptoms I should watch for? Is this an avoidable issue for me?
12. I travel a great deal and scuba dive. Will I need to wear a compression sleeve for the rest of my life to avoid lymphedema?
13. Am I lymph node and estrogen positive or negative? Please explain.
14. What are the chances of a recurrence in my right breast? How about an occurrence in the left? Do calcifications change these chances or statistics?
15. How fast are new tumors likely to grow?

16. Explain all of the cancer stages. How accurate are the tests for staging? What stage am I at?
17. What tests are needed prior to surgery (bone density, chest X-ray, abdominal X-ray, Breast MRI, and full body MRI)? Anything else needed prior to surgery?
18. Will you do the sentinel node test under twilight sleep or anesthesia?
19. How soon must I have surgery?
20. Do I need to be catheterized during surgery?
21. How soon after surgery can I go home?
22. Will I have a surgical drain? How many drains are needed? How is it removed? When? How do I handle at-home care?
23. Can I wear a tooth guard during surgery, as I've just had expensive dental work?
24. Do I need to be intubated? Can we just do the IV thing instead like at a dentist's office?
25. Will medication for nausea be added to the anesthesia so I wake up from surgery without that potential issue?
26. Treatment after surgery: radiation, chemo, or both? Detail both processes, please.
27. Chemo: Do you suggest that a port be implanted? Can the port for chemo be placed while you are doing the lumpectomy or mastectomy to avoid another surgery? Explain the risks. I hear there are several risks, as opposed to chemo through a vein in your arm via an IV.
28. Radiation: Explain the shorter length radiation option called the MammoSite radiation therapy system. Am I a candidate?
29. Mastectomy only: Explain the pros and cons of a "TRAM flap" versus implants and expanders.
30. Mastectomy: Can we do your surgery then reconstructive surgery and implant the chemo port all at the same time? Why or why not?
31. Lumpectomy: are you able to manipulate the breast tissue to fill the cavity left behind by the tumor, therefore providing a more normal appearance? (This is called oncoplastic immediate

lumpectomy reconstruction.) One doctor's opinion was that the moved tissue would dissolve with radiation while another tells me it is a very good option if the sizes of my tumors are less than one-third of my total breast size.

32. Will the MammoSite balloon (a twice-a-day-for-five-days radiation treatment of the direct site) interfere with this manipulation or final look in any way? How about with traditional radiation?

33. Due to my calcifications, is total radiation of the entire breast a more appropriate process for me?

34. How long after surgery do I start chemo or radiation treatment?

35. How often and how long are each treatment and the overall treatment? How much time should be allowed for setup, etc., at each visit?

36. What are the side effects to each treatment?

37. Can I drive myself for treatments or must someone be with me?

38. What problems should be reported to you and what problems are normal?

39. Recognizing that this is a teaching hospital, I understand that I might not see *just* you. I don't want to be the breast du'jour; is it possible that I will be able to stay with you throughout the journey? Can we limit my exposure to a lot of students?

40. What restrictions do I have after surgery (showering, driving, sex, exercise) and for how long?

41. Will I need to take cancer drugs like Tamoxofin, Aromasin or Arimidex after surgery? Which one and why is that selection better for me? For how long will I need to take them? What are the side effects? Are there other drugs that would respond to my cancer so I don't need to worry about uterine cancer, hot flashes, new calcification developing or lung clots with Tamoxofin?

42. What clinical trial drugs are available? Am I a candidate? What are the side effects? How long are these trials? Are there any clinical trials that I should be involved in?

43. Should I take vitamins? How do you feel about Co-Q-10? Vitamin D? Soy?

44. How do you feel about bio-identical progesterone? (I am estrogen and progesterone positive.)

45. How should my diet change? (I don't like meat except chicken and fish.) Is eating Italian or spicy cuisine, risky?

46. Should I be tested for the BRAC1 and BRAC2 disease? Her2?

47. Is there a possibility that you would begin surgery with a lumpectomy protocol and then determine, mid-surgery, that a mastectomy would have been better? How do you proceed at that point? Should we decide in advance of this potential what to do?

48. When do I get to meet your team? Which "ologists" are included? Will you coordinate with them or must I?

49. What specifically do I need to tell my mom, sister and nieces when they go for a mammogram so that they can be checked early and more carefully?

50. Is there a blood test that my family can get now to determine the likelihood of a potential cancer, as there is for men for prostate cancer?

51. Do I have travel restrictions before and after surgery? How about before and after treatment?

52. What will my insurance cover?

53. Am I a better candidate for MammoSite or traditional radiation treatment due to the fact that my tumor is so high and deep within the chest wall?

54. Please confirm that the sentinel node test, the wire insertion and the lumpectomy or mastectomy are all done on the same day and in the same surgery while I am asleep.

55. Do you have a radiologist, oncologist, plastic surgeon and pathologist on your team or do you work with a network of people outside of your office? Are they the same people all of the time?

56. When can I meet with you and the team prior to the surgery to go over a list of questions and concerns?

57. What is the most common problem you encounter with my type of surgery?
58. Have you ever needed to re-operate? Why?
59. Can you save my nipple?
60. Stitches, staples, dissolving stitches or surgical glue for this surgery?

Questions for the Breast Surgeons (Post-Surgery)

1. How many nodes were removed?
2. How many were cancerous?
3. Has the cancer spread? Where?
4. How and when will we know if it has metastasized?
5. Did you get clear margins?
6. When can I drive again?
7. I had uncontrollable shivers, sweats and lung pain when lying down for the first three days (Thursday to Saturday). Is that normal? Reaction to drugs?
8. What restrictions do I have until chemo starts (sex, working out)? Is there anything to be careful of, expect or avoid?
9. The landscape under my arm has changed. Will that go back to where it was before?
10. The landscape in my back has changed. Will that go back as well?
11. What stage am I at? What does that mean?
12. When can the drain(s) be removed?
13. When can I begin to take a shower?
14. When can I begin to use lotions and creams?
15. What massaging techniques do you recommend to keep the scar tissue at bay?
16. Is the number of nodes recovered, of any importance? Have all the lymph nodes been removed on that side?
17. What are the signs of lymphedema?
18. Is it better, worse or makes no difference to have found cancer in one axillary lymph node versus several nodes?
19. What is my prognosis and what do you base it on?

20. Is it better, worse or makes no difference to have found cancer in one axillary lymph node versus several nodes?

Questions for the Chemo Oncologist

1. Chemo treatment will begin on _____ and will go until _____ and will be ____ times per _____.
2. How often and how long will each treatment be, including blood tests? How much time should be allowed for setup, etc., during each visit?
3. Can I drive myself for treatments or must someone be with me?
4. What problems should be reported to you and what issues are normal? Who should I call and what are their hours? What about weekends?
5. What are the names of the drugs in the chemo cocktail?
6. How long after chemo starts will I begin to lose my hair? Any idea how long it takes to return? Any chance I won't lose it? Will color or texture change?
7. How sick should I expect to get? For how long?
8. Are there any restrictions with chemo (travel, driving, exercise, sex)?
9. Explain the stage that I have been given (2B, TIC, N1 and MO). What does this mean in terms of my survival? Is there a chance my breast cancer could come back faster due to this stage?
10. Will chemo change the landscape of my spared skin?
11. What are the signs of lymphedema?
12. Is lymphedema a concern for me? What about scuba diving? Air travel?
13. Do I need to wear a compression sleeve for exercise and for travel in the air and scuba diving? For how long will this be necessary?
14. Are any other tests needed prior to treatment (bone density, chest X-ray, abdominal X-ray, breast MRI, Mugascan, and full body MRI)?

Questions for Follow-up Chemo Appointments

1. A friend has told me that she was given a blood test to test for cancer markers for her breast cancer follow-up. Is that testing available for me? Why or why not?
2. I have also read that John Hopkins has a new blood test to detect cancers such as breast, colon, lung and prostate. Do you know of these tests and are they the same or different as noted in No. 1 above? Please explain. I am concerned about my left breast and everyone around me seems to be able to get a test to check some marker for breast cancer.
3. My reconstruction surgery is scheduled for June 5th. When do I stop taking Tamoxifen prior to surgery and when should I start back up? Are there any other drugs or vitamins that I should stop taking prior to surgery?
4. Is there anything that I can do to reduce my long-term risk of leukemia and heart damage from chemo?
5. Now that I have had cancer, am I no longer a candidate to be an organ donor in my will and on my license?
6. HELP! I am as dry as the Sahara desert when having sex!
7. What is my prognosis and what do you base it on?
8. What is your opinion on the new study on women and drinking, and the link to breast cancer?
9. I am also having laser surgery for my eye in early May (narrow angle glaucoma iridotomy). During chemo, I noticed a major change in my eyes. Have you heard similar concerns from others clients? It is out-patient and does not require anesthesia? May I continue with Tamoxifen before and after this procedure?
10. Lingering side effects I have had since treatment began: sleeping issues, nausea and occasionally throwing up (mornings and late at night; no pattern), eye issues (blurry, tear a lot). Is there anything I can do to eliminate these things?
11. What is the most common problem you encounter with your patients after chemo?

Questions after Chemo

1. Tell me about aromatase inhibitors. Do they apply to me? Why? Pros and cons? Risk factors?
2. Is it better, worse or makes no difference to have found cancer in one axillary lymph node versus several nodes?
3. When do I start Tamoxofin? For how long will I need to take it? What are the side effects? Are there other drugs that would respond to my cancer so I don't need to worry about uterine cancer, hot flashes, new calcification developing or lung clots with Tamoxofin? Compare and contrast Tamoxofin with Latrozole and other new drugs currently available.
4. After Tamoxofin, will I need to take Arimidex or Aromasin or some other new drug available at the time? Why? For how long? Side effects?
5. What is involved in the test to see if I am cancer-free? (Is that the CA-125 test?) When do I take that test?
6. Do I need to wear the compression sleeve for the rest of my life? What about when scuba diving?
7. Why is my weight in triage always different from what is noted on the yellow drug document?
8. If issues develop after chemo, do I call you or Dr. Connelly (breast surgeon)? (Sleep issues, odd pains, fever, etc.)
9. Are any other tests needed (PET scan, bone density scan, Chest X-ray, abdominal X-ray, breast MRI, and full body MRI)? Why or why not?
10. How long can I wait before beginning radiation? How much does my life and the quality of my life depend on this decision to have radiation or not to have it?
11. What else are my leftover drugs good for? (Steroids? Anti-nausea?)
12. Why can't you provide an opinion on radiation? All I speak to suggest I listen to your advice, as you are the lead oncologist for my case.
13. Would it be wise to have a PET scan to check for hot spots to see if radiation is even needed?

Questions for the Radiation Oncologist

1. Will radiation be required? Why? For how long? Pros and cons? Side effects; long-term and short-term? Is there another treatment that I could have instead?
2. Why do you recommend radiation when I was margin negative, and with a T-1 node?
3. What about risk of skin burns, lymphedema and limitations for the future if radiation is needed then?
4. What about lymphangiosarcoma? How often have you experienced this in your practice?
5. Will any radiation be directed to my armpit?
6. What are the risks of not doing radiation? I am told and have read that radiation is only used in advanced breast cancer cases or in cases with high risk for recurrence (more than one node positive) and that for me, radiation may not be necessary. Do you agree? Why or why not?
7. How will radiation therapy affect my risk of a local recurrence, distant metastasis or a new breast cancer?
8. What side effects should I expect? How long will they last? What symptoms need medical attention?
9. Do I need to stay away from bras or bathing suits during treatment?
10. What other cautions or restrictions should I be aware of?
11. What problems should be reported to you?
12. Who do I contact with questions or concerns? Over the weekend?
13. Will radiation change the landscape of my spared skin (tissues feel firmer, breast may shrink, swell, small red marks on skin due to tiny broken blood vessels, skin turns darker)?
14. Will radiation affect my chances of having a successful reconstruction surgery?
15. How long after radiation do I need to wait for reconstruction surgery?
16. Are any reconstruction options closed to me due to radiation? I've read that tissue expansion surgery may not be possible.

17. Does my body produce or retain more calcium than necessary and is that why I have had calcifications? Where do they come from? Can they be avoided in the future?
18. Which exact area(s) will be treated?
19. What equipment will be used? What radiation volume or specifications? Who has and what is the latest technology or does the University of Chicago have the latest?
20. Can you tell me about complication rates, five-year survival rates, quality of life measures for just chemo and for chemo and radiation combined?
21. What are the chances of skin rashes? Rib fractures? Heart injury? Radiation pneumonitis? Changes in DNA?
22. How often will checkups and tests be required after treatment is completed? What specialist manages this care? How is follow-up care handled?
23. How do we know if and when radiation has been successful? Is there a test?
24. Would it be wise to have a PET scan to check for hot spots to see if radiation is even needed?
25. Do any local hospitals, closer to my home, have the same equipment? Which is the better facility (equipment, doctors, technicians)?
26. Will insurance cover the entire treatment?
27. What are the chances of contracture? Fibrosis? Lung Issues?
28. Can you bend the radiation away from major organs?
29. Can you stay away from under my arm (axillary area) due to lymphedema potentials? Will that make the treatment less effective?
30. Will you radiate the intramamory lymph node chain? Why or why not?
31. How long can I wait before beginning radiation due to my schedule?
32. How long should I allow for each treatment?
33. What recipe of radiation will you use?

34. What do you feel the impact of radiation treatment is on survival for someone with my cancer type, brand and stage?
35. What about radiation therapy and systemic recurrences?
36. What about radiation therapy and cardiotoxicity?
37. Is ductal carcinoma more deadly than lobular? Are recurrences the same?
38. What are your personal observations or statistics with long term side effects (lymphedema, heart problems, lung problems, rib fracture, radiation pneumonitis, and brachial plexopathy).
39. What do you see as a percentage of people who have a local recurrence with those who have had radiation versus those who have not? Same question with a distant recurrence?
40. What is the most common problem you encounter with patients after radiation?
41. What is my prognosis and what do you base it on?

Questions for the Reconstruction Surgeon

Initial Consultation Questions

1. How many steps are involved with each procedure? What are they?
2. What do you suggest as the best options for me? Why
3. What are the risks and complications for each option I have? How common are those risks?
4. How long will it take to complete my reconstruction from start to finish?
5. How much experience do you have with each procedure?
6. How many were failures? What happened?
7. How long have you been doing the procedure that I will have?
8. Do you have "before" and "after" photos that I can look at for each procedure?

9. What results are reasonable for me? (I asked to see pictures immediately after surgery, then three months later, six months and twelve months.)

10. May I speak to a few patients that you performed the same surgery on?

11. What are the risks and benefits of your selection for me?

12. Do you remove the scar tissue left from surgery and radiation?

13. What can be done to my current breast to be sure it looks the same as the new one? Is the nipple left alone if a lift is done? Will I have feeling with my normal breast after a lift?

14. May I see photographs at several stages (right after surgery, three months, five months, nine months, one year)? May I see pictures of those that didn't work out so well?

15. May I talk with some of your patients about the procedure?

16. How long will the reconstruction surgery last?

17. How long will I be in the hospital?

18. How much pain should I expect?

19. How long is the recovery period?

20. What are the restrictions after reconstruction surgery and for how long?

21. Will I go home with drains?

22. What will my breast look and feel like right after surgery? In six months? One year?

23. If you operate while I am lying on a table how do you know if the breasts are even, symmetrical, will fall naturally and look the same when I am sitting up?

24. Will I ever have feeling in either breast since I need to reconstruct one and lift one? How about the nipple?

25. Can nipple reconstruction be done at the same time? What about the areola? How is this all done?

26. What type of implants do you recommend? Why? How long will they last?

27. How do you feel about the various type flap surgeries that are available? Can you do the perforator flap to save taking muscle? (The doctor dissects out the arteries that perforate

through the muscle to the skin and thus spares the muscle.) How much experience do you have in microvascular surgeries?

28. Silicone has health problems associated with it. What are they?
29. What are the after-care requirements for the reconstruction option that you feel is best?
30. How are mammograms done on a reconstructed breast?
31. How much will it cost? What is covered by insurance?
32. Stitches, staples, dissolving stitches or surgical glue for this surgery?
33. I would like to see pictures of a DIEP flap that you have done. Do you have pictures that are immediately after one month later, three months later, six months later and one year later?
34. I would also like to see pictures of the scars I will have.
35. Do you check to see if an SIEA is possible before performing the DIEP?
36. How do you compensate for a moving belly button?
37. Pre-op suggestions for skin care.
38. Post-op suggestions for skin care.
39. Have you ever heard of a pain ball that is used at home after surgery for pain management? Are they effective?
40. I imagine I will need to be catheterized for urine. Will you wait to do that until after I am in la-la land?
41. How long will the drains be with me?
42. I know that pictures are taken to show progress and the before and after and to show other patients but is there a need for them during surgery? Please explain
43. Right below my collarbone it looks as if I had a horse step on me. Will that be filled out?
44. Is there a possibility that once you open me up that you would discover cancer or something else that would require the surgery to stop? Has that ever happened?
45. Will you have a clear view of the intramamory lymph nodes? Will you check to be sure they are not inflamed or sickly looking? If they are what is your next step?

46. How is the flap monitored after reconstruction surgery for proper blood flow? How do I monitor it at home?
47. Travel restrictions after reconstruction surgery?
48. Workout restrictions after reconstruction surgery?
49. What kind of changes can I expect in my breast?
50. What are my options if I am dissatisfied with the cosmetic outcome?
51. What is the estimated cost of reconstruction, tattoo, nipple and breast lift for my other breast or implant?
52. What should I consider for lefty—implant or lift?
53. What does my insurance cover? Will they cover any complications due to surgery?
54. How much pain or discomfort will I feel and for how long?
55. Will I need a blood transfusion?
56. What is the most common problem you encounter with my type of surgery?
57. Have you ever needed to re-operate?
58. What kind of changes can I expect in my breast?
59. What are my options if I am dissatisfied with the cosmetic outcome?

Questions for the Previous Patients of the Reconstruction Surgeon

1. On a scale of 1-10, how was the pain in the hospital after surgery?
2. On a scale of 1-10, how was the pain once home from the hospital?
3. How long did it take you to feel normal?
4. Did you have any infections or other issues?
5. How long has it been since you were finished?
6. How does it look now?
7. How does it feel now?
8. What made you decide on this type of surgery over the others available?
9. Why did you pick this doctor and hospital?

10. Do you have any advice for at home care?
11. Do you have any other advice?
12. What do the scars look like now? Are they noticeable?
13. What was the largest issue or problem you faced after surgery?
14. Does the tattoo for the areola look realistic?
15. Did you do the tattoo at the hospital or somewhere else?
16. Does the nipple look real?
17. Did you have radiation? Chemo?

Questions to Ask the Reconstruction Surgeon about the Nipple and Breast Lift Surgeries (See Chapter 84 for information on the tattoo procedure)

1. How do you excise the "dog-eared" skin left on the incisional scar on my abdomen to provide a flat profile?
2. How is that skin then used for the nipple?
3. How long are both procedures?
4. Please detail both procedures.
5. What is the after care for both surgical sites?
6. How long will after care be required?
7. Is color added to the nipple during this surgery or weeks later?
8. Can I be placed in twilight sleep for surgery?
9. How long will it take for a complete healing?
10. What are my restrictions after surgery and for how long?
11. What is the largest issue that can be expected post-surgery?
12. Will there be scars? Where?
13. Will you use dissolvable stitches?
14. May I see pictures of nipples you have constructed in the past? Breast lifts?
15. Should I expect any changes in my nipple after surgery
16. Will there be any change in sensation due to the breast lift?
17. Will the skin and fat be removed and discarded or stuffed back into the breast to create a firmer result as righty has?

18. How do you attain the fuller look at the top of the breast like righty has?
19. Will I have a drain?
20. My left breast still falls to the left when lying down while righty is front and center. What can be done about that?
21. Will my reconstructed breast need any revisions?

The Language Of Breast Cancer

Adjuvant Therapy Adjuvant therapy is treatment that is added to increase the effectiveness of a primary therapy—like chemo, radiation, biologic or hormonal therapy either alone or in combination after surgery. This therapy increases the chances of curing the cancer or prolonging a remission.

Alopecia A partial or complete loss of hair from natural or other causes. Many, but not all cancer drugs cause total or partial alopecia.

Androgen A hormone that produces male characteristics.

Antiangiogenesis Therapy The use of drugs or other substances to inhibit or prevent cancerous tumors from developing new blood vessels.

Antiemetic A drug that prevents or relieves nausea and vomiting which are common side effects of chemotherapy.

Antiestrogen A substance for example, the drug Tamoxifen that blocks the effects of the female hormone estrogen on tumors. Antiestrogens are used to treat some cancers that depend on estrogen for growth, such as hormonally responsive breast cancer.

Areola The area of pigment around the nipple.

Aromatase Inhibitor A drug that inhibits the aromatase enzyme, which is critical to the production of the female hormone estrogen; especially after menopause. The growth of many breast cancers is fueled by estrogen.

A-Typical Cell A mild to moderately abnormal cell.

Axilla The area of the armpit.

Axillary Lymph Nodes Lymph nodes located in the armpit area.

Benign Tumor An abnormal mass of tissue that is not cancerous and will not invade nearby tissue or spread to other parts of the body.

Bilateral Involving both sides (both breasts).

Biomarker A measurable biological property that is used to identify women at risk.

Biopsy Removal of tissue.

Bisphosphonates for Metastatic Cancer A class of drugs that can effectively prevent or slow down loss of bone that occurs from metastatic lesions, reduce the risk of fractures, and decrease pain. Bisphosphonate drugs work by inhibiting bone resorption, or breakdown, which may increase when cancer has metastasized to the bones.

Bone Marrow The soft inner part of large bones that produce blood cells.

Bone Scan Is a test to determine if there are signs of cancer in the bones.

Brachytherapy A radiation treatment that travels very short distances. For example, radioactive material or "seeds" can be placed inside or near cancerous tissue to attack the cancer most efficiently.

Calcifications Small calcium deposits in the breast tissue that can be seen by mammography.

Cancer in Situ Cancer limited to the surface of tissue with no invasion of adjacent tissue.

Carcinoma Cancer arising in the epithelial tissue (skin, glands and the lining of internal organs). Most cancers are classified as carcinomas.

Chemoembolization A procedure in which the blood supply to the tumor is blocked mechanically by injecting chemotherapy-loaded particles into the blood vessel supply with the intent of clogging blood vessels and delivering high concentrations of chemotherapy.

Chemotherapy Treatment of disease using certain chemicals. The term generally refers to *cytotoxic* drugs given for cancer treatment.

Conformal Radiation A form of radiation therapy in which the radiation beams are shaped in three dimensions to match the shape of the tumor. The shaping is accomplished by special equipment and special computer programs. It is also called 3-D-CRT

Cord (a.k.a. axilary web syndrome) is a painful condition, which has been identified as a complication of axilary lymph node dissection

Core Biopsy A type of needle biopsy where a small core of tissue is removed from a lump without surgery.

Cytotoxic Causing the death of cells. The term usually refers to drugs used in chemotherapy.

DIEP Flap See chapter 73 for a complete definition

Dose Density Delivery of the same dose of chemotherapy in shorter intervals.

Ductal Carcinoma INSITU Ductal cancer cells that have not grown outside of their site of origin, sometimes referred to as pre-cancerous.

Edema Swelling caused by a collection of fluids in the soft tissue.

Enzyme Inhibitor A drug that restricts production of certain proteins (enzymes) in cells that allow rapid growth of cancer cells.

Estrogen Female sex hormones that are produced by the ovaries, adrenal gland, placenta and fat.

Estrogen Receptor Protein found on some cells to which estrogen molecules will attach. If a tumor is positive for estrogen receptors, it is sensitive to hormones.

Excisional Biopsy Taking the entire lump out.

Fat Necrosis Is an area of dead fat that generally follows some kind of trauma or surgery, a cause of lumps.

Fine Needle Aspiration A procedure performed under local anesthesia in which a needle is inserted into the body to obtain a sample for the evaluation of suspicious tissue or too drain accumulated fluids from the body.

GAP Flap See chapter 73 for a complete definition

Hematoma Collection of blood in the tissues. Hematomas can occur in the breast after surgery.

HER2 status Breast cancers that overexpress a gene called HER2 are often more aggressive than HER2-negative cancers, but can be targeted with specific drugs, including Herceptin and Tykerb.

Hormone Status Breast cancer cells may or may not have receptors for the hormones estrogen and progesterone. Hormone receptor-positive cancers often grow more slowly than hormone negative cancers, and hormone receptor-positive status means doctors can make use of hormone therapy. Some of those drugs include Tamoxifen and Arimidex.

Hormone Therapy Treatment with hormones or drugs to interfere with hormone production or hormone action, or the surgical removal of hormone producing glands. Hormone therapy may kill cancer cells or slow their growth.

Hyperfractionated Radiation Therapy Is a method of delivering smaller than usual single doses of radiation two to three times a day. This method can allow for a greater overall dose while shortening the total duration of radiation.

Immune System Is the most complex group of cells and organs that defend the body against infection and disease.

Immunocompromised Having a weakened immune system—for any reason. This condition is sometimes present in the very young and they very old, in patients with HIV, and in patients who have received a bone marrow transplant or those undergoing chemotherapy.

Immunotherapy The use of agents that stimulate or augment the body's immune response against cancer or other diseases.

Infiltrating Cancer An invasive cancer that penetrates beyond the layer of cells it is sitting on.

Infusion A continuous drip of fluids or medications into the blood, usually through a vein.

INSITU Mass In the site of. When speaking of cancer, insitu refers to tumors that haven't grown beyond their site of origin and invaded neighboring tissue.

Internal Radiation The placement of radioactive material inside the body (as close as possible to the cancer)

Invasive A cancer that has moved beyond its place of origin, usually the milk ducts or lobule lining, to invade surrounding breast tissue.

Investigational New Drug A drug approved by the U.S. Food and Drug Administration (FDA) to be used in clinical trials, but not yet approved for commercial marketing.

LAT Flap Latissimus flap is an area of skin, muscle and tissue taken from your upper back and used for reconstruction after a mastectomy or a partial mastectomy. See chapter 73 for a complete definition

Lidocaine a drug most commonly used for local anesthesia.

Localized Restricted to the site if origin without evidence of spread.

Lump A mass of tissue that may or may not be cancerous.

Lumpectomy The surgical excision of a tumor without removing large amounts of surrounding tissue.

Lymphadenectomy A surgical procedure in which the lymph nodes are removed and examined to see if they contain cancer.

Lymphangiosarcoma Is a tumor in the lymphatic system.

Lymphedema Swelling in the arms or legs caused when too much lymph fluid collects in tissue. It can happen after lymph nodes and vessels are removed by surgery or treated by radiation. It can occur immediately in the post-surgical period or begin unexpectedly several years later. This is an infrequent complication of a lumpectomy.

Lymph Fluid Is an almost colorless fluid that is collected from tissue in all parts of the body and travels through the lymphatic system, carrying cells that help fight infection and disease.

Lymph Nodes Small, bean shaped structures that are part of the immune system and store special cells or bacteria traveling through the body.

Lymph Node Status Breast fluid drains into your lymph nodes, so stray cells from a cancer that is beginning to spread may be caught in the nodes. The so-called Sentinel nodes are mostly directly linked to the breast. If these nodes are positive, more lymph nodes are removed and dissected to determine how many nodes the cancer has reached, and to help in assessing risk and determining treatment.

Lymphatic system Composed of capillaries, vessels and nodes collecting lymph and depositing it into the circulatory system. This process transports proteins, fat, water and removes impurities. It also produces cells of the immune system, called lymphocytes, which are vital in fighting bacteria.

Malignant Tumor Is a cancerous or life threatening mass of cells, tending to become progressively worse. Cancer can invade and destroy nearby tissue and spread to other parts of the body.

Metastasis The spread of cancer from one part of the body to another. Cells in the metastatic (secondary) tumor are like those in the original (primary) tumor.

Metastasize When cancer has spread from where it started to another area of the body.

Microcalcification Tiny calcifications in the breast tissue usually seen only on a mammogram. When clustered they can be a sign of Ductal carcinoma insitu.

Micrometastases A very small amount of cancer that has spread from its original location and cannot be detected with currently available tests.

Multimodality Therapy The combined use of more than one method of treatment, for example, surgery, chemotherapy or radiation therapy.

Mutation an alternation of the genetic code.

Myocutaneous Flap Is a flap of skin, muscle and fat taken from one part of the body to fill in an empty space in another part of the body.

Necrosis Dead tissue.

Needle Biopsy Removal of fluid, cells or tissue with a needle for examination under a microscope. There are two types: fine needle aspiration and core needle biopsy.

Neoadjuvant Therapy Treatment given before the primary treatment, usually surgery, to shrink the tumor. It can be chemotherapy, radiation therapy or hormone therapy.

Neuropathy Damage to nerves, usually in the context of treatment related damage generally, in the hands and or feet.

Neutropenia An abnormally low count of infection fighting white blood cells in the body. This is a common side effect of many chemotherapy drugs.

Nodal Status Indicates whether a cancer has spread (node-positive) or not spread (node-negative) to the lymph nodes. The number and site of positive nodes can help predict the risk of cancer recurrence.

Node Negative Cancer that has not spread to the lymph nodes.

Node Positive Cancer that has spread to the lymph nodes.

Nonmetastatic Cancer that has not spread from the original site to other sites in the body.

Nonrandomized Study A clinical trial in which all patients receive the same investigational treatment.

Oncologist A doctor who is specially trained in the diagnosis and treatment of cancer. Medical oncologists specialize in the use of chemotherapy and other agents—such as antibodies, hormones, etc.—to treat cancer. Radiation oncologists specialize in the use of x-rays (radiation) to kill tumors. Surgical oncologists specialize in performing operations to treat cancer.

Oncology the study of cancer.

Oncoplastic immediate lumpectomy reconstruction In some cases after a lumpectomy, plastic surgeons can immediately intervene prior to radiation to help reshape the breast into a more aesthetically appealing shape.

Oconotype DX and MammaPrint These are genetic tests that measure the levels of a suite of genes expressed by a tumor.

Researchers hope that these and other tests will help them understand how dangerous a cancer might be and why some cancers respond to certain treatments while others do not.

Palliative Treatment Therapy that relieves symptoms, such as pain, but is not expected to cure cancer. Its main purpose is to improve the patient's quality of life.

Palmar—Plantar Erythrodysesthesia This is more commonly called hand and foot syndrome. This is a side effect of chemotherapy. It is characterized with peeling, itching, burning and reddened skin on the palms of the hands and the soles of the feet.

Pathologist Doctor who specializes in examining tissue and diagnosing disease.

Placebo An inert, inactive substance that is not distinguishable in appearance from the active substance that may be used in clinical trials to compare the effects of a given treatment with no treatment.

Precancerous Abnormal cellular changes that are potentially capable of becoming cancerous.

Progesterone Hormone produced by the ovary involved in the normal menstrual cycle.

Prognosis The probable outcome or course of a disease; the chance of recovery.

Prophylactic Mastectomy Removal of all breast tissue to avoid the risk of developing breast cancer.

Radiation Therapy Treatment with high energy rays to kill cancer cells.

Radioactive dye a liquid material injected into your veins so that specific things they are looking at show up while be viewed through special machines

Red Blood Cells Red blood cells carry oxygen from the lungs to the rest of the body by using a red pigment called hemoglobin.

Relapse A return of the disease after it has been in remission following treatments.

Remission Disappearance of the signs and symptoms of cancer. When this happens, the disease is said to be "in remission". Remission can be temporary or permanent, partial or complete.

Resection Surgical removal or excision of tissue.
Residual Disease Cancer cells that remain after attempts have been made to eradicate the disease.

Risk Factor Is something that increases a person's chance of developing a disease.

Sentinel Lymph Node The lymph node that is first in the drainage system of an organ to entrap cancer cells. If the sentinel lymph node is found free of cancer, the likelihood of other nodes being full of cancer goes down tremendously, eliminating the need for their surgical removal and complications thereof.

SIEA See chapter 73 for a complete definition.

Stage The extent of the spread of cancer.

Stage 1 The tumor measures less than 2 centimeters. Although cancer cells have invaded fatty or connective tissue, the cancer has not spread outside the breast including lymph nodes.

Stage 2 A stage 2A tumor can be as large as 5 centimeters without lymph node involvement or less than 2 centimeters but has spread to nearby lymph nodes under the arm. A stage 2B tumor is between 2 and 5 centimeters and cancer has invaded one to three nearby nodes; the tumor can be larger than 5 centimeters as long as it has not invaded axilary nodes.

Stage 3 A large tumor with positive lymph nodes or a tumor with "grave" signs

Stage 4 A tumor with obvious metastasis.

Standard Treatment A treatment currently in use and considered to be the best known form of therapy on the basis of past studies.

Stereotactic Radiosurgery A special focal form of radiation therapy that uses a large number of narrow, precisely aimed, high-dose beams of ionizing radiation. The beams are aimed from many directions and meet at a specific point; the tumor. The treatment is delivered in one session. Stereotactic radiotherapy or fractional stereotactic radiosurgery is stereotactic radiosurgery delivered in multiple fractions over a period of time.

Steroid Therapy Treatment with corticosteroid drugs to reduce swelling, pain and other symptoms of inflammation.

Supportive Therapy Therapy that relieves the symptoms, such as nausea and vomiting, that are associated with cancer treatments. Its primary purpose is to improve the quality of life.

Systemic Therapy Treatment that reaches and affects cells throughout the body.

TAP thoracodorsal artery perforator flap See Chapter 73 for a complete definition.

Three Dimensional Conformal Radiation Therapies A promising new technique in radiation therapy that decreases the exposure of normal tissue to radiation. Using computerized tomography (CT) scans and other imaging techniques, radiation oncologists have developed methods for determining the three dimensional size and shape of the cancer. This allows high-dose external beam radiation therapy to be delivered with less damage to normal cells.

Tumor An abnormal mass of tissue caused by excessive cell growth and division. Tumors perform no useful body function and are either benign (not cancerous) or malignant (cancerous).

Ultrasound Ultrasound uses high-frequency sound waves and their echoes to create an image.

Unresectable When something is unable to be surgically removed.

White Blood Cells One of the sub types of blood cells that helps fight infection.

About The Author

Before Cancer

Suzanne Zaccone is currently Executive Vice-Chairman and formerly President and co-owner of Graphic Solutions International, LLC (GSI), a global, ISO QS9000, certified custom print house. She founded the business twenty-four years ago with her brother, Bob Zaccone, Executive Vice-President. What was once a small company of three quickly grew, and now employs 110 people and produces over $25 million in annual revenue. It is now called GSI Technologies, LLC.

As a member of the Tag & Label Manufacturers Institute, Suzanne served a term as President, the first female in its seventy-five year history, was the Chair of the Communications committee for seven years, and held a seat on the Board of Directors for thirteen years.

Currently, she has a seat on the Board of Directors of the DiTrolio Flexographic Institute and has been its President since 2005. She is listed in "Who's Who in Finance and Industry," "Who's Who of Emerging Leaders in America," "Who's Who of American Women," "Who's Who in the Midwest," "Who's Who in the World," and "Who's Who among Young American Professionals."

After Cancer

Suzanne Zaccone, semi-retired, remains happy and continues to laugh, drink vodka and smoothies and definitely maintains her attitude. She is now a Cancer Survivor and is available at any time of the day or night to talk to anyone diagnosed with any cancer.

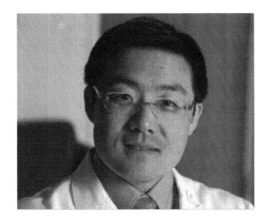

About Dr. Song
(Dr. Song's Corner)

David H. Song, MD, MBA, FACS, is an internationally recognized expert in plastic surgery with additional training in reconstructive microsurgery. He is a Professor of Surgery, Vice-Chairman of the Department of Surgery, Chief of Plastic Surgery and Residency program director at the University of Chicago Medical Center. At the age of thirty-four, he was the youngest appointed Chief and Program Director of a major academic plastic surgery program in the country. He specializes in breast reconstruction and oconoplastic surgery.

Dr. Song is well-recognized for his extensive experience with perforator breast reconstruction procedures, including deep inferior epigastric perforator flap (SGAP), superficial inferior epigastric artery flap (SIEA), thoracodorsal artery perforator flap (TAP) and the uses of Acellular Dermal Matrix (Alloderm) to enhance breast implant reconstruction and reconstruct abdominal wall defects. Additionally, he has pioneered several techniques for the repair and reconstruction of chest wall defects. Dr. Song's research interests focus on outcome improvement in lumpectomy and mastectomy reconstruction.

He is involved in several clinical trials exploring advancements in these procedures. For his work, he received the prestigious Arthur G. Michel award, given annually by the Breast Cancer Network of Strength (formerly Y-Me) for the clinician of the year.

In addition, Dr. Song serves on the board of Medical Aid for Children of Latin America (MACLA), an organization that provides free surgical care for children with congenital deformities in the Dominican Republic. He is also immediate past-president of the Chicago Society of Plastic Surgeons, and a board member of the American Society of Plastic Surgeons (ASPA) and the Association of Academic Chairmen of Plastic Surgery (AACPS). Dr. Song recently received his M.B.A. from the University of Chicago Booth School of Business, which he plans to utilize for the advancement of healthcare delivery with an emphasis on breast cancer awareness, treatment and prevention.

"Suzanne writes with wit and warmth. Between the lines is an important message that is relevant to all women who have shared in her experience. Suzanne took the time to research, ask questions, and take excellent care of herself—before, during and after her treatment. She listened to her doctors, and to herself. She radiates health from the inside out. Her story will help others to radiate their special health, too."

~Anne Ritke McCall, M.D., FACRO
Fox Valley Radiation Oncology, LLC
Edward Cancer Center

"Suzanne was diagnosed with breast cancer many months ago. This courageous lady kept a virtual diary of every detail, of every moment of her care. You get the feeling that you are in the room with her as she describes procedures, medication and counseling with the various doctors and nurses.

"Ever wonder what it is like to have breast cancer; the fears, the laughter, the love, the faith, the fleeting thoughts of vulnerability, the concerns? They are expressed here by a real survivor. The author, in a humorous and whimsical way, describes her fight with cancer, and how she refused to accept that she would be any—thing but cured when this journey was ended. Her faith, her intelligence and her unique writing skills jump off each page as you take this adventure with her."

~Ron Harper
Founder, Harper Corporation of America

5674171R0

Made in the USA
Lexington, KY
03 June 2010